Understanding Animal Disorders:
A Clinical Approach

Understanding Animal Disorders:
A Clinical Approach

Editor: Herbert Dunda

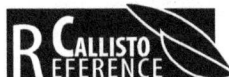

R CALLISTO
REFERENCE

www.callistoreference.com

Callisto Reference,
118-35 Queens Blvd., Suite 400,
Forest Hills, NY 11375, USA

Visit us on the World Wide Web at:
www.callistoreference.com

ISBN: 978-1-64116-152-7 (Hardback)

Cataloging-in-Publication Data

Understanding animal disorders : a clinical approach / edited by Herbert Dunda.
    p. cm.
Includes bibliographical references and index.
ISBN 978-1-64116-152-7
1. Animals--Diseases. 2. Veterinary medicine. 3. Veterinary therapeutics. I. Dunda, Herbert.
SF745 .U53 2019
636.089--dc23

Table of Contents

Preface

Every book is initially just a concept; it takes months of research and hard work to give it the final shape in which the readers receive it. In its early stages, this book also went through rigorous reviewing. The notable contributions made by experts from across the globe were first molded into patterned chapters and then arranged in a sensibly sequential manner to bring out the best results.

The prevention, diagnosis and treatment of all animal disorders is under the domain of veterinary medicine. Animals suffer from a variety of diseases and psychological disorders. Farm animals, laboratory animals and pet animals are prone to disorders. Some common eating disorders in animals are activity anorexia, thin sow syndrome and pica. The understanding of behavioral disorders is difficult due to a lack of comprehension of animal communication and psychology. Obsessive compulsive disorder, addiction, depression, stress, self-aggression, etc. are examples of behavioral disorders. Besides these, animals also suffer from a variety of diseases mediated by different pathogens such as virus, bacteria and fungi. Genetic diseases in animals include complex vertebral malformation, hyperkalemic periodic paralysis, foal immunodeficiency syndrome, etc. The topics covered in this extensive book deal with the core aspects of animal disorders. It presents researches and studies performed by experts across the globe. Students, researchers, experts and all associated with this field will benefit alike from this book.

It has been my immense pleasure to be a part of this project and to contribute my years of learning in such a meaningful form. I would like to take this opportunity to thank all the people who have been associated with the completion of this book at any step.

Editor

Expression, purification and immunochemical characterization of recombinant OMP28 protein of *Brucella* species

Y. Manat[1,*], A.V. Shustov[2], E. Evtehova[1] and S.Z. Eskendirova[1]

[1]*Laboratory of Cell Biotechnology, National Centre for Biotechnology, Astana, 010000, Republic of Kazakhstan*
[2]*Laboratory of Genetic Engineering, National Centre for Biotechnology, Astana, 010000, Republic of Kazakhstan*

Abstract

Brucellosis is the lion's share of infectious disease of animals and it has a particular socio-economic importance for the Republic of Kazakhstan. Sixty percent of epizootic outbreaks of brucellosis identified in the Commonwealth of Independent States (CIS) originated from Kazakhstan in recent years. Definitive diagnosis of brucellosis remains a difficult task. Precisely for this reason, we evaluated a purified recombinant out membrane protein 28 (rOMP28) of *Brucella* species (*Brucella* spp.) produced in *Escherichia coli* (*E. coli*) as a diagnostic antigen in an Indirect ELISA (I-ELISA) for bovine brucellosis. The gene encoding OMP28 was synthesized using a two-round PCR procedure. In order to produce the rOMP28, the *de novo* synthesized DNA was cloned into the expression vector pET-22b(+). Then, the rOMP28 was expressed in *E. coli* system and characterized in the present study. We further estimated the diagnostic potential of purified rOMP28 of *Brucella* spp. for screening bovine sera. To determine if rOMP28 has a valuable benefit for use in the serodiagnosis of bovine brucellosis, rOMP28-based I-ELISA was performed. *Brucella* spp. positive (n=62) and *Brucella* spp. negative (n=28) samples from tube agglutination test (TAT) were positive (n=59) and negative (n=27) by I-ELISA, respectively. These findings show that the rOMP28 of *Brucella* spp. could be a good candidate for improving serological diagnostic methods for bovine brucellosis.
Keywords: *Brucella* spp., Brucellosis, I-ELISA, rOMP28, Western blot.

Introduction

Brucellosis caused by Gram-negative, facultative, intracellular bacteria belonging to the genus *Brucella*. It is an emerging zoonosis, and an economically important infection of humans and animals with a worldwide distribution. Owing to its heterogeneous and poorly specific clinical symptomatology, the diagnosis of brucellosis always requires laboratory confirmation, either by isolation of the pathogen or by demonstration of specific antibodies. The slow growth of *Brucella* in culture may delay diagnosis for more than seven days. Furthermore, handling of these microorganisms poses a high risk to laboratory personnel, since *Brucella* spp. are class III pathogens (Christopher *et al.*, 2010; Poester *et al.*, 2010; Smirnova *et al.*, 2013).

The conventional serological tests, of which the most frequently used are the Rose Bengal test (RBT), the tube agglutination test (TAT) and the complement fixation test (CFT), principally measure antibodies against the immunodominant smooth lipopolysaccharide (S-LPS) of the bacterial cell membrane. The traditional serological test for diagnosing brucellosis in cattle in Kazakhstan is TAT. However, agglutination tests sometimes give false-positive results due to cross-reactions with other microorganisms. In addition, serological tests based on anti-LPS antibodies give false positives because of cross-reactivity with other Gram-negative bacteria such as *Yersinia enterocolitica* O:9, *Salmonella* spp. and *Escherichia coli* (Christopher *et al.*, 2010; Smirnova *et al.*, 2013).

Outer membrane proteins (OMPs) of *Brucella* spp. have been the focus of vaccine development and the diagnosis of brucellosis (Cloeckaert *et al.*, 2001; Gupta *et al.*, 2010; Ko *et al.*, 2012). OMP28 is considered as one of the outer membrane proteins of *Brucella* (Cha *et al.*, 2012) and has been identified as an important diagnostic antigen in brucellosis (Seco-Mediavilla *et al.*, 2003; Poester *et al.*, 2010). OMP28 is highly conserved among *B. abortus*, *B. suis*, *B. ovis*, *B. canis*, *B. neotomae* and *B. melitensis*. Recombinant OMP28 was sensitive and specific for diagnosis of *Brucella* infection in animals by indirect enzyme-linked immunosorbent assay (I-ELISA) (Kumar *et al.*, 2008; Gupta *et al.*, 2010; Thavaselvam *et al.*, 2010; Liu *et al.*, 2011; Dong-Bao *et al.*, 2012; Lim *et al.*, 2012; Qiu *et al.*, 2012; Azizpour *et al.*, 2013; Kim *et al.*, 2013; Xin *et al.*, 2013).

Materials and Methods

Reagents and equipment

All primers were synthesized by Invitrogen corporation (Invitrogen, USA). A Bio-Rad T100™ Thermal Cycler was used for PCR. *E.coli* laboratory strain BL21 (DE3) was obtained from Novagen. HisTrap FF crude was sourced from GE Healthcare life sciences. Bovine serum samples [positive (62) and negative (28) well known serum samples of bovine infected with *Brucella*

*Corresponding Author: Manat Yesbol. Laboratory of Cell Biotechnology, National Centre for Biotechnology, Astana, 010000, Republic of Kazakhstan. E-mail: manatyesbol@gmail.com

spp.] were obtained from the RSE "Republican Veterinary Laboratory," the Ministry of Agriculture of RK. All chemicals used in this study were of analytical grade and purchased from Sigma (Str. Louis, MO).

De novo synthesis of OMP28 gene

The gene encoding the OMP28 was synthesized in a constructive PCR using long oligonucleotides as primers. First, amino acid sequences of the OMP28 protein of *Brucella* spp. were downloaded from Genbank and compared in a multiple alignment.

The *in silico* designed sequence for the OMP28 is shown in Fig. 1. This gene was codon-optimized for expression in *E.coli*. The vector NTI suite was used for reverse translation coupled with codon-optimization for heterologous species (*E.coli* K12).

The DNAWorks v3.2.2 was used to calculate sequences of primers for the *de novo* synthesis of DNA fragments. The primers used for the *de novo* gene synthesis are listed in Table 1. These primers were designed for use in PCR with annealing temperature of 62°C in presence of 50 mmol/L Na$^+$ and 2 mmol/L Mg^{2+}. In the constructive PCR procedure, these primers were divided into two groups and designated as "internal" or "flanking" primers. Each of the internal primers was 100% homologous to the corresponding region in the sequence to be synthesized. Internal primers were interleaved in the sense-antisense-sense-antisense manner. The whole set of internal primers covered the entire length of the DNA fragment to be synthesized except for the very 5'- and 3'-terminal linkers. The terminal linkers with restriction sites for subsequent cloning were included in the flanking primers.

The *de novo* synthesis of OMP28 gene was performed as a two-round PCR. Phusion HotStart DNA polymerase (Thermo Scientific) was used to avoid PCR errors. The mixture of 20 internal primers (each at 0.4 pmol/L final concentration) was subjected to the first round of PCR.

The external template was not added to reactions in the first round. A total 30 cycles were carried out as following: denaturation at 95°C for 1 min, annealing at 60°C for 1 min and extension at 72°C for 1 min. The PCR products of the first round were diluted 1:10 with water and 1 μL of the first round PCR product was used in the second round of PCR amplification. For the second round of PCR, a pair of flanking primers (each at 2 pmol/L final concentration) was used. The product of the second round PCR was expected to be 787 bp in length. The PCR products were subjected to electrophoresis in 1% agarose gels, cloned into pGEM-T using the pGEM-T Easy Cloning kit (Promega) and sequenced. Double strand automated sequencing was performed for confirmation of the identity of the cloned fragment to the designed sequence of the gene.

Protein expression and purification

E.coli BL21(DE3) were transformed with the plasmid pET-22b(+) carrying the gene of OMP28 and grown on solid LB/ampicillin (100 μg/mL) plates at 37°C overnight. A single colony was selected to grow a 5mL starter culture overnight at 37°C. The starter culture was inoculated into 500mL LB/ampicillin (100 μg/mL) and incubated at 37°C with shaking until the OD$_{600}$ reached 0.6. Expression of recombinant OMP28 was induced by addition of IPTG to a final concentration of 0.5 mmol/L and expression was continued for 12 h at 25°C. Finally cells were harvested and collected by centrifugation (at 6000xg for 10 min at 4°C) and washed twice with distilled water (20 mL).

In order to ascertain the localization of the expressed recombinant protein, cells were resuspended in 20 mL lysis buffer (20% sucrose; 20mM HEPES pH 7.5; 5mM EDTA; 0.1% Triton X-100), [10mL lysis buffer per gram wet weight cells], followed by the addition of 2mL lysozyme (final concentration is 1mg/mL), 20 μl DNase (final concentration is 0.01mg/mL)and 200 μl

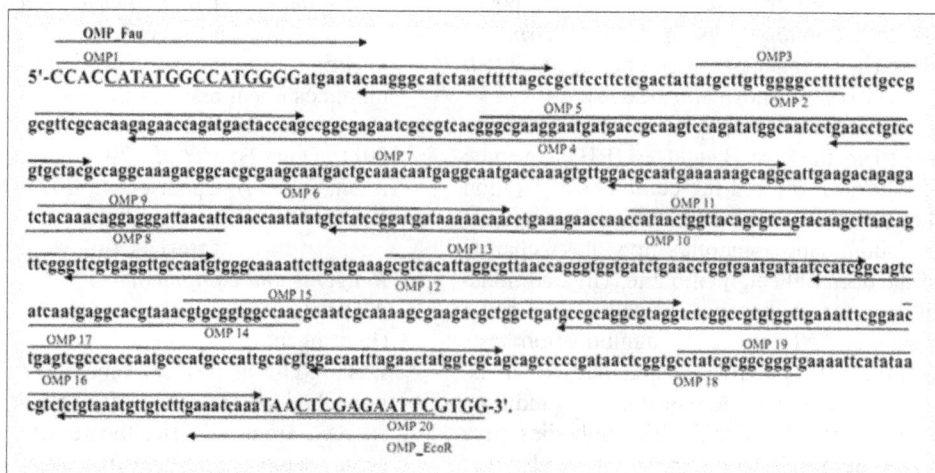

Fig. 1. The nucleotide sequence of OMP28 used for the internal (OMP1-OMP20) and flanking (OMP_Fau and OMP_EcoR) primers. The DNA sequences used for primer design are shown by arrows.

Table 1. Primers for synthesis of OMP28 gene.

Name	Sequence (5'-3')	Internal or flanking
OMP1	CCACCATATGGCCATGGGGATGAATACAAGGGCAT CTAACTTTTTAGCC	Internal
OMP2	AAAAGGCCCCAACAAGCATAATAGTCGAGAAGGA AGCGGCTAAAAAGTTAGATGCCCTTG	Internal
OMP3	ATGCTTGTTGGGGCCTTTTCTCTGCCGGCGTTCG CACAAGAGAACCAGATGACTACCCAG	Internal
OMP4	GGTCATCATTCCTTCGCCCGTGACGGCGATTCTC GCCGGCTGGGTAGTCATCTGGTTCTC	Internal
OMP5	GGGCGAAGGAATGATGACCGCAAGTCCAGATA TGGCAATCCTGAACCTGTCCGTGCTACG	Internal
OMP6	TCATTGTTTGCAGTCATTGCTTCGCGTGCCGTCT TTGCCTGGCGTAGCACGGACAGGTTC	Internal
OMP7	AGCAATGACTGCAAACAATGAGGCAATGACCAA AGTGTTGGACGCAATGAAAAAAGCAGG	Internal
OMP8	AATGTTAATCCCTCCTGTTTGTAGATCTCTGTCTT CAATGCCTGCTTTTTTCATTGCGTC	Internal
OMP9	CTACAAACAGGAGGGATTAACATTCAACCAATA TATGTCTATCCGGATGATAAAAACAAC	Internal
OMP 10	CTGACGCTGTAACCAGTTATGGTTGGTTCTTTC AGGTTGTTTTTATCATCCGGATAGACA	Internal
OMP 11	CCATAACTGGTTACAGCGTCAGTACAAGCTTAA CAGTTCGGGTTCGTGAGCTTGCCAATG	Internal
OMP 12	GTTAACGCCTAATGTGACGCTTTCATCAAGAAT TTTGCCCACATTGGCAAGCTCACGAAC	Internal
OMP 13	GCGTCACATTAGGCGTTAACCAGGGTGGTGATC TGAACCTGGTGAATGATAATCCATCGG	Internal
OMP 14	GTTGGCCACCGCACGTTTACGTGCCTCATTGAT GACTGCCGATGGATTATCATTCACCAG	Internal
OMP 15	CGTGCGGTGGCCAACGCAATCGCAAAAGCGAAGA CGCTGGCTGATGCCGCAGGCGTAGGT	Internal
OMP 16	CATTGGTGGGCGACTCAGTTCCGAAATTTCAAC CACACGGCCGAGACCTACGCCTGCGGC	Internal
OMP 17	CTGAGTCGCCCACCAATGCCCATGCCCATTGCAC GTGGACAATTTAGAACTATGGTCGCA	Internal
OMP 18	CACCCGCCGCGATAGGCACCGAGTTATCGGGG GCTGCTGCGACCATAGTTCTAAATTGTC	Internal
OMP 19	CCTATCGCGGCGGGTGAAAATTCATATAACGT CTCTGTAAATGTTGTCTTTGAAATCAAA	Internal
OMP 20	CCACGAATTCTCGAGTTATTTGATTTCAAAGA CAACATTTACAGA	Internal
OMP_Fau	CCACCATATGGCCATGGGGATGAATAC	Flanking
OMP_EcoR	CCACGAATTCTCGAGTTATTTGATTTC	Flanking

RNase (final concentration is 0.1mg/mL). IPTG was added to a final concentration of 0.2 mM and further incubated at room temperature for 1 hr. The bacterial cell suspension was then sonicated for 10 min with a pulse interval of 5 s (OMNI-Ruptor 4000) in an ice-water bath. The lysate was centrifuged at 6000xg for 30 min at 4°C, supernatant discarded and the pellet was resuspended in 5mL of lysis buffer, then sonicated for 7 min with a pulse interval of 5 s. The sonicated extract was centrifuged at 6000xg for 10 min at 4°C. In this way, inclusion bodies were obtained, followed by resuspention of the inclusion body with buffer A (20mM

Na$_3$PO$_4$ pH 7,4; 500mM NaCl; 20mM imidazole, 8 M urea), sonicated 50 % level 4-5, one pulse, incubated for 1 hr at room temperature, then centrifuged at 8000xg for 30 min, carefully collected the supernatant (discarded the pellet). The supernatant and inclusion bodies, with appropriate controls and molecular mass markers, were analyzed by 12% SDS-PAGE, as described by Laemmli (1970). After confirmation of the solubility, purification of the rOMP28 from inclusion bodies was carried out using a HisTrap FF crude with a native purification protocol as specified by the manufacturer: removed the snap-off end at the column outlet, then washed the column with 5 column volumes of distilled water (5mL). Equilibrated the column with 5 column volumes of binding buffer (buffer A containing 8M urea), then applied pretreated sample using a syringe and collected in a separate tube as Flowthrough, followed by washing with buffer A (5mL). Column and buffers (buffer A, buffer B) were then connected to the GE Healthcare chromatography system and equilibration started. The purified protein was checked by 12% SDS-PAGE followed by Coomassie blue staining, and protein concentration was estimated by the Bradford method.

Immunoreactivity of rOMP28 Brucella proteins to bovine sera using Western blot and indirect ELISA

The presence of specific antibodies against rOMP28 in bovine sera was demonstrated by Western blot and indirect ELISA. Briefly, purified rOMP28 preparations were run in 12% SDS-PAGE gels and transferred onto nitrocellulose membranes. The membranes were then blocked with 1% bovine serum for 2 h at 37°C and washed five times with PBS (0.01 mol/L, pH 7.2) containing 0.05% Tween 20 (PBST). Membranes were then incubated with serum samples for 10 h at 4°C (serum: PBST at 1:100). The membranes were washed with PBST and incubated with HRP-conjugated goat anti-bovine IgG antibody (1:5000 dilution) for 1 h at 37°C. Finally, the membranes were washed with PBST and the colors developed by adding 4-chloro-1-naphthol in the presence of hydrogen peroxide.

Antibody responses were also measured in indirect ELISA against rOMP28 of *Brucella* spp. in bovine sera. Briefly, 96-well microtitre plate (Nunc-Maxisorp, Denmark) was coated overnight with 100 µl of purified rOMP28 antigen (2 µg/mL) in Phosphate-buffered saline (PBS, pH 7.4) at 4°C. Next day, plate was washed three times with PBS-T and blocked with bovine serum albumin (1%) in PBS-T for 1 h at 37°C. After 3 – 4 washings with PBS-T, the plate was incubated with positive sera at a 1/100 dilution, at 37°C for 2 h. After 3 – 4 washings of the plate, anti-bovine HRP conjugate (100 µl/well) was added (1/10000) and incubated at 37°C for 1 h. After incubation, the plate was washed 3 – 4 times and 100 µl of freshly prepared substrate solution (10 mg OPD/10mL substrate buffer with 100 µl of 3% H$_2$O$_2$) was added to each well and

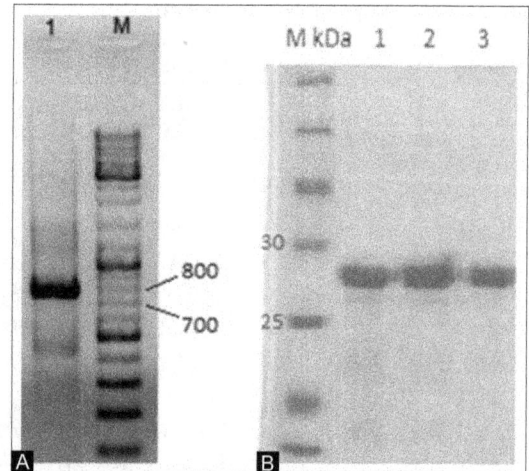

Fig. 2. (A) Agarose electrophoresis of second round PCR product (lane 1), M: DNA molecular weight marker. (B) SDS-PAGE analysis of Purified rOMP28; M: Protein marker; 1, 2, 3: rOMP28. The proteins were separated by 12% SDS-PAGE and stained with Coomassie brilliant blue.

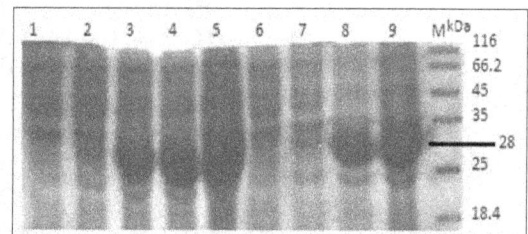

Fig. 3. SDS–PAGE analysis of rOMP28 in pET-22(b+) expression vector with modified buffers under denaturing conditions. 1: Uninduced clone (total); 2: Clear lysate of 2 h induction; 3: Lysate of 4 h induction; 4: Lysate of 6 h induction; 5: Lysate of overnight induction; 6: inclusion body without induction; 7: inclusion body after 2 h induction; 8: inclusion body after 4 h induction; 9: inclusion body induction overnight, M: protein molecular weight marker (Thermo scientific).

incubated for 10 - 15 min in the dark. The reaction was stopped by addition of 100 µl of H$_2$SO$_2$ (2M) per well. The absorbance was measured using ELISA reader (Bio-Rad) at 490 nm.

Results and Discussion

The outer membrane proteins (OMPs) of *Brucella* spp. were initially identified in the early 1980s and have been extensively characterized as potential immunogenic and protective antigens. However, research about the location of OMP28 has not been consistent so far. Lindler *et al.* (1996) found the OMP28 located in the outer membrane and bleb. Rossetti *et al.* (1996) localized this protein in the periplasm. Contrarily, Cloeckaert *et al.* (2001) considered this protein as a soluble protein by using certain monoclonal antibodies. Making a correct diagnosis of brucellosis in animals is not always possible due to the reduced efficiency of the bacteriological methods and serological reactions, therefore, these methods need to be further improved. One of the potential attempts to increase the sensitivity and specificity of serologic tests is by using the recombinant analogs of immunodominant proteins of pathogenic *Brucella* which have been extensively studied.

The de novo synthesis of OMP28 gene and purification of recombinant OMP28 antigen

Amino acid sequences of the OMP28 protein of *Brucella* spp. were downloaded from Genbank and compared in a multiple alignment. The gene encodes OMP28 of *Brucella* spp. was *de novo* synthesized. The *de novo* synthesis of OMP28 gene was performed as a two-round PCR. The product of the second round PCR showed a band of the expected length in (787 bp) (Fig. 2A). DNA sequencing results confirmed that the *de novo* synthesized OMP28 gene had the correct orientation to the designed sequence of the gene.

In order to overproduce the 28 kDa outer membrane protein (OMP28) of *Brucella* spp., the synthesized DNA was cloned into the expression vector, pET-22b(+) (Life Technology, USA). Expression of rOMP28 was achieved with *E. coli* BL21(DE3). The SDS-PAGE analysis of the cell lysate and various eluates showed the expression of the expected 28 kDa recombinant protein. Purification of the rOMP28 from inclusion bodies was carried out using a HisTrap FF crude with a native purification protocol as specified by the manufacturer. The different eluates were analysed by SDS-PAGE and the highly purified protein concentration was calculated and was estimated at 3.2 mg/mL (Fig. 2B and Fig. 3).

Immunoreactivity of rOMP28 of Brucella spp.

The diagnostic potential of rOMP28 of Brucella *spp.* was further evaluated for screening positive (n=62) and negative (n=28) bovine serum samples (determined by TAT). The immunochemical reactivity of highly purified rOMP28 was studied in I-ELISA assay compared to a tube agglutination test (TAT). The cut off value for I-ELISA was determined at 0.096 which was double the average OD_{492} value of negative serum 0.042 ±0.003 at a 1:100 dilution. I-ELISA absorbance values of *Brucella* positive sera using rOMP28 had a strong positive reaction in comparison to the TAT value (Fig. 4). The immunoreactivity of rOMP28 based ELISA relative to the reference method (TAT) is shown in Table 2. Totally, 59 (95.1%) and 3 (4.9%) of the 62 TAT-positive sera were rOMP28 antigen based I-ELISA positive and negative, respectively. In addition, it also detected one of the TAT- negative samples as positive (3.6%) and the remaining 27 samples (96.4%) as negative.

The potency of purified rOMP28 was studied in field sera for diagnosis of brucellosis using Western blot (Fig. 5). The immunoreactivity of the expressed protein was confirmed by Western blot. The protein band at 28kDa specifically reacted with bovine brucellosis sera. No reaction was observed with the negative serum samples.

In the present study, we selected the outer membrane protein (Omp28) of *Brucella* spp. as a candidate antigen to be further evaluated. The coding gene for *Brucella* spp. OMP28 was *de novo* synthesized, expressed in the *E.coli* system and used to develop rOMP28 I-ELISA in an attempt to increase the sensitivity and specificity for diagnosing bovine brucellosis. Our study has shown that I-ELISA, using rOMP28 protein, yielded high sensitivity and specificity for detection of *Brucella* antibodies in bovine sera, as shown in Table 2. Furthermore, these results contradict previously published data, which described this antigen as of no diagnostic value (Xin *et al.*, 2013). However, data from other studies (Cloeckaert *et al.*, 2001; Liu *et al.*, 2011; Cha *et al.*, 2012) showed that the OMP28-based I-ELISA had high sensitivity and specificity in the diagnosis of brucellosis in bovine sera, conforming to our results.

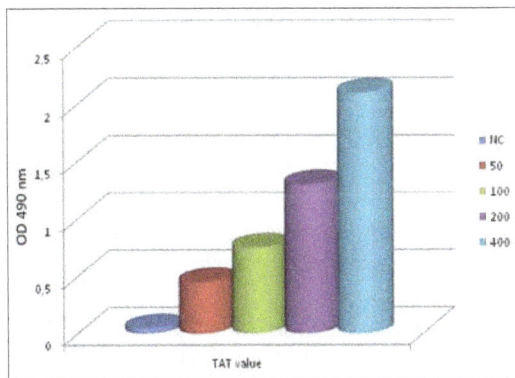

Fig. 4. ELISA absorbance values of bovine sera using rOMP28 compared to a TAT. ELISA absorbance values of *Brucella* positive and negative sera were estimated using 2 μg/mL of rOMP28 antigen. The Brucella positive sera were composed of TAT; 50 (n=5), TAT; 100 (n=23), TAT; 200 (n=24) and TAT; 400 (n=7). Immunoassay plates were charged with sera at a dilution of 1:100.

Table 2. Diagnostic values of rOMP28 antigen based I-ELISA compared to a TAT.

Diagnostic values ELISA	TAT positive (n=62)	TAT negative (n=28)	Chi-Square distribution	Sensitivity	Specificity
ELISA positive	59	1	72.8 (P>0.999)	59:62·100% =95,1%;	27:28·100% =96,4%;
ELISA negative	3	27			

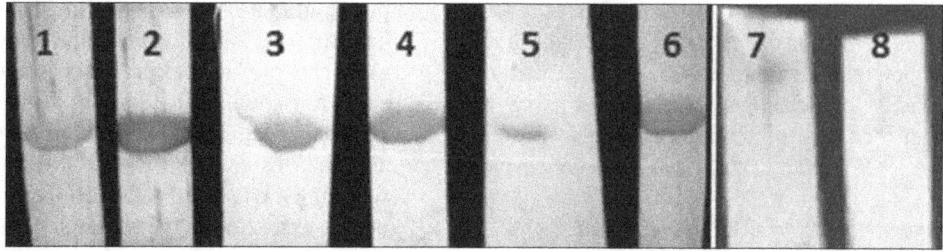

Fig. 5. Analysis of the immunoreactivity of the recombinant protein by Western blot. The immunoreactivity of rOMP28 was elucidated with *Brucella* positive and negative bovine serum. Samples: 1-6 (positive for brucellosis); 7-8 (negative for brucellosis).

In conclusion, the outer membrane protein OMP28 of *Brucella* spp. is identified as a major immunodominant antigen and a potential antigen for developing serological tests for bovine brucellosis.

References

Azizpour, M., Hosseini, S., Akbary, N., Basiri, H., Nezamabadi, M. and Sarikhani, M. 2013. Amplification, cloning, and expression of *Brucella melitensis* BP26 gene isolated from Markazi province in order to produce BP26 recombinant protein. Arak Med. Univ. J. 16, 62-70.

Cha, S.B., Rayamajhi, N., Lee, W.J., Shin, M.K., Jung, M.H., Shin, S.W., Kim, J.W. and Yoo, H.S. 2012. Generation and envelope protein analysis of internalization defective Brucella abortus mutants in professional phagocytes, RAW 264.7. FEMS Immunol. Med. Microbiol. 64, 244-254.

Christopher, S., Umapathy, B.L. and Ravikumar, K.L. 2010. Brucellosis: rewiew on the recent trends in pathogenicity and laboratory. J. Lab. Physicians 2, 55-60.

Cloeckaert, A., Baucheron, S., Vizcaino, N. and Zygmunt, M.S. 2001. Use of Recombinant OMP28 protein in Serological Diagnosis of *Brucella melitensis* infection in Sheep. Clin. Diagn. Lab. Immunol. 8, 772-775.

Dong-Bao, X., Ming-Chun, G., Di-Fei, C., Xiao-Dong, W. and Jun-Wei, W. 2012. Identification of Linear B-cell Epitope of Structural Protein OMP28 of Brucella abortus. Acta Vet. Zoo. Sin. 43, 1444-1448.

Gupta, V.K., Kumari, R., Vohra, J., Singh, S.V. and Vihan, V.S. 2010. Comparative evaluation of recombinant OMP28 protein for serological diagnosis of *Brucella melitensis* infection in goat. Small Ruminant Res. 93, 119-125.

Kim, D., Park, J., Kim, S., Son, Y. and Song, J. 2013. Brucella Immunogenic OMP28 Forms a Channellike Structure. J. Mol. Biol. 425, 1119-1126.

Ko, K.Y., Kim, J.W., Her, M., Kang, S., Jung, S.C., Cho, D.H. and Kim, J.Y. 2012. Immunogenic proteins of Brucella abortus to minimize cross reactions in brucellosis diagnosis. Vet Microbiol. 156, 374-380.

Kumar, S., Tuteja, U., Kumar, A. and Batra, H.V. 2008. Expression and purification of the 26 kDa periplasmic protein of *Brucella abortus*: a reagent for the diagnosis of bovine brucellosis. Biotechnol. Appl. Biochem. 49, 213-218.

Laemmli, U.K. 1970. Cleavage of structural proteins during the assembly of the head of bacteriophage T4. Nature 227, 680-685.

Lim, J., Kim, D., Lee, J., Min, W., Chang, H. and Kim, S. 2012. Evaluation of recombinant 28kDa outer membrane protein of Brucella abortus for the clinical diagnosis of bovine brucellosis in Korea. J. Vet. Med. Sci. 74, 687-691.

Lindler, L.E., Hadfield, T.L., Tall, B.D., Snellings, N.J., Rubin, F.A., Van De Verg, L.L., Hoover, D. and Warren, R.L. 1996. Cloning of a Brucella melitensis group 3 antigen gene encoding Omp28, a protein recognized by the humoral immune response during human brucellosis. Infect. Immun. 64(7), 2490-2499.

Liu, W.X., Hu, S., Qiao, Z.J., Chen, W.Y., Liu, L.T., Wang, F.K., Hua, R.H., Bu, Z.G. and Li, X.R. 2011. Expression, purification and improved antigenic specificity of a truncated recombinant OMP28 protein of Brucella melitensis M5-90: a potencial antigen for differencial serodiagnosis of brucellosis in sheep and goats. Biotechnol. Appl. Biochem. 58, 32-38.

Poester, F.P., Nielsen, K., Samartino, L.E. and Yu, W.L. 2010. Diagnosis of Brucellosis. Open Vet. Sci. J. 4, 46-60.

Qiu, J., Wang, W., Wu, J., Zhang, H., Wang, Y., Qiao, J., Chen, C., Gao, G.F., Allain, J.P. and Li, C. 2012. Characterization of Periplasmic Protein OMP28 Epitopes of Brucella melitensis Reacting with Murine Monoclonal and Sheep Antibodies. PloS One *7*(3), e34246. http://doi.org/10.1371/journal.pone.0034246.

Rossetti, O.L., Arese, A.I., Boschiroli, M.L. and Cravero, S.L. 1996. Cloning of Brucella abortus gene and characterization of expressed 26-kilodalton periplasmic protein: potential use for diagnosis. J. Clin. Microbiol. 34(1), 165-169.

Seco-Mediavilla, P., Verger, J-M., Grayon, M., Cloeckaert, A., Marín, C.M., Zygmunt, M.S.,

Fernández-Lago, L. and Vizcaíno, N. 2003. Epitope mapping of the Brucella melitensis OMP28 immunogenic protein: usefulness for diagnosis of sheep brucellosis. Clin. Diagn. Lab. Immunol. 10, 647-651.

Smirnova, E.A., Vasin, A.V., Sandybaev, N.T., Klotchenko, S.A., Plotnikova, M.A., Chervyakova, O.V., Sansyzbay, A.R. and Kiselev, O.I. 2013. Current Methods of Human and Animal Brucellosis Diagnostics. Adv. Infec. Dis. 3, 177-184.

Thavaselvam, D., Kumar, A., Tiwari, S., Mishara, M.

and Prakash, A. 2010. Cloning and expression of the immunoreactive Brucella melitensis 28 kDa outer-membrane protein (Omp28) encoding gene and evaluation of the potential of Omp28 for clinical diagnosis of brucellosis. J. Med. Microbiol. 59, 421-428.

Xin, T., Yang, H., Wang, N., Wang, F., Zhao, P., Wang, H., Mao, K., Zhu, H. and Ding, J. 2013. Limitations of the BP26 protein-based indirect enzyme-linked immunosorbent assay for diagnosis of Brucellosis. Clin. Vaccine Immunol. 20(9), 1410-1417.

2

Histopathological alterations in spleen of freshwater fish *Cyprinus carpio* exposed to sublethal concentration of sodium cyanide

M. David* and R.M. Kartheek

Environmental and Molecular Toxicology Laboratory, Department of PG Studies and Research in Zoology, Karnatak University, Dharwad, Karnataka, India- 580003

Abstract

Aquatic ecosystems in areas with intense mining activity are often subject to cyanide contamination; the present study was aimed to evaluate the harmful effects of sodium cyanide on histoarchitechtural aspect of spleen of freshwater fish *Cyprinus carpio* using an *in vivo* approach. The fishes were exposed to a sublethal concentration of 0.2 mg/L of sodium cyanide for duration of 10 and 20 days and were further allowed to undergo recovery for 14 days in a toxicant free medium. From the present investigation findings like occurrence of haemosiderin pigment, melanomacrophage centers, vacuolation and necrotic eosinophils were evident in all the fishes exposed to sodium cyanide. However, changes were more pronounced in fish subjected to 10 days of exposure, which was followed by 20 days of exposure and 14 days of recovery. The study revealed that there seemed to be the presence of homeostatic mechanism in fish that allows them to stabilize and overcome stress, which in present case is caused by sublethal concentration of sodium cyanide. Since the recovery phenomenon may be adaptive and even strategic, the present investigation also throws a light on adaptive behaviour of fish under stressful environments.

Keywords: Histopathology, Melanomacrophage center, Recovery studies, Sodium cyanide, Spleen.

Introduction

One of the most important and poisonous substances known to man is cyanide. Cyanide is a noxious substance and possesses a property of killing both target and non-target organisms when discharged into the environment (Dube and Hosetti, 2011). The toxicity of cyanide is due to its influence as a respiratory poison in almost all forms of life (Yen *et al.*, 1995). Acute doses of cyanide are usually lethal, due to marked susceptibility of the nerve cells of the respiratory centre leading to hypoxia (Greer and Jo, 1995). Chronic cyanide intoxication has been implicated in numerous anomalies such as ataxic neuropathy (Osuntokun, 1981), goitre (Cliff *et al.*, 1986) and histopathology (Dixon and Leduc, 1981).

Sodium cyanide being extremely toxic is also very functional in various fields and hence is used in large scale by the international mining community to purify gold and other precious metals through milling of high grade ores and heap leaching of low grade ores. This process adequately needs cycling of millions of gallons of alkaline solutions containing high concentrations of potentially toxic sodium cyanide, free cyanide and metal cyanide complexes, which then openly access the aquatic ecosystems. The discharge of toxic pollutants into water bodies may perhaps result in the chronic toxicity in fish (LeBlanc and Bain 1997).

Cyanide and cyanogenic compounds are crucial toxic components which commonly exist in the environment and cyanide toxicity to the fish can be influenced by a variety of factors including concentration, environmental temperature and dissolved oxygen content (Ballantyne, and Marrs 1987). Earlier studies suggest that the toxicity of cyanide is categorically linked to variations in the enzyme activities of liver (Ma and Pritsos, 1997), and is also associated with the aetiology of goitre (Cliff *et al.*, 1986), tropical ataxic neuropathy (Osuntokun, 1981) and epidemic spastic paraparesis (Howlett *et al.*, 1990). However, the possible toxic consequence of cyanide on histoarchitechtural aspect of the immunological organ spleen is very limited.

Spleen being a major peripheral lymphoid organ plays an important role in antigen trapping (Hansen, 1997). Spleen serves as one of the primary haemopoitic organs, as teleost fish have no modulatory cavity in their bones (Agius and Roberts, 2003). Lymphocytes and the macrophages are the mainly concentrated areas in earlier histopathoogical studies as they are important for the defence system of the fishes (Fournie *et al.*, 2001; Kurtovic *et al.*, 2008). Although spleen is known for its vital role in the immune system regulation, comparatively, less attention is attributed to its structure and microanatomy.

A large number of studies have indicated the toxic effect of cyanide on different organs of *Cyprinus carpio* (David and Kartheek, 2014a,b,c). However, little is known about the direct effect of cyanide exposure on spleen. Therefore the present study is

*Corresponding Author: Prof. Muniswamy David. Department of PG Studies and Research in Zoology, Karnatak University, Dharwad, Karnataka, India- 580003. Email: mdavid.kud@gmail.com

undertaken to evaluate the toxicological impact of sodium cyanide to immunological organ spleen using histopathological studies.

Materials and Methods

Collection and maintenance of fish

Healthy *Cyprinus carpio* were procured from the State Fisheries Department, Neersagar, Dharwad, Karnataka, India and were acclimatized to laboratory conditions for 15 days at 24 °C. Further they were held in dechlorinated tap water in large cement tanks which were previously washed with potassium permanganate to free the walls from any microbial growth. Fish were fed regularly and 12–16 h of photoperiod was maintained daily during acclimatization. Water was renewed daily, and its physico-chemical characteristics were analyzed following standard methods as suggested by American Public Health Association (APHA, 2005).

Grouping of Experimental Fish

The fishes were set apart into four different groups namely; Group 1 (control), Group 2 (10 day exposure), Group 3 (20 day exposure) and Group 4 (14 day recovery). Each group was maintained in triplicate and consisted of 10 fishes.

Preparation of stock and exposure of fishes

Sodium cyanide of 95% purity was procured from Loba Chemie Pvt. Ltd., Mumbai, India. Stock solution was prepared by dissolving sodium cyanide in double distilled water in a standard volumetric flask. Water was renewed every day over test periods. Henceforth, the replacement of the water medium was followed by the addition of the desired dose of the test compound. The fish were exposed in batches of 10 to a fixed concentration of sodium cyanide with 20 L of water in three replicates for each concentration. One tenth (0.1 mg/L) of the 96 h LC_{50} (1mg/L) was selected as sub lethal concentration for studies and the durations of exposure were 10 and 20 days. Further, the fish were allowed to undergo a recovery period of 14 days. This study was conducted under the guidelines issued by Organization for economic co-operation and development (OECD, 1992) for static-renewal test conditions. At the end of 10 and 20 days of exposure and that of 14 days of recovery, the fish were sacrificed and sampled for histopathological studies.

Histopathological analysis

For the histopathological examination, the method was followed as described by Humason (1972). The animal was dissected and the organ of interest (spleen) was isolated under aseptic conditions. The sample was fixed in Bouin's fluid for 24 to 48 h. Later, the tissue was processed in a series of graded alcohol and embedded in paraffin which was filtered thrice. Organs in paraffin were sectioned into 5 μm thick ribbons by using semi-automated microtome (LeicaRM 2255) and sections were stained primarily with haematoxylin and counter stained with eosin (H & E) for light microscopic examination (Lille, 1969). The sections were observed under 200X magnification. The microscopic view was photographed using an Olympus phase contrast microscope (Olympus BX51, Tokyo, Japan) with attached photography machinery (ProgResC3, Jenoptic-Germany). The photographed images were further observed for differences and the findings were recorded. The studies were carried out at Department of PG studies and research in Zoology after the approval from Committee for the Purpose of Control and Supervision of Experiments on Animals (CPCSEA).

Results

The present investigation revealed histopathological alterations in splenic section of fish exposed to sublethal concentration (0.2 mg/L) of sodium cyanide (Group 2 & 3) and relatively less number of lesions was noted in fish that were allowed to recover (Group 4). However, no lesions were observed in sections of spleen of control fish (Group 1).

The water analysis was carried out prior to the exposure studies and the results for the same were found as follows, temperature, 25 ± 2 °C; pH, 7.6 ± 0.2; dissolved oxygen, 7.7 ± 0.8 mg/L; total hardness, 30.4 ± 3.1 mg as CaCO3/L; salinity, nil; specific gravity, 1.003; conductivity less than 14 μS/cm; calcium, 17.86 ± 0.92 mg/L; phosphate, 0.4 ± 0.004 μg/L and magnesium, 0.8 ± 0.3 mg/L. The findings in the section of spleen of fish exposed to sodium cyanide are illustrated in Figure 1 (200x) and Figure 2 (400x). Various findings like haemosiderosis, melanomacrophage centers (MMC), vacuolation, necrotic eosinophils were observed in the spleen sections of all fish exposed to sodium cyanide. Furthermore, the severity of the findings in Group 2 was the highest followed by Group 3 and Group 4 which were exposed to a period of 10 and 20 days of exposure and 14 days of recovery, respectively.

Discussion

Over the years, spleen structure and function in many vertebrate species, including fish, has been studied due to its importance of involvement in immunity related role. In spleen of fish, white pulp proliferation, lymphocyte depletion, as well as an increase in the size of spleen, haemosiderosis and increase in melanomacrophage centers has often been associated with environmental contamination (Schwaiger et al., 1996; Gogal et al., 1999; Montero et al., 1999; Garcia-Abiado et al., 2004).

One of the important physiological features is melanomacrophage centers (MMC) which are seen in the fish spleen (Agius and Roberts, 2003). They are assumed to be the functional substitutes of the germinal centers of spleen (Ellis, 1980).

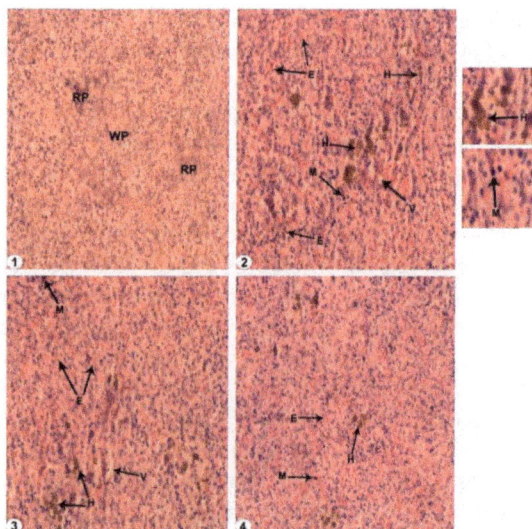

Fig. 1. Section of spleen showing: **1:** Normal architechture, Red pulp (RP), White pulp (WP); **2:** Necrotic eosinophils (E), Melanomacrophage (M), Vacuolation (V), Haemosiderin (H); **3:** Necrotic eosinophil (E), Melanomacrophage (M), Haemosiderin (H), Vacuolation (V); **4:** Necrotic eosinophil (E), Melanomacrophage (M) and Haemosiderin (H). H & E, 200X.

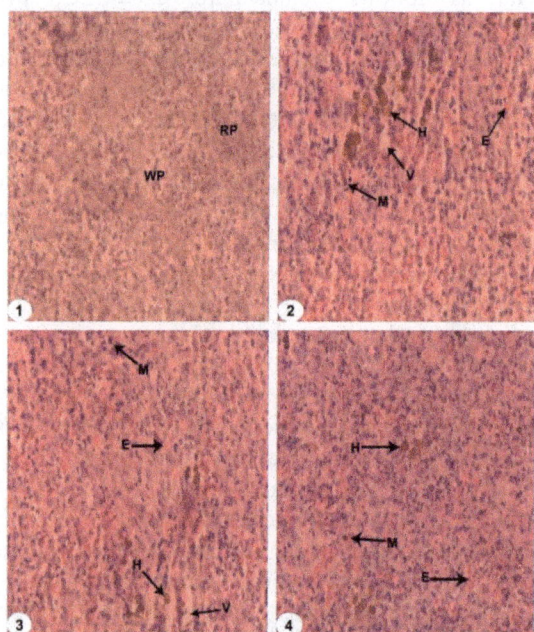

Fig. 2. Section of spleen showing: **1:** Normal architechture, Red pulp (RP), White pulp (WP); **2:** Necrotic eosinophils (E), Melanomacrophage (M), Vacuolation (V), Haemosiderin (H); **3:** Necrotic eosinophil (E), Melanomacrophage (M), Haemosiderin (H), Vacuolation (V); **4:** Necrotic eosinophil (E), Melanomacrophage (M) and Haemosiderin (H). H & E, 400X.

MMC may contain four types of brown pigments: melanin, lipofuscin, ceroid and hemosiderin (Couillard *et al.*, 1999). Stressful conditions to the animal often

result in increased number of its splenic MMC's (Montero *et al.*, 1999), which is in agreement with the present investigation as a large number of MMC's are observed in splenic sections of fish exposed to sublethal concentration of sodium cyanide. Earlier reports by Prashanth and Neelgund (2007), David *et al.* (2008), Dube and Hosetti (2011) and David and Kartheek (2014a,b,c) have suggested the potential biochemical and histopathological toxicity of sodium cyanide towards different freshwater fishes.

Haemosiderin is one of the breakdown products of Hb from senescent and degenerated erythrocytes (Zapata and Cooper, 1990). Haemosiderosis is a pathological condition occurring due to the deposition of haemosiderin. Haemosiderosis is related to an increased rate of erythrocyte destruction in the spleen (Hibiya, 1982) which in present case is perhaps a consequence of sublethal cyanide exposure to the fish *Cyprinus carpio*. This in turn may result in decreased haemoglobin content which is usually attributed to RBC destruction and irregular movement of haemoglobin from the spleen in fishes (Scott and Rogers, 1981). Similar deposition of haemosiderin pigments has been observed in the spleen of fishes exposed to sodium cyanide in the present study. Therefore, it can be said that the findings from previous study and the observations of the present investigation are in a positive accord.

Kaleeswaran *et al.* (2010) suggested the increased severity in the MMC as a homeostatic mechanism of the fish spleen to phagocytose the increasing deposits of haemosiderin and other debris resulting from the destruction of tissues. This matches with the present study wherein the occurrence of MMC could be seen in splenic sections of exposed fish. The present investigation is also in agreement with the findings of Fournie *et al.* (2001) who associated the density of splenic macrophage aggregates in estuarine fishes to exposure to degraded environments. In another study, *Oreochromis niloticus* upon exposure to 1 µg/l of Chlorpyrifos, the sections of pronephros exhibited increased diameter of MMC, the study was reported by Holladay *et al.* (1996) and the reports obtained are in agreement with the present investigation.

The findings obtained in the present investigation are in agreement with reports of Spazier *et al.* (1992) who observed vacuolation in splenic tissue of European eel *Anguilla anguilla* following stress and resulting in impairment of normal physiology of fish. Immune suppression in present case may be a consequence of reduced number of mature lymphocytes. The data is in agreement with Anderson *et al.* (1989) who reported the study on immune-suppression in splenic section of rainbow trout upon exposure to different concentrations of chemical toxicant. Since alterations of the spleen can occur in some pathological conditions (Gogal *et al.*, 1999; Garcia-Abiado *et al.*, 2004), it can be inferred that exposure to sodium cyanide in sublethal doses affects the histoarchitechture of spleen of *C. carpio*. But recovery in later periods may be a revitalization phenomenon as every organism strives to overcome the stress to prove its existence. Recovery phenomenon in the present case may be adaptive and even strategic. The findings obtained in the present investigation may also therefore contribute for the future studies in the field of immunotoxicology of fishes.

Conclusion

From the observations made in the present investigation, it may be inferred that sodium cyanide is highly toxic to freshwater fish *C. carpio* when exposed to a sublethal concentration of 0.2mg/L for 10 and 20 days. However, allowing the fishes to recover in toxicant free medium for 14 days may help to overcome stress and restore histoarchitechture of spleen to some extent. We concluded that the histopathological study may prove to be an important biomarker to characterize the toxicological impacts in the environment.

Acknowledgments

The authors thank the University Grants Commission (UGC), New Delhi, India for the financial assistance through UGC Major Research Project scheme [F. No. 41-103/2012]. We also thank the state fisheries department, Neersagar for their kind help in procuring the fishes for our experiments.

Conflict of interest

The authors declare no conflict of interest.

References

Agius, C. and Roberts, R.J. 2003. Melano-macrophage centres and their role in fish pathology. J. Fish Dis. 26, 499-509.

Anderson, D.P., Swiciki, A.K. and Dixon, O.W. 1989. Immuno-stimulation by levamisole in rainbow trout (*Salmo gairdneri*) in vivo. In Viruses of Lower Vertebrates (W. Ahne & E. Kurstak, eds): pp: 469-478. New York: Sringer-Verlag.

APHA. 2005. Standard Methods for the examination of water and waste water. 21st Ed. Washington DC.

Ballantyne, B. and Marrs, T.C. 1987. Eds. Clinical and experimental toxicology of cyanides. John Wright, Bristol, England. pp: 41-126.

Cliff, J., Essers, S. and Rosling, H. 1986. Ankle clonus correlating with cyanide intake from cassava in rural children from Mozambique. J. Trop. Pediatr. 32(4), 186-189.

Couillard, C.M., Williams, P.J., Courtenay, S.C. and Rawn, G.P. 1999. Histopathological evaluation of Atlantic tomcod (*Microgadus tomcod*) collected at estuarine sites receiving pulp and paper mill effluent. Aquat. Toxicol. 44, 263-278.

David, M., Munaswamy, V., Halappa, R. and Marigoudar, S.R. 2008. Impact of sodium cyanide on catalase activity in the freshwater exotic carp, *Cyprinus carpio* (Linnaeus). Pestic. Biochem. Physiol. 92, 15-18.

David, M. and Kartheek, R.M. 2014a. Sodium cyanide induced histopathological changes in kidney of fresh water fish *Cyprinus carpio* under sublethal exposure. Int. J. Pharm. Chem. Boil. Sci. 4(3), 634-639.

David, M. and Kartheek, R.M. 2014b. Sodium cyanide induced biochemical and histopathological changes in fresh water fish Cyprinus carpio under sublethal exposure. Int. J. Toxicol. Appl. Pharmacol. 4(4), 64-69.

David, M. and Kartheek, R.M. 2014c. Biochemical changes in liver of freshwater fish *Cyprinus carpio* exposed to sublethal concentration of sodium cyanide. Indo Am. J. Pharm. Res. 4(9), 3669-3675.

Dixon, D.G. and Leduc, G. 1981. Chronic cyanide poisoning of Rainbow trout and its effects on growth respiration and liver histopathology. Arch. Environ. Contam. Toxicol. 10, 117-131.

Dube, P.N. and Hosetti, B.B. 2011. Inhibition of ATPase activity in the freshwater fish *Labeo rohita* (Hamilton) exposed to sodium cyanide. Toxicol. Mech. Methods 21(8), 591-595.

Ellis, A.E. 1980. Antigen-trapping in the spleen and kidney of the plaice, *Pleuronectes platessa* (L.). J. Fish Dis. 3, 413-426.

Fournie, J.W., Summers, J.K., Courtney, L.A., Engle, V.D. and Blazer, V.S. 2001. Utility of splenic marcrophage aggregates as an indicator of fish exposure to degraded environment. J. Aquat. Anim. Health 13(2), 105-116.

Garcia-Abiado, M.A., Mbahinzireki, G., Rinchard, J., Lee, K.J. and Dabrowski, K. 2004. Effect of diets structure in tilapia, Oreochromis sp., reared in a recirculating system. J. Fish Dis. 27, 359-368.

Gogal, R.M., Smith, B.J., Robertson, J.L., Smith, S.A. and Holladay, S.D. 1999. Tilapia (*Oreochromis niloticus*) dosed with azathrioprine display immune effects similar to those seen in mammals, including apoptosis. Vet. Immunol. Immunopathol. 68, 209-227.

Greer, J.J. and Carter, J.E. 1995. Effects of cyanide on neural mechanism controlling breathing in neonatal rat in vivo. Neurotoxicology 16, 211-215.

Hansen, J.D. 1997. Characterization of Rainbow trout terminal deoxynucleotidyl transferase structure and expression. TdT and RAG1 co-expression define the trout primary lymphoid tissues. Immunogenetics 46, 367-375.

Hibiya, T. 1982. An atlas of fish histology. Normal and pathological features. Kodansha Ltd., Tokyo.

Holladay, S.D., Smith, S.A., El-Habback, H. and

Caceci, T. 1996. Influence of chlorpyrifos, an organophosphate insecticide on the immune system of Nile tilapia. J. Aquat. Anim. Health 8, 104-110.

Howlett, W.P., Brubaker, G.R., Mlingi, N. and Rosling, H. 1990. Konzo, an epidemic upper motor neuron disease studied in Tanzania. Brain 113, 223-235.

Humason, G.L. 1972. Animal tissue techniques. 3rd edition. WH Freeman and Company.

Kaleeswaran, B.S., Ilavenil, S. and Ravikumar, S. 2010. Changes in biochemical, histological and specific immune parameters in *Catla catla* (Ham.) by *Cynodon dactylon* (L.). J. King Saud Univ. - Sci. 24, 139-152.

Kurtovic, B., Teskerelzi, E. and Teskerelzi, Z. 2008. Histological comparison of spleen and kidney tissue from farmed and wild European sea bass (*Dicentrachus labrax L.*). Acta adriat. 49(2), 147-154.

LeBlanc, G.A. and Bain, L.J. 1997. Chronic toxicity of environmental contaminants: Sentinels and biomarkers. Environ. Health Perspect. 105, 65-80.

Lille, R.D. 1969. Biological Stains. 8 Ed. The Williams and Wilkiins CO., Baltimore, USA.

Ma, J. and Pritsos, C.A. 1997. Tissue specific bioenergetic effects and increased enzymatic activities following acute sublethal preoral exposure to cyanide in the mallard duck. Toxicol. Appl. Pharmacol. 142, 297-302.

Montero, D., Blazer, V.S., Socorro, J., Izquierdo, M.S. and Tort, L. 1999. Dietary and culture influences on macrophage aggregate parameters in gilthead seabream (*Sparus aurata*) juveniles. Aquaculture 179, 523-534.

OECD. 1992. Guidelines for Testing of Chemicals (No.203; Adopted: 17th July, 1992).

Osuntokun, B.O. 1981. Cassava diet, chronic cyanide intoxication and neuropathy in Nigerian Africans. World Rev. Nutr. Diet. 36, 141-173.

Prashanth, M.S. and Neelgund, S.E. 2007. Free cyanide- induced Biochemical changes in Nitrogen metabolism of the Indian Major carp, *Cirrhinus mrigala*. J. Basic Clin. Physiol. Pharmacol. 8(4), 277-287.

Schwaiger, J., Fent, K., Stecher, H. and Negele, R.D. 1996. Effects of sublethal concentrations of triphenyltinacetate on Rainbow trout (*Oncorhynchus mykiss*). Arch. Environ. Contam. Toxicol. 30, 327-334.

Scott, A.L. and Rogers, W.A. 1981. Hematological effects of prolonged sublethal hypoxia on channel catfish *Ictalurus punctatus* (Rafinesque). J Fish Biol. 18, 591-601.

Spazier, E., Storch, V. and Braunbeck, T. 1992. Cytopathology of spleen in eel, *Anguilla anguilla*, exposed to a chemical spill in the Rhine River. Dis. Aquat. Organisms 14, 1-22.

Yen, D., Tsai, J., Kao, W., Hu, S., Lee, C. and Deng, J. 1995. The clinical experience of acute CN-poisoning. Am. J. Emerg. Med. 13, 524-528.

Zapata, A.G. and Cooper, E.L. 1990. The immune system: comparative histopathology. John Wiley and Sons, Chichester, England, Zool. Soc. Bengalis. 1, 67-70.

3

Urinary capillariosis in six dogs from Italy

A. Mariacher[1,2,*], F. Millanta[2], G. Guidi[2] and S. Perrucci[2]

[1]Istituto Zooprofilattico Sperimentale delle Regioni Lazio e Toscana, Viale Europa 30, 58100 Grosseto, Italy
[2]Dipartimento di Scienze Veterinarie, Viale delle Piagge 2, 56124 Pisa, Italy

Abstract
Canine urinary capillariosis is caused by the nematode *Pearsonema plica. P. plica* infection is seldomly detected in clinical practice mainly due to diagnostic limitations. This report describes six cases of urinary capillariosis in dogs from Italy. Recurrent cystitis was observed in one dog, whereas another patient was affected by glomerular amyloidosis. In the remaining animals, the infection was considered an incidental finding. Immature eggs of the parasite were observed with urine sediment examination in 3/6 patients. Increased awareness of the potential pathogenic role of *P. plica*. and clinical disease presentation could help identify infected animals.
Keywords: Cystitis, Dog, Glomerular amyloidosis, Urinary capillariosis.

Introduction

Urinary capillariosis in dogs is caused by *Pearsonema plica* (Trichurida, Capillariidae), a nematode that infects domestic and wild carnivores worldwide. Clinical cases of canine urinary capillariosis have been reported in the United States (Senior *et al.*, 1980; Kirkpatrick and Nelson, 1987) and Europe, including France (Cazelles *et al.*, 1989), Switzerland (Spillmann and Glardon, 1989; Basso *et al.*, 2014), Holland (van Veen, 2002), Poland (Studzińska *et al.*, 2015) and Italy (Callegari *et al.*, 2010; Maurelli *et al.*, 2014). Adult parasites live superficially attached to the mucosa of the urinary bladder, while the ureters and renal pelvis are seldom affected (Bork-Mimm and Rinder, 2011).

P. plica has an indirect life cycle that involves earthworms (*Lumbricina*) as intermediate hosts (Senior *et al.*, 1980) and domestic and wild carnivores as definitive hosts (Anderson, 2000). *P. plica* is most often reported in dogs with access to outdoor environments, especially hunting dogs and kenneled dogs (Senior *et al.*, 1980; Callegari *et al.*, 2010). The red fox (*Vulpes vulpes*) is considered the wild reservoir of *P. plica* for domestic animals in Europe (Davidson *et al.*, 2006; Magi *et al.*, 2014), but the wolf (*Canis lupus*) is emerging as an additional reservoir (Bagrade *et al.*, 2009; Mariacher *et al.*, 2015). Despite the high prevalence in the red fox, urinary capillariosis has been rarely reported in dogs in Italy (Callegari *et al.*, 2010; Maurelli *et al.*, 2014) and the real occurrence of the disease is probably underestimated.

Indeed, urinary capillariosis has often been regarded as having minor clinical and pathological significance, due to frequent subclinical presentations and limitations in its diagnosis (Otranto, 2015). However, in heavy parasite loads, *P. plica* may be responsible for severe lower urinary tract maladies, both in domestic (Rossi *et al.*, 2011; Basso *et al.*, 2014) and wild carnivores (Fernández-Aguilar *et al.*, 2010; Bork-Mimm and Rinder, 2011; Alić *et al.*, 2015). These urinary disorders generally include pollakiuria, dysuria and hematuria, may have chronic or recurrent clinical forms and do not improve after symptomatic or empirical antibiotic treatments (Senior *et al.*, 1980; van Veen, 2002; Rossi *et al.*, 2011).

Diagnosis of *P. plica* infection is based on examination of the urine sediment, an assessment seldom performed in the routine parasite diagnoses of dogs and cats (Otranto, 2015) as it is mostly reserved for symptomatic patients. Moreover, false negative results may commonly occur even when *P. plica* infection is established and symptomatic, due to a long prepatent period, irregular elimination of low numbers of eggs and difficulties in detecting immature or atypical eggs (Senior *et al.*, 1980; Rossi *et al.*, 2011; Basso *et al.*, 2014; Maurelli *et al.*, 2014). This study describes six cases of urinary capillariosis in dogs, and highlights the variability of its clinical presentation.

Case details

Six cases of urinary capillariosis were examined in two different veterinary facilities in Italy. Diagnoses were based on the detection of mature and immature *P. plica* eggs in the urinary sediment of the six dogs. Eggs were identified as *P. plica* based on: 1) mature eggs are barrel-shaped, colorless and operculated, show a slightly pitted wall and bipolar plugs and measure 55-68 μm x 24-29 μm (Basso *et al.*, 2014); and/or 2) immature eggs are smaller, lack a shell and show rudimentary polar plugs (Basso *et al.*, 2014). Clinical details and findings at urine sediment examination are summarised in Tables 1 and 2 respectively.

*Corresponding Author:** Alessia Mariacher. Istituto Zooprofilattico Sperimentale delle Regioni Lazio e Toscana, Viale Europa 30, 58100 Grosseto, Italy. Email: *alessia.mariacher@izslt.it*

Table 1. Breed, gender, age and clinical data of six dogs with urinary capillariosis.

Case ID	Season (month/year)	Geographic origin	Breed	Gender	Age (yrs)	Household	Presenting complaint	Physical examination	Final diagnosis	Treatment regimen	Follow-up
Case 1	Winter (02/2012)	Pisa (CI)	Maremma hound	MI	5	In+Out (boar hunting)	Weight loss, polyuria-polydipsia	Pale mucous membranes	Glomerular amyloidosis	Fenbendazole 50 mg/Kg orally once a day for 7 days	Negative
Case 2	Spring (05/2012)	Siena (CI)	MB	MI	4	In+Out (game bird hunting)	Leishmaniasis evaluation	Slightly enlarged peripheral lymph nodes	Leishmaniasis	Fenbendazole 50 mg/Kg orally once a day for 7 days	Negative
Case 3	Autumn (09/2015)	Pisa (CI)	MB	MI	4	Out (dog shelter)	Leishmaniasis evaluation	Normal	Leishmaniasis	Fenbendazole 50 mg/Kg orally once a day for 7 days	Negative
Case 4	Winter (12/2014)	Udine (NI)	MB	MI	8	In	Recurrent cystitis; hematuria	Hematuria	n.a.	---	---
Case 5	Winter (01/2015)	Udine (NI)	Lhasa Apso	MI	3	In	Lethargy	Fever	Fever of unknown origin	---	---
Case 6	Winter (01/2015)	Udine (NI)	American Staffordshire	FN	9	In	Urinary tenesmus	Urinary tenesmus	Pelvic hemangiosarcoma	---	---

Season: Season of presentation; CI: Central Italy; NI: Northern Italy; MB: Mixed-breed; FN: Neutered female; MI: Intact male; Yrs: Years; In: Indoor; Out: Outdoor; n.a.: Not available; Follow-up: Follow up at 7 and 14 days after treatment, by urinary sediment examination; ---: Not treated/lost to follow-up

Case 1

Case 1 was an intact male Maremma hound aged five. The dog had access to rural and forest environments during hunting season. The dog was referred for polyuria/polydipsia and was diagnosed with chronic kidney disease at stage III (International Renal Interest Society, 2013) and nephrotic syndrome. Urinary capillariosis was diagnosed based on the presence of mature *P. plica* eggs in the urinary sediment; a slight pyuria was also present. Serological tests were negative for *Leishmania* sp. and tick-borne diseases, except for a low positive IgG titer (1:40) for *Ehrlichia canis*. The dog was treated with ramipril (VASOTOP; MSD Animal Health), dietary protein restriction, and fenbendazole (50 mg/Kg orally once a day for seven days). Urine sediment examination was repeatedly negative for parasite eggs starting seven days after treatment. Due to worsening proteinuria, a renal biopsy was performed a month later. Histopathology showed glomerular amyloidosis (Fig. 1), chronic interstitial nephritis, and scattered foci of tubular necrosis.

Case 2

Case 2 was an intact male mixed-breed dog aged four. The dog had access to rural and forest environments during hunting season. This patient was referred for leishmaniasis, with no history of urinary signs and renal function parameters were in their normal range. Typical mature eggs of *P. plica* were identified in the urine sediment (Fig. 2), along with a slight pyuria. Urinary capillariosis was treated with fenbendazole (50 mg/Kg orally once a day for seven days), and the urine sediment was negative for parasite eggs at seven and fourteen days after treatment.

Case 3

Case 3 was an intact male mixed-breed dog aged four, who was recently rescued from a dog shelter. The dog was presented for an evaluation of leishmaniasis, he had no history of urinary signs and renal function parameters were in their normal range. Mature eggs of *P. plica* were identified in the urine sediment, along with slight pyuria and hematuria. Urinary capillariosis was treated with fenbendazole (50 mg/Kg orally once a day for seven days), and the urine sediment was negative for parasite eggs at seven and fourteen days after treatment.

Case 4

Case 4 was an intact male mixed-breed dog aged eight, who lived indoors in an urban setting. The patient had a history of recurrent cystitis and hematuria. At physical examination the dog showed gross hematuria, and at urine sediment examination severe hematuria, moderate pyuria and rare immature eggs of *P. plica* were observed. Because only immature eggs were found the infection was not promptly identified in this case, and the dog only received symptomatic treatment

Table 2. Findings at urine sediment examination in six dogs with urinary capillariosis.

Case ID	SG	pH	PU/CU	WBC	RBC	Hyaline casts	Crystals	Bacteria	Epithelial cells
Case 1	1010	6.5	9.56	+	0	0	0	0	+
Case 2	1030	8.0	0.25	+	0	0	0	0	+
Case 3	1060	7.0	0.18	+	+	0	Struvite +++	0	++
Case 4	1050	6.0	n.a.	++	++++	+	0	0	+++
Case 5	1060	5.0	n.a.	+	0	0	0	0	+
Case 6	1030	8.0	n.a.	+	++++	0	Struvite +	0	+

SG: Specific gravity; PU/CU: Protein/creatinine ratio; WBC: White blood cells, RBC: Red blood cells; n.a.: Data not available. Normal ranges for these parameters are as follows: SG: 1030-1040, pH: 5.5-7.0, PU/CU: 0.1-0.5, WBC: 0, RBC: 0, casts: 0, crystals: 0, bacteria: 0, epithelial cells: 0/+

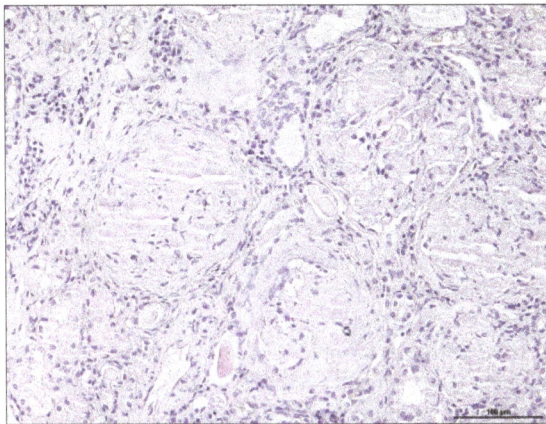

Fig. 1. Canine kidney (case 1): renal glomeruli showing the presence of amorphous hyaline and eosinophilic extracellular material suggestive of amyloid deposition (H&E, Bar = 100 μm).

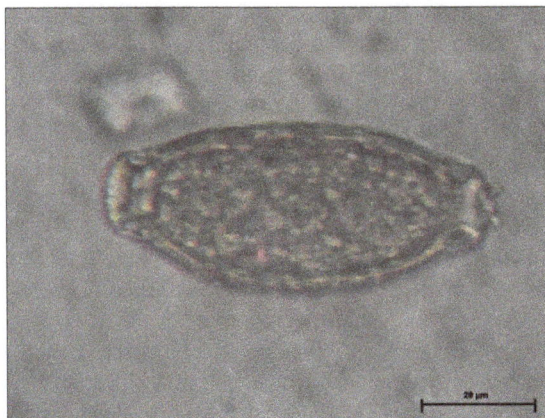

Fig. 2. Urine sediment examination. *Pearsonema plica* mature egg, showing a thick wall and bipolar plugs (Bar = 20 μm).

with non-steroidal anti-inflammatory drugs. Six months after the initial examination, the dog was presented for a routine health control and the resulting urine sediment examination was negative for *P. plica*.

Case 5

Case 5 was an intact male Lhasa Apso aged three, who lived indoors in an urban setting. The dog was presented for lethargy and fever. Immature eggs of *P. plica* were identified in the urine sediment, along with a slight pyuria. Physical examination and clinical laboratory tests did not identify a specific cause of disease and a fever of unknown origin was eventually diagnosed. The dog did not receive any specific treatment for urinary capillariosis and was later lost to follow-up.

Case 6

Case 6 was a neutered female American Staffordshire aged nine, who lived indoors in an urban setting. The patient was presented with urinary tenesmus. At urine sediment examination severe hematuria, slight pyuria and immature eggs of *P. plica* were observed. A pelvic hemangiosarcoma compressing the urethra was diagnosed with computed tomography and histopathology. Because of the poor prognosis, the owners consented to perform euthanasia.

Discussion

Of the six cases of urinary capillariosis presented here, one dog showed characteristic clinical signs, consisting of recurrent episodes of hematuria and cystitis (case 4). This patient was asymptomatic six months after the initial diagnosis and its urine sediment was negative for capillariid eggs, despite not receiving any antiparasitic treatment. This finding could be explained by the gradual decrease in the excretion of eggs in the urine, which can occur within a couple of months from the onset of the patent infection (Senior *et al.*, 1980).

The fact that self-limiting infections may occur must not lead to neglecting urinary capillariosis in terms of diagnosis and therapy. There are reports of cases that feature severe clinical signs that may be in relation to a high number of adult parasites and to the chronicity of the infection (Rossi *et al.*, 2011; Basso *et al.*, 2014). Furthermore, it cannot be excluded that urinary capillariosis may contribute to the onset or worsening of renal disease.

Indeed, one of the infected animals (case 1) showed considerable similarities to a dog previously described by Callegari *et al.* (2010) that was affected by glomerular amyloidosis and chronic interstitial nephritis. Since in both cases common infectious diseases were ruled out, *P. plica* infection was considered to be a contributing factor to the deposition of amyloid substance, via a chronic antigenic and inflammatory stimulus (Callegari *et al.*, 2010).

In the remaining four cases, the detection of eggs in the sediment was considered an incidental finding. The absence of clinical signs, in these cases, may be due to a low number of adult parasites in the urinary tract or to their only very superficial attachment to the bladder mucosa (Kruger and Osborne, 1993; Bowman *et al.*, 2002).

In all the cases presented, urine sediment examination showed slight pyuria in absence of bacteria, while hematuria was not a constant finding with 2/6 dogs exhibiting both gross and microscopic hematuria.

In cases 4, 5 and 6, only immature eggs, lacking the outer shell and with rudimentary opercules, were detected in the urine sediment. The regular presence of immature, along with mature, *P. plica* eggs in the urinary sediment of an infected dog has been reported in a previous study (Basso *et al.*, 2014). Data from this study confirm this finding and indicate that in infected dogs the detection of immature *P. plica* eggs may be rather frequent. In this study, two of the three infected dogs in which only immature eggs were isolated, showed no typical signs of urinary capillariosis. This may be due to a low parasite load, or it is possible that finding only immature eggs may be more likely when the number of eggs in the urinary sediment is low. Moreover, this result also indicates that a specific parasitological experience is needed to diagnose the infection in similar cases.

Cases 4, 5 and 6 lived exclusively indoors and were only walked outside on a lead by their owners. This finding suggests that contact with infected intermediate hosts can easily occur even in urban environments. Therefore, *P. plica* infection should always be included in the differential diagnosis of diseases of the lower urinary tract, even when the patient does not live outdoors. The spread of foxes into urban and periurban areas is a common phenomenon occurring in many European countries (Sréter *et al.*, 2003) and this could result in an increased risk of infection for pets. Two other cases (cases 1 and 2) involved hunting dogs working in rural and forest environments, where they were most likely exposed to settings contaminated by wild reservoir hosts (foxes and wolves). Case 3 was recently rescued from a dog shelter, an environment where infection by *P. plica*

is known to be easily maintained and spread (Senior *et al.*, 1980).

Interestingly, 5/6 infected animals were intact males, but sex predilection was not observed in a previous study by Senior *et al.* (1980) involving a larger number of animals.

Treatment of *P. plica* infection can be challenging and over time it has been attempted with off-label use of different drugs such as: benzimidazoles, avermectines and levamisole. However, to date there are no approved drugs for treating dogs with urinary capillariosis (Senior *et al.*, 1980; Kirkpatrick and Nelson, 1987; van Veen, 2002; Basso *et al.*, 2014; Studzińska *et al.*, 2015). Treatment with fenbendazole performed on three animals in this study appeared to be effective; however, it was recently pointed out that standard urinary sediment examination is not the most adequate way to monitor treatment effectiveness, and more sensitive methods should be used (Otranto, 2015).

In conclusion, data from the present study emphasize the importance of including urinary capillariosis in the differential diagnosis of both chronic and recurrent lower urinary tract and renal disease. Clinicians should be aware that false negative results can be obtained at urinary sediment examination in symptomatic patients, due to low sensitivity of the technique and to parasite biology. Moreover, infection may run asymptomatic, so routine parasitological examination of the urine sediment is advisable in dogs, regardless of the presence or absence of urinary clinical signs. Recently, FLOTAC and Mini-FLOTAC were found to be more sensitive than the classic sedimentation technique in detecting *Pearsonema* eggs in urine specimens (Maurelli *et al.*, 2014). Furthermore, in infected dogs ultrasonographic examination may reveal hyperechogenicity and thickening of the bladder wall, while endoscopic examination of the urine bladder may detect viable *P. plica* worms attached to the mucosa (Basso *et al.*, 2014).

Development and adoption of more sensitive techniques would be welcome in order to help clinicians diagnose and monitor urinary capillariosis.

Conflict of interest

The authors declare that there is no conflict of interest.

Acknowledgements

The authors wish to thank Dr. Francesca Ceccotto and her colleagues at Clinica Veterinaria Serenissima (Sacile, UD; Italy) who provided data for this study.

References

Alić, A., Hodxić, A., Kadrić, M., Besirović, H. and Prasović, S. 2015. *Pearsonema plica* (*Capillaria plica*) infection and associated urinary bladder pathology in red foxes (*Vulpes vulpes*) from Bosnia and Herzegovina. Parasitol. Res. DOI: 10.1007/s00436-015-4382-6.

Anderson, R.C. 2000. *Nematode parasites of vertebrates: their development and transmission.* CABI Publishing, UK.

Bagrade, G., Kirjušina, M., Vismanis, K. and Ozoliņš, J. 2009. Helminth parasites of the wolf *Canis lupus* from Latvia. J. Helminthol. 83, 63-68.

Basso, W., Spänhauer, Z., Arnold, S. and Deplazes, P. 2014. *Capillaria plica* (syn. *Pearsonema plica*) infection in a dog with chronic pollakiuria: challenges in the diagnosis and treatment. Parasitol. Int. 63, 140-142.

Bork-Mimm, S. and Rinder, H. 2011. High prevalence of *Capillaria plica* infections in red foxes (*Vulpes vulpes*) in Southern Germany. Par. Res. 108, 1063-1067.

Bowman, D.D., Hendrix, C.M., Lindsay, D.S. and Barr, S.C. 2002. Feline Clinical Parasitology. Iowa State University Press, Ames, Iowa, USA.

Callegari, D., Kramer, L., Cantoni, A.M., Di Lecce, R., Dodi, P.L. and Grandi, G. 2010. Canine bladderworm (*Capillaria plica*) infection associated with glomerular amyloidosis. Vet. Parasitol. 168, 338-341.

Cazelles, C., Bourdeau, P. and Vidal, J. 1989. Capillariose vesicale chez un chien: a propos d'un cas. Point Vet. 21, 41-44.

Davidson, R., Gjerde, B., Vikoren, T., Lillehaug, A. and Handeland, K. 2006. Prevalence of *Trichinella* larvae and extra intestinal nematodes in Norwegian red foxes (*Vulpes vulpes*). Vet. Parasitol. 136, 307-316.

Fernández-Aguilar, X., Mattsson, R., Meijer, T., Osterman-Lind, E. and Gavier-Widén, D. 2010. *Pearsonema* (*syn Capillaria*) *plica* associated cystitis in a Fennoscandian arctic fox (*Vulpes lagopus*): a case report. Acta Vet. Scand. DOI: 10.1186/1751-0147-52-39.

International Renal Interest Society. 2013. http://www.iris-kidney.com [accessed 01 February, 2015].

Kirkpatrick, C.E. and Nelson, G.R. 1987. Ivermectin treatment of urinary capillariasis in a dog. J. Am. Vet. Med. Assoc. 191, 701-702.

Kruger, J.M. and Osborne, C.A. 1993. The role of uropathogens in feline lower urinary tract disease. Clinical implications. Vet. Clin. North Am. Small Anim. Pract. 23, 101-123.

Magi, M., Guardone, L., Prati, M.C., Mignone, W. and Macchioni, F. 2014. Extraintestinal nematodes of the red fox (*Vulpes vulpes*) in north-west Italy. J. Helminthol.11, 1-6.

Mariacher, A., Eleni, C., Fico, R., Ciarrocca, E. and Perrucci, S. 2015. *Pearsonema plica* and *Eucoleus böhmi* infections and associated lesions in wolves (*Canis lupus*) from Italy. Helminthologia 52, 364-369.

Maurelli, P.M., Rinaldi, L., Rubino, G., Lia, R., Musella, V. and Cringoli, G. 2014. FLOTAC and mini-FLOTAC for uro-microscopic diagnosis of *Capillaria plica* (syn. *Pearsonema plica*) in dogs. BMC Res. Notes 7, 591.

Otranto, D. 2015. Diagnostic challenges and the unwritten stories of dog and cat parasites. Vet. Parasitol. 212, 54-61. DOI: 10.1016/j.vetpar.2015.06.002.

Rossi, M., Messina, N., Ariti, G., Riggio, F. and Perrucci, S. 2011 Symptomatic *Capillaria plica* infection in a young European cat. J. Feline Med. Surg.13, 793-795.

Senior, D.F., Solomon, G.B., Goldschmidt, M.H., Joyce, T. and Bovee, K.C. 1980. *Capillaria plica* infection in dogs. J. Am. Vet. Med. Assoc. 176, 901-905.

Spillmann, S.K. and Glardon, O.J. 1989. Welche diagnose stellen sie? - Welche therapeutischen massnhamen schlagen sie vor? Schweiz. Arch. Tierheilkd. 131, 213-214.

Sréter, T., Széll, Z., Marucci, G., Pozio, E. and Varga, I. 2003. Extraintestinal nematode infections of red foxes (*Vulpes vulpes*) in Hungary. Vet. Parasitol. 115, 329-334.

Studzińska, M.B., Obara-Gałek, J., Demkowska-Kutrzepa, M. and Tomczuk, K. 2015. Diagnosis and therapy of *Capillaria plica* infection: report and literature review. Acta Parasitol. 60, 563-566.

van Veen, L. 2002. Bladder infection with *Capillaria plica* in a male dog. Tijdschrift voor diergeneeskunde. 127, 393-394.

4

Cellular and molecular etiology of hepatocyte injury in a murine model of environmentally induced liver abnormality

M.A. Al-Griw[1,*], R.O. Alghazeer[2], S.A. Al-Azreg[3] and E.M. Bennour[4]

[1]*Division of Developmental Biology, Zoology Department, Faculty of Science, University of Tripoli, Tripoli, Libya*
[2]*Chemistry Department, Faculty of Science, University of Tripoli, Tripoli, Libya*
[3]*Department of Pathology and Clinical Pathology, Faculty of Veterinary Medicine, University of Tripoli, Tripoli, Libya*
[4]*Department of Internal Medicine, Faculty of Veterinary Medicine, University of Tripoli, Tripoli, Libya*

Abstract

Exposures to a wide variety of environmental substances are negatively associated with many biological cell systems both in humans and rodents. Trichloroethane (TCE), a ubiquitous environmental toxicant, is used in large quantities as a dissolvent, metal degreaser, chemical intermediate, and component of consumer products. This increases the likelihood of human exposure to these compounds through dermal, inhalation and oral routes. The present *in vivo* study was aimed to investigate the possible cellular and molecular etiology of liver abnormality induced by early exposure to TCE using a murine model. The results showed a significant increase in liver weight. Histopathological examination revealed a TCE-induced hepatotoxicity which appeared as heavily congested central vein and blood sinusoids as well as leukocytic infiltration. Mitotic figures and apoptotic changes such as chromatin condensation and nuclear fragments were also identified. Cell death analysis demonstrates hepatocellular apoptosis was evident in the treated mice compared to control. TCE was also found to induce oxidative stress as indicated by an increase in the levels of lipid peroxidation, an oxidative stress marker. There was also a significant decrease in the DNA content of the hepatocytes of the treated groups compared to control. Agarose gel electrophoresis also provided further biochemical evidence of apoptosis by showing internucleosomal DNA fragmentation in the liver cells, indicating oxidative stress as the cause of DNA damage. These results suggest the need for a complete risk assessment of any new chemical prior to its arrival into the consumer market.

Keywords: Apoptosis, DNA damage, Environmental toxicant, Liver, Oxidative stress.

Introduction

The extensive use of chemicals has been recently criticized due to their persistence in the environment and their accumulation in the tissues of organisms. One of the most concerned issues in the modern society is evaluating the toxicity of environmental (pollutant) chemicals, such as cadmium, mercury, bisphenol A (BPA), dioxin and trichloroethane (TCE). Some of these toxicants show immediate effect whereas others can result in subtle alterations that are delayed in their expression (Wang *et al.*, 2013). TCE is considered as ubiquitous environmental toxicant and it is a volatile organic solvent that has been used in large quantities as an industrial dissolvent, a metal degreaser, a chemical intermediate, and as a component of consumer products (Warren *et al.*, 1998; Wang *et al.*, 2013). TCE has been originally produced as a safer alternative to other chlorinated solvents; as its acute and chronic toxicities are relatively low (EPA, 2007). However, the exposure to high concentrations of TCE could result in toxic effects especially to those who are subjected to TCE either in the workplace or to those who recreationally abuse the solvent (Warren *et al.*, 1998; ATSDR, 2006).

In humans, epidemiological studies showed that acute exposure have produced an impaired performance in the tests of manual dexterity, eye-hand coordination, perceptual speed and reaction time (Mackay *et al.*, 1987; Warren *et al.*, 1998). While severe exposures to TCE have resulted in sensitization of the heart to epinephrine-induced arrhythmias and mild hepatorenal effects (ATSDR, 2006).

Liver function can be affected through several cellular and molecular mechanisms. Numerous studies have suggested oxidative alterations in hepatocytes such as mitochondrial dysfunction, membrane injury and denaturation of DNA and other cell components (Kurose *et al.*, 1997). Excessive production of reactive oxygen species (ROS), such as the superoxide anion O_2^- and hydroxyl radicals (HO·) can lead to altered enzyme activity, decreased DNA repair, impaired utilization of oxygen, glutathione depletion, and lipid peroxidation. Some of these alterations induced by oxidative stress have been recognized to be characteristic features of necrosis (Gujral *et al.*, 2001, 2002). ROS has been involved in the pathogenesis of diseases and a variety of ROS-mediated modifications of proteins have been

*Corresponding Author: Dr. Mohamed A. Al-Griw. Division of Developmental Biology, Zoology Department, Faculty of Science, University of Tripoli, P.O. Box 13160, Tripoli, Libya. E-mail: m.algriw@uot.edu.ly

reported in various diseases (Khan *et al*., 2001; Morgan *et al*., 2005; Oates, 2010; Wang *et al*., 2013). Proteins perform crucial functions within living cells, but even a relatively minor structural modification of proteins often leads to a marked change (generally lowering) in their functions (Orengo *et al*., 1999). Increasing evidence suggests that ROS-modified proteins such as protein carbonyls and lipid peroxidation-derived aldehydes [LPDAs, including malondialdehyde (MDA) and 4-hydroxynonenal (HNE)]-protein adducts may elicit an autoimmune response and contribute to disease pathogenesis (Ben Mansour *et al*., 2010). Indeed, higher levels of MDA-/HNE-modified proteins and protein carbonyls have been seen in autoimmune disease patients (Ben Mansour *et al*., 2010; Wang *et al*., 2010), illustrating a role for these oxidative modified proteins in autoimmune diseases. Oxidative stress can affect cell integrity only when antioxidant mechanisms are no longer able to cope with free radical generation. The cell death could be either through apoptosis or necrosis. The apoptosis is a permanent cell death where nucleus undergoes fragmentation, whereas the necrosis results from reversible cellular changes, as under favorable condition necrotic cells become a normal cell (Chattopadhyay and Wahi, 2009). During injury, cells die by a combination of several mechanisms including intracellular oxidant stress, exposure to external cytotoxic mediators, and prolonged ischemia. Cell death of hepatocytes following liver injury is characterized by swelling of cells and their organelles, release of cell contents, eosinophilia, karyolysis, and induction of inflammation (Chattopadhyay *et al*., 2007). These morphological features are characteristic of oncotic necrosis. It was postulated that most liver cells actually die by apoptosis (Chattopadhyay *et al*., 2007; Chattopadhyay and Wahi, 2009), which is morphologically characterized by cell shrinkage, formation of apoptotic bodies with intact cell organelles and the absence of inflammation (Chattopadhyay and Wahi, 2009). It has been documented that 50-80% of liver endothelial cells and hepatocytes die through apoptosis during the first three to six hours following injury (Gujral *et al*., 2001). Immediate cell contents release and inflammation are not consistent with apoptosis as the only mode of cell death and interventions such as overexpression of BCL-2 can prevent both apoptotic and necrotic cell injury (Gujral *et al*., 2001, 2002). Previously, many laboratories reported evidence for apoptotic cell death after liver injury (Gujral *et al*., 2002). According to these studies, 50-70% of endothelial cells and 40-60% of hepatocytes undergo apoptosis during ischaemic reperfusion (Gujral *et al*., 2002). A high percentage of apoptotic hepatocytes were also identified in human liver allografts (Gujral *et al*., 2001, 2002). Although there is morphological evidence of apoptosis for individual

cells, the quantitation of apoptosis in the tissue was mainly based on the TUNEL assay (Gujral *et al*., 2001, 2002). In addition to these parameters, DNA laddering and moderate caspase-3 activation were also reported (Gujral *et al*., 2001, 2002).

As little data is available regarding the molecular and cellular etiology of TCE-mediated liver abnormality, therefore, the aim of this study was to investigate, through an *in vivo* murine model, the possible contribution of oxidative stress, DNA damage and apoptosis in TCE-mediated hepatotoxicity.

Materials and Methods

Animals and housing

All efforts were made to fulfill the ethical experimentation standards such as minimizing the pain during animal handling and experiments as well as reducing the number of animals used. A total of twenty four Swiss albino mice, with an age range of three to five weeks and weight range of 21-24 g, were used in this study. They were bred in the animal house of the Zoology Department (Faculty of Science, University of Tripoli, Tripoli, Libya) and housed under natural conditions of light (12 hour cycle), temperature $(24 \pm 2°C)$ and $55 \pm 5\%$ relative humidity. Food and drinking water were available *ad libitum*.

Experimental design

Animals were divided into four groups of six mice each. These groups were: Two TCE-treated groups, sham control group and vehicle control group. Various concentrations of TCE (Baxter International) were dissolved in corn oil and administered to mice intraperitoneally with repeated doses (100 or 400 µg/kg BW TCE twice weekly for three weeks). The doses were calculated and delivered in 80-100 µl of corn oil based on their body weight (Melani *et al*., 2003; Wang *et al*., 2013). TCE doses were selected as they considered safe by Environmental Protection Agency (EPA) (Lane *et al*., 1982). Mice serving as vehicle control received just the corn oil. However, the sham control group neither receive the toxicant (TCE) nor the vehicle (corn oil). The exposure window was selected because this is the critical development window in the mouse (Wang *et al*., 2014).

Clinical assessment

All the animals were regularly observed for the signs of toxicity and survival rate was recorded during the entire study. Two independent observers confirmed the cause of death to exclude TCE-nonrelated mortality. The body weight of each animal was recorded at the initiation of study and once a week during the study, as well as prior to sacrifice.

Tissue processing and histopathology

For necropsy, mice were deeply anesthetized then euthanized. The livers were dissected immediately and washed with normal saline. Then, saline was soaked on blotting paper and liver weight was recorded for each individual animal and the liver was immediately preserved in 10% formalin. For histological examination, slides were prepared as described by Bancroft and Cook (1984). The liver architecture was observed and imaged using low- and high-power objectives under a light microscope (Leica, Germany).

Scoring of cell death

To assess cell death, images of H&E-stained liver sections were examined by using ImageJ software (version 1.45) and a manual count was performed. Cell numbers were expressed as a percentage of the number present for each treatment group and an overall percentage obtained by averaging the data for all cells within a treatment group. Apoptotic cells were identified by morphological criteria such as cell shrinkage, chromatin condensation and margination, and apoptotic bodies (Gujral et al., 2001), while hepatocytes undergoing necrosis were identified using the criteria as increased eosinophilia, cell swelling and lysis, loss of architecture, karyolysis and karyorrhexis. The percent of apoptosis was estimated by evaluating the number of microscopic fields with apoptosis compared to the entire histologic section. The scoring scale was set from 0 to 5, with the following criteria: (0): No necrosis; (1): Mild; (2): Mild to moderate; (3): Moderate; (4): Moderate to severe; and (5): Severe. For each liver section, the eight scores were averaged, and this average was considered as a replicate. All histopathology work was done in randomly selected animals by two independent examiners.

DNA isolation and electrophoresis

For genomic analysis, hepatic tissues of control and TCE-treated mice were kept deeply frozen. DNA was isolated using a QIAamp DNA MiniKit (Qiagen). In brief, up to 25 mg of tissue samples were ground into small pieces and homogenized in DNA lysis buffer and proteinase K (2 mg/mL) and incubated in the same buffer overnight at 56° C. Samples were treated with RNase A (20 mg/mL), purified on spin column and eluted with Tris/EDTA buffer. The extracted DNA was measured by UV spectrophotometry (BioPhotometer, eppendorf), with an absorbance of A260/A280 nm ratios at pH 8.0. To determine the integrity of the extracted DNA, three micrograms of each DNA extract were fractionated by electrophoresis on 1.5% agarose gel. The gel was stained with GelRed™ (Sigma) and the DNA bands were visualized under UV light source.

Lipid peroxidation (LPO) assay

The thiobarbituric acid reactive substances (TBARS) assay, which measures MDA (an end product of lipid peroxidation) concentration, has been used as a measure of oxidative stress (Dalle-Donne et al., 2006). Briefly, 0.2 ml of liver homogenate (10% W/V in Phosphate buffered saline) was added to 100 μl BHA to prevent further oxidation and 500 μl of 25% HCl and 500 μl 1% TBA. The mixture was vortexed for 20 sec and incubated in a water bath at 90 °C for 1 h and cooled down to 20° C. The mixture was measured for absorbance at 532 nm using a spectrophotometer (Jenway UV-6305, Essex, England). The calibration curve was obtained using different concentrations of 1, 1, 3, 3-tetramethoxypropane as standard to determine the concentration of TBA-MDA adducts in samples as nmol/ml (Utley et al., 1967).

Statistics

Statistical significance was determined using analysis of variance or t-test, as appropriate (SPSS, version 20). Data are presented as means ± standard error of the mean (SEM).

Results

Impact of TCE on animal survival

The TCE treatment did not affect the survival/mortality rate of the animals as compared to control during the experiment.

TCE exposure increases liver weight but not body weight

The body and liver weights in the different groups have been monitored in order to investigate the impact of TCE on such parameters. The results showed that TCE insult had no significant effect on the overall body weight (Table 1). There was a significant increase in the liver weight of 400 μg/kg TCE-treated group compared to control ($P = 0.01$). The vehicle had no significant effect on the body and liver weights when applied under normoxic conditions (Table 1). No significant changes were observed in the liver weight of 100 μg/kg TCE-treated groups (Table 1) indicating that TCE at the dose of 100 μg/kg bw is a No Observed Adverse Effective Level (NOAEL) for mice in this study.

TCE induces vascular and degenerative changes in hepatic architecture

At necropsy, no gross pathological changes have been noticed on the livers of control and TCE-treated mice. The histopathological examination of liver tissues of sham control group exhibited normal architecture of hepatocytes, blood sinusoids, and portal areas including hepatic portal vein, hepatic artery, and bile ducts (Fig. 1a). The liver sections of TCE-treated mice revealed different histopathological changes represented by mild congestion of hepatic blood vessels, perivascular aggregation of lymphocytes in

Table 1. The impact of TCE on body and liver weights.

Groups	Body weight (g)	Liver weight (g)
Sham	27.91±0.71	1.26±0.23
Vehicle	28.56±1.19	1.27±0.13
100 μg/kg TCE	28.25±0.67	1.43±0.04
400 μg/kg TCE	31.08±0.86	1.89±0.21*

Data are represented as mean±SEM (n=6-8 per group) *Significantly different from control ($P \leq 0.05$).

portal area and hydropic degeneration of hepatocytes in centrolobular zone. Furthermore, sections exhibited some hepatocytes with mitotic figures and activated Kuffer cells. In 100 µg/kg TCE-treated mice, the histological examination of hepatic tissues showed a mild vascular congestion and dilation, perivascular cloudy swelling and hydropic degeneration, mild biliary proliferation, and interstitial and periportal aggregation of lymphocytes (Fig. 1b). The hepatic tissues of mice received 400 µg/kg TCE treatment showed a vascular congestion and cellular degeneration evidenced by cloudy swelling of hepatocytes with proliferation of bile ductules (Fig. 1c). Moreover, there were a large number of regenerative hepatocytes with hyperchromatic nuclei (Fig. 1c).

TCE induces nuclear alterations and hepatocellular apoptosis

Cell death, which could be induced in hepatic tissues by early exposure to TCE, was evaluated. The results showed that there was an increased hepatocyte cell death after TCE induced hepatic injury. Cell death analysis demonstrated that a large majority of hepatocytes undergone apoptosis in response to TCE treatment. Hepatocytes in TCE-treated mice displayed distinct morphological alterations in their nuclei, compared to control, represented by a prominent chromatin condensation and vacuole formation (Fig. 2a). In most cells, nuclear changes were accompanied by other degenerative changes. Most of the hepatocytes with cytoplasmic and/or nuclear degenerative changes maintained an intact plasma membrane. Limiting the counting of total hepatocyte nuclei to areas with true cross sections of hepatocytes made it possible to selectively count only the nuclei which were clearly were within a hepatocyte. The quantitative analysis of cell death revealed that the TCE-treated mice had a significant increase in the number of apoptotic hepatocytes compared to control (Fig. 2b). The vehicle control group had only rare apoptotic cells, and there was no significant difference between sham and vehicle groups. Moreover, there was no significant difference in the percentage of apoptotic hepatocytes between 100 µg/kg and 400 µg/kg TCE-treated groups (Fig. 2b). To substantiate our histological evidence for liver abnormality, a biomarker of hepatocyte count (DNA concentration and content) was used. Internucleosomal DNA fragmentation by endonuclease cleavage is a well-defined biochemical marker of cells undergoing apoptosis which results in DNA fragments, as compared to necrosis that causes nonspecific degradation of DNA into random-sized fragments (Wyllie, 1981). Nuclear DNA from control and TCE-treated mice was analyzed by agarose gel electrophoresis. DNA fragmentation was markedly induced in the TCE-treated groups when compared to that in control (Fig. 3a). A smear pattern resulting from random DNA degradation suggested

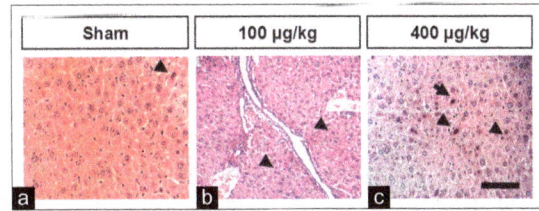

Fig. 1. Representative light photomicrograph of hepatic tissue sections from control and TCE-treated mice (H&E 100X). (a) Hepatic tissues of sham control mice with normal hepatic lobules and hepatocytes. (b) Hepatic tissues of 100 µg/kg TCE-treated mice with mild steatosis and inflammatory infiltrates. (c) Hepatic tissues of 400 µg/kg TCE-treated mice with severe steatosis and inflammatory infiltrates. Fibrotic and hepatocyte alterations can be seen in the TCE-treated tissues. The arrows in panel a, b, and c indicate a cell with vacuolated and pale-staining cytoplasm and alterations in nuclear morphology respectively. n=6. Scale bar = 250 µm.

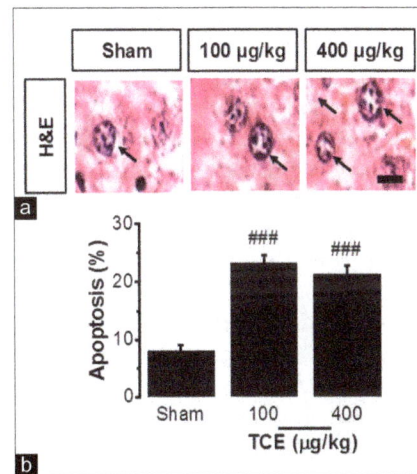

Fig. 2. Quantification of hepatocytes with fragmented DNA. (a) Representative photomicrographs of hepatic tissues from control and TCE-treated mice (H&E 400X). Control mice nucleus showed no or little histopathological changes (normal nuclear appearance). Hepatocytes were partly lost and some cells exhibited necrotic characteristics after TCE exposure (arrows). In TCE-treated mice, the nuclei also exhibited typical apoptotic morphology as condensed and fragmented (arrows). Scale bar = 30 µm. (b) Quantification of hepatic cell death in control and TCE-treated mice. Data are expressed as the mean ± SEM (n = 6). #Significantly different from control ($P < 0.05$).

that necrosis might have occurred concurrently with apoptosis. Also there was a reduction in the DNA concentration of the TCE-treated mice (Fig. 3b). These data are consistent with the increase in the hepatocellular apoptosis. In addition, the vehicle had no significant effect on the DNA concentration when applied under normoxic conditions (Fig. 3c).

TCE increases lipid peroxidation in the hepatic tissues

TCE has been shown to generate free radicals and induce oxidative stress both *in vivo* and *in vitro* (Wang *et al.*, 2013). To further evaluate the role of lipid peroxidation/oxidative stress in induction of TCE mediated hepatotoxicity, formation of MDA in the liver homogenates of control and TCE-treated mice was quantified. MDA is a marker of oxidative lipid damage and a major oxidative product of peroxidized polyunsaturated fatty acids (Zhang *et al.*, 2004). The present results showed that MDA levels in the liver homogenates were higher in both 100 µg/kg bw and 400 µg/kg bw TCE-treated groups compared to that in control (Fig. 4a), suggesting an overall increase in oxidative stress. Moreover, vehicle had no significant effect on the MDA level when applied under normoxic conditions (Fig. 4b).

Discussion

The exposure to environmental toxic chemicals can cause several detrimental effects in biological cell systems (Topham, 1980; House *et al.*, 1996; Snyder and Andrews, 1996; Griffin *et al.*, 2000; Wang *et al.*, 2007, 2013; Al-Griw *et al.*, 2015a,b,c). TCE, a widely used industrial agent and a ubiquitous environmental contaminant, is non-carcinogenic (group 3) because there is inadequate evidence for carcinogenicity in both human and animals according to EPA and National Toxicology Program (NTP) technical report (NTP, 2000; EPA, 2007). In addition, according to WHO toxicological report, TCE is not considered as toxic, and not necessary to drive a health risk based on the guideline standards (WHO, 2003). However, the Agency for Toxic Substances and Disease Registry (ATSDR) indicated that TCE affects many internal organs and systems such as cardiovascular and nervous system (Lawrence, 2006). TCE has been implicated in the development of autoimmune disorders in humans (Cooper *et al.*, 2009) and induces autoimmune response in experimental animals (Wang *et al.*, 2007, 2013; Cooper *et al.*, 2009). However, the mechanisms by which TCE induces/accelerates the autoimmune disease pathogenesis are still unclear.

The present study showed that oxidative stress and apoptosis, a form of genetically programmed cell death, as a potential mechanism mediating hepatocyte cell death after exposure to low dose of TCE. A combination of techniques has been used to obtain morphological and biochemical evidence for oxidative stress and apoptosis, including biochemical markers, histopathological examination with diverse staining techniques and DNA gel electrophoresis. Although other forms of cell death might have occurred, our data suggest that both oxidative stress and apoptosis contributed to the loss of hepatocytes after TCE induced liver injury. *In vivo* experimental studies are crucial to evaluate environmental chemicals with adverse risk to health at birth or later in life. The *in vivo* study of the toxicity of chemicals is of great importance because animal systems are extremely complicated, and the interaction

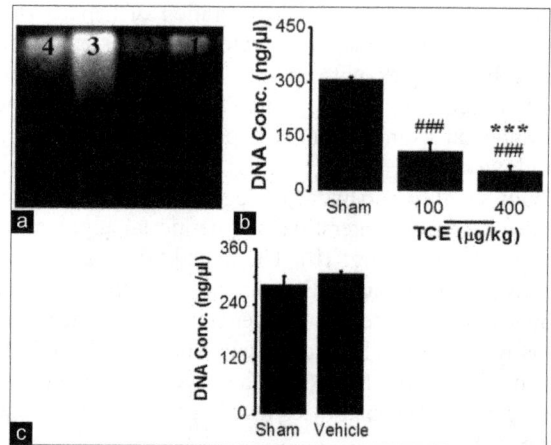

Fig. 3. DNA biomarker for hepatocytes (DNA content, quality and integrity) in control and TCE-treated mice. (a) Agarose gel electrophoresis of DNA isolated from liver of control and TCE-treated mice; sham control (lane1), vehicle control (lane2), 100 µg/kg TCE-treated mice (lane3) and 400 µg/kg TCE-treated mice (lane4). Almost no or little DNA degradation was detected in controls. DNA ladder with internucleosomal DNA fragmentation fragments appeared with a smear pattern in TCE treatment groups. (b) Quantification of DNA concentration in control and TCE-treated groups. Data are presented as the mean ± SEM. (c) Quantification of DNA concentration in sham and vehicle groups. Data are presented as the mean ± SEM (n = 6). *Significantly different from sham control ($P \leq 0.05$). #Significantly different from 100 µg/kg TCE-treated group ($P \leq 0.05$).

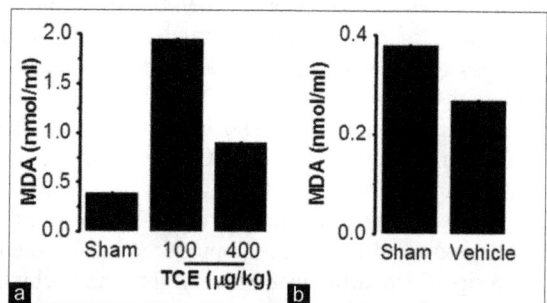

Fig. 4. Levels of oxidative stress biomarker MDA (nmol/ml) in the murine livers. (a) Quantification of levels of MDA (nmol/ml) in the livers of control and TCE-treated groups. (b) Quantification of levels of MDA (nmol/ml) in the livers of sham and vehicle groups. The values are presented as means ± SEM (n = 6).

of chemical compounds with biological components could lead to unique biodistribution, clearance, immune responses and metabolism. The results of this study revealed that TCE insult could increase the liver weight and cause its injury. The observation detected by H&E staining showed that the control livers presented normal features with normal hepatic lobule and normal hepatocytes, while in the TCE-treated groups, hepatocyte damage was manifested by severe steatosis and inflammatory infiltrates. When compared to control group, liver sections of TCE treated groups showed widely distributed pyknotic nuclei and morphological alterations in their nuclei. When referring to the TCE toxicity, prior studies (Quast et al., 1984, 1988) reported that TCE exposure have no impact on weights of body and livers in rats but can induce liver damage and affect hepatocyte counts. In contrast, we detected dominant changes in the liver, but not body, weights. The increase in the liver weight may be attributable to the inflammatory events generated due to TCE exposure as appeared in the histopathological sections of liver.

Classically, hepatocyte cell death during liver injury was indicated by either programmed (apoptosis), or accidental, uncontrolled cell death (necrosis). Growing evidence from our current understanding of the biochemical and molecular mechanisms involved in cell demise has provided an expanding view of various modes of cell death that can be triggered during both acute and chronic liver damage such as necroptosis, pyroptosis, and autophagic cell death. The complexity of noninvasively assessing the predominant mode of cell death during a specific liver insult in either experimental in vivo models or in humans is highlighted by the fact that in many instances there is significant crosstalk and overlap between the different cell death pathways (Eguchi et al., 2014).

Several studies reported evidence for apoptotic cell death during liver injury. In this study, a combination of techniques has been used to obtain morphological and biochemical evidence for apoptosis, including histopathological examination with diverse staining techniques. Light microscopy showed alterations in the nuclear morphology of hepatocytes in TCE-treated groups, which were characterized by prominent chromatin condensation and vacuole formation. Hence, we demonstrated nuclear morphological alterations in TCE hepatocytes, but not in the control groups. In most cells, nuclear changes were accompanied by other degenerative changes. Most of the hepatocytes with cytoplasmic and/or nuclear degenerative changes maintained an intact plasma membrane. Our study demonstrated that apoptosis, a form of genetically programmed cell death, is a potential mechanism mediating hepatocyte death. Although other forms of cell death might have occurred, our data suggest that apoptosis might contribute to the loss of hepatocytes in response to TCE exposure. However, the results of this study strongly suggested that the main mode of cell death after injury was necrosis, although we cannot exclude potential switch in the mode of cell death from necrosis to apoptosis.

In recent years, free radical-mediated reactions as the potential mechanism in the pathogenesis of autoimmune diseases have drawn increasing attention (Khan et al., 2001). TCE is known to generate free radicals, and cause increased lipid peroxidation in both in vivo and in vitro models (Khan et al., 2001; Wang et al., 2007). Several lines of evidence in lupus-prone mice showed that increased generation of ROS was correlated with increased autoantibodies production, illustrating a potential role of oxidative stress in TCE induced autoimmune response (Wang et al., 2007, 2010). Although there is a large body of literature addressing immune responses during environmental chemicals exposure, the TCE immunotoxicity is poorly understood. Even though TCE is known to generate free radicals, causes increased oxidative stress and induces autoimmune response (Wang et al., 2007, 2013), potential mechanisms by which TCE induced ROS generation lead to an autoimmune response and their contribution to disease pathogenesis remains largely unknown.

To further support these findings and offer new mechanistic evidence for the role of oxidative stress in TCE-induced injury, we first examined the markers of oxidative stress in TCE-treated mice. TCE- treated groups showed a significant increase in the liver MDA level in comparison to untreated groups. TCE insult also led to increased formation of MDA in sera, spleens and kidneys, major organs where TCE is known to generate free radicals and induce autoimmune disorders (Griffin et al., 2000; Wang et al., 2013), further confirming earlier findings of the potential of TCE in inducing increased lipid peroxidation. It was found that the TCE treatment can result in hepatotoxicity by elevating the oxidative stress markers MDA, hydroxynonenal (HNE)-protein, and protein oxidation (carbonylation) (Wang et al., 2013). Consistent with these findings, our results also unravel the same changes. The increase in the oxidative stress markers in the liver is attributed to the damage of hepatocytes, which is supported by the histopathological picture of the hepatic tissues.

In conclusion, our findings demonstrated that early exposure to TCE could cause serious hepatotoxicity, oxidative stress, lipid peroxidation and degeneration/apoptosis of hepatocytes in mouse at later in life. Histopathological examination of liver tissues exposed to TCE showed heavily congested central vein and blood sinusoids, widespread pyknotic nuclei in the hepatic tissue, and leukocyte infiltration. The results also showed that TCE exposure leads to a significant induction of MDA and increases protein oxidation (carbonylation) in the liver, suggesting the potential of TCE to induce an overall increase in oxidative stress. Taken together, the results of this study suggest that oxidative stress and apoptosis might play a crucial role in hepatotoxicity of TCE. These results also provide important insights into mechanisms of TCE-elicited toxicity and call for further research regarding protective measures against TCE-induced hepatocyte damage.

Acknowledgments
This work was supported in part by the Division of Developmental Biology, Zoology Department, Faculty of Science, University of Tripoli, Tripoli, Libya.
Conflict of Interest
The authors declare that they have no competing interests.

References

Al-Griw, M.A., Salama, N.M., Treesh, S.A., Algadi, L.N. and Elnfati, A.H. 2015a. Cell Death in Mouse Brain following Early Exposure to Trichloroethane (TCE). Int. J. Adv. Res. 3(6), 1424-1430.

Al-Griw, M.A., Elnfati, A.H., Salama, N.M., Maamar, M.S., Treesh, S.A. and Shaibi, T. 2015b. Mode of Cell Death in Mouse Brain Following Early Exposure to Low-Dose Trichloroethane: Apoptosis or Necrosis. Am. J. Biol. Life Sci. 3(6), 232-240.

Al-Griw, M.A., Salama, N.M., Treesh, S.A. and Elnfati, A.H. 2015c. Transgenerational Genetic Effect of Trichloroethane (TCE) on Phenotypic Variation of Acrosomal Proteolytic Enzyme and Male Infertility Risk. Int. J. Genet. Genomics 3(5), 43-49.

ATSDR. 2006. Toxicological Profile for 1,1,1-trichloroethane (update). U.S. Department of Health and Human Services, Public Health Service. Agency for Toxic Substances and Disease Registry. https://www.atsdr.cdc.gov/toxprofiles/tp70.pdf.

Bancroft, J.D. and Cook, H.C. 1984. Manual of Histological Techniques. Churchill Livingstone, Edinburgh, London, Melbourne, New York.

Ben Mansour, R., Lassoued, S., Elgaied, A., Haddouk, S., Marzouk, S., Bahloul, Z., Masmoudi, H., Attia, H., Aïfa, M.S. and Fakhfakh, F. 2010. Enhanced reactivity to malondialdehyde modified proteins by systemic lupus erythematosus autoantibodies. Scand. J. Rheumatol. 39, 247-253.

Chattopadhyay, P., Sharma, A.K. and Wahi, A.K. 2007. Folic acid protects hepatobiliary function in ischemic reperfusion of rat liver. Indian J. Gastroentrol. 26, 95-96.

Chattopadhyay, P. and Wahi, A.K. 2009. Hepatocyte Deaths Occur by Apoptosis After Ischemia-Reperfusion Injury in the Rat Liver Transplantation Model. Trends Biomater. Artif. Organs 23, 1-5.

Cooper, G.S., Makris, S.L., Nietert, P.J. and Jinot, J. 2009. Evidence of autoimmune-related effects of trichloroethylene exposure from studies in mice and humans. Environ. Health Perspect. 117, 696-702.

Dalle-Donne, I., Rossi, R., Colombo, R., Giustarini, D. and Milzani, A. 2006. Biomarkers of oxidative damage in human disease. Clin. Chem. 52, 601-623.

Eguchi, A., Wree, A. and Feldstein, A.E. 2014. Biomarkers of liver cell death. J. Hepatol. 60, 1063-1074.

EPA. 2007. Toxicological Review of 1,1,1-Trichloroethane (CAS No. 71-55-6). In Support of Summary Information on the Integrated Risk Information System (IRIS). EPA/635/R-03/013. U.S. Environmental Protection Agency, Washington, DC. https://cfpub.epa.gov/ncea/iris/iris_documents/documents/toxreviews/0197tr.pdf.

Griffin, J.M., Blossom, S.J., Jackson, S.K., Gilbert, K.M. and Pumford, N.R. 2000. Trichloroethylene accelerates an autoimmune response by Th1 T cell activation in MRL+/+ mice. Immunopharmacology. 46, 123-137.

Gujral, J.S., Bucci, T.J., Farhood, A. and Jaeschke, H. 2001. Mechanism of Cell Death During Warm Hepatic Ischemia-Reperfusion in Rats: Apoptosis or Necrosis? Hepatology. 33, 397-405.

Gujral, J.S., Knight, T.R., Farhood, A., Bajt, M.L. and Jaeschke, H. 2002. Mode of cell death after acetaminophen overdose in mice: Apoptosis or oncotic necrosis? Toxicol. Sci. 67, 322-328.

House, R.A., Liss, G.M., Wills, M.C. and Holness, D.L. 1996. Paresthesias and sensory neuropathy due to 1,1,1-trichloroethane. J. occup. environ. Med. 38, 123-124.

Khan, M.F., Wu, X. and Ansari, G.A. 2001. Anti-malondialdehyde antibodies inMRL+/+mice treatedwith trichloroethene and dichloroacetyl chloride: Possible role of lipid peroxidation in autoimmunity. Toxicol. Appl. Pharmacol. 170, 88-92.

Kurose, I., Higuchi, H., Miura, S., Saito, H., Watanabe, N., Hokari, R., Hirokawa, M., Takaishi, M., Zeki, S., Nakamura, T., Ebinuma, H., Kato, S. and Ishii, H. 1997. Oxidative stress-mediated apoptosis of hepatocytes exposed to acute ethanol intoxication. Hepatology. 25, 368-378.

Lane, R.W., Riddle, B.L. and Borzelleca, J.F. 1982. Effects of 1,2-dichloroethane and 1,1,1-trichloroethane in drinking water on reproduction and development in mice. Toxicol. Appl. Pharmacol. 63, 409-421.

Lawrence, S.J. 2006. Description, properties, and degradation of selected volatile organic compounds detected in ground water—A Review of Selected Literature: Atlanta, Georgia, U. S. Geological Survey, Open-File Report 2006-1338, 62 pages, a Web-only publication at: http://pubs.usgs.gov/ofr/2006/1338/.

Mackay, C.J., Campbell, L., Samuel, A.M., Alderman, K.J., Idzikowski, C., Wilson, H.K. and Gompertz, D. 1987. Behavioral changes during exposure to 1,1,1-trichloroethane: Time-course and relationship to blood solvent levels. Am. J. Ind.

Med. 11, 223-239.

Melani, A., Pantoni, L. and Bordoni, F. 2003. The selective A2A receptor antagonist SCH 58261 reduces striatal transmitter outflow, turning behavior and ischemic brain damage induced by permanent focal ischemia in the rat. Brain Res. 959, 243-250.

Morgan, P.E., Sturgess, A.D. and Davies, M.J. 2005. Increased levels of serum protein oxidation and correlation with disease activity in systemic lupus erythematosus. Arthritis Rheum. 52, 2069-2079.

NTP. 2000. NTP technical report on the toxicity studies of 1,1,1-trichloroethane administered in microcapsules in feed to F344/N rats and B6C3F1 mice. National Toxicology Program. (41) NIH 004402. www.michigan.gov/./deq-rrd-chem-111-TrichloroethaneDatasheet_527455_7.pdf.

Oates, J.C. 2010. The biology of reactive intermediates in systemic lupus erythematosus. Autoimmunity 43, 56-63.

Orengo, C.A., Todd, A.E. and Thornton, J.M. 1999. From protein structure to function. Curr. Opin. Struct. Biol. 9, 374-382.

Quast, J.F., Calhoun, L.L. and Frauson, L.E. 1988. 1,1,1-trichloroethane formulation: A chronic inhalation toxicity and oncogenicity study in Fischer 344 rats and B6c3F1 mice. Fundam. Appl. Toxicol. 11, 611-625.

Quast, J.F., Calhoun, L.L. and McKenna, M.J. 1984. Chlorothene VG: A chronic inhalation toxicity and oncogenicity study in rats and mice (part 1 and 2) with cover letter dated 08/21/1984. The Dow Chemical Company, Midland, MI. Submitted under TSCA Section 4; EPA Document No. 40-8424496; NTIS No. OTS0510656. https://cfpub.epa.gov/ncea/iris/iris_documents/documents/subst/0197_summary.pdf.

Snyder, R. and Andrews, L.S. 1996. Toxic effects of solvents and vapors. In: Klaassen, CD; ed. Casarett and Doull's Toxicology: The Basis Science of Poisons, 5th ed. New York: McGraw-Hill, pp: 133-186.

Topham, J.C. 1980. Do induced sperm-head abnormalities in mice specifically identify mammalian mutagens rather than carcinogens? Mutat. Res. 74, 379-387.

Utley, H.G., Bernheim, F. and Hochstein, P. 1967. Effect of sulfhydryl reagents on peroxidation in microsomes. Arch. Biochem. Biophys. 118, 29-32.

Wang, G., Cai, P., Ansari, G.A.S. and Khan, M.F. 2007. Oxidative and nitrosative stress in trichloroethene-mediated autoimmune response. Toxicology 229, 186-193.

Wang, G., Pierangeli, S.S., Papalardo, E., Ansari, G.A. and Khan, M.F. 2010. Markers of oxidative and nitrosative stress in systemic lupus erythematosus: Correlation with disease activity. Arthritis Rheum. 62, 2064-2072.

Wang, G., Wang, J., Ma, H., Ansari, G.A.S. and Khan, M.F. 2013. N-Acetylcysteine protects against trichloroethene-mediated autoimmunity by attenuating oxidative stress. Toxicol. Appl. Pharmacol. 273, 189-195.

Wang, W., Hafner, K.S. and Flaws, J.A. 2014. In utero bisphenol A exposure disrupts germ cell nest breakdown and reduces fertility with age in the mouse. Toxicol. Appl. Pharmacol. 276, 157-164.

Warren, D.A., Reigle, T.G., Muralidhara, S. and Dallas, C. 1998. Schedule-controlled operant behavior of rats during 1,1,1-trichloroethane inhalation: Relationship to blood and brain solvent concentrations. Neurotoxicol. Teratol. 20, 143-153.

WHO. 2003. 1,1,1-Trichloroethane in Drinking-water. Background document for development of WHO Guidelines for Drinking-water Quality. World Health Organization WHO/SDE/WSH/03.04/65., 16. www.who.int/water_sanitation_health/dwq/chemicals/111-Trichloroethane.pdf

Wyllie, A. 1981. Cell death: A new classification separating apoptosis from necrosis. In: Bowen ID LR, ed. Cell death in biology and pathology. Chapman and Hall: London, England, pp: 9-34.

Zhang, Y.T., Zheng, Q.S., Pan, J. and Zheng, R.L. 2004. Oxidative damage of biomolecules in mouse liver induced by morphine and protected by antioxidants. Basic Clin. Pharmacol. Toxicol. 95, 53-58.

5

Metabolic and adaptive immune responses induced in mice infected with tissue-dwelling nematode *Trichinella zimbabwensis*

N. Onkoba[1,2,*], M.J. Chimbari[1], J.M. Kamau[2,3,4] and S. Mukaratirwa[4]

[1]*College of Health Sciences, School of Nursing and Public Health, University of KwaZulu-Natal (UKZN), Howard Campus, Durban, South Africa*
[2]*Tropical Infectious Diseases, Institute of Primate Research, Karen, Nairobi, Kenya*
[3]*School of Medicine, Department of Biochemistry, University of Nairobi, Kenya*
[4]*School of Life Sciences, University of KwaZulu-Natal, Westville Campus, Durban, South Africa*

Abstract

Tissue-dwelling helminths are known to induce intestinal and systemic inflammation accompanied with host compensatory mechanisms to counter balance nutritional and metabolic deficiencies. The metabolic and immune responses of the host depend on parasite species and tissues affected by the parasite. This study investigated metabolic and immuno-inflammatory responses of mice infected with tissue-dwelling larvae of *Trichinella zimbabwensis* and explored the relationship between infection, metabolic parameters and Th1/Th17 immune responses. Sixty (60) female BALB/c mice aged between 6 to 8 weeks old were randomly assigned into *T. zimbabwensis*-infected and control groups. Levels of Th1 (interferon-γ) and Th17 (interleukin-17) cytokines, insulin and blood glucose were determined as well as measurements of body weight, food and water intake. Results showed that during the enteric phase of infection, insulin and IFN-γ levels were significantly higher in the *Trichinella* infected group accompanied with a reduction in the trends of food intake and weight loss compared with the control group. During systemic larval migration, trends in food and water intake were significantly altered and this was attributed to compensatory feeding resulting in weight gain, reduced insulin levels and increased IL-17 levels. Larval migration also induced a Th1/Th17 derived inflammatory response. It was concluded that *T. zimbabwensis* alters metabolic parameters by instigating host compensatory feeding. Furthermore, we showed for the first time that non-encapsulated *T. zimbabwensis* parasite plays a role in immunomodulating host Th1/Th17 type responses during chronic infection.
Keywords: Enteric phase, Insulin, Larval migration, Th1 and Th17, *Trichinella zimbabwensis*.

Introduction

Trichinella zimbabwensis is a non-encapsulated zoonotic nematode that is prevalent and widely distributed in Southern Africa where it infects a wide variety of animals (Mukaratirwa and Foggin, 1999; Pozio *et al.*, 2002; Mukaratirwa *et al.*, 2008, 2013; La Grange *et al.*, 2009, 2010). The parasite has potential of causing future outbreaks of human trichinellosis in sub-Sharan Africa due to its capability to infect non-human primates and increase in risk factors like poor animal rearing systems, increased animal product movements and human-wildlife-livestock interactions (Murrell *et al.*, 2005; Mukaratirwa *et al.*, 2008, 2013; Gottstein *et al.*, 2009).

Trichinella infection is acquired through ingestion of raw or undercooked meat infected with *Trichinella* muscle larvae (Nöckler *et al.*, 2000). During the enteric phase of infection, the adult female worm releases up to 1500 new born larvae (NBL) in the intestines which penetrate the intestinal mucosa and migrate to the muscles (Despommier, 1998; Appleton *et al.*, 2001; Gagliardo *et al.*, 2002). The NBL cause temporary enteric and tissue inflammation during migration to the sites of predilection (Bruschi and Chiumiento, 2011). The migrating larvae stimulate both mucosal and systemic immune responses where the parasite utilizes host cell-biological systems to establish its parasitism (Pozio *et al.*, 2004) without causing an overt inflammatory reaction specifically during an asthmatic reaction (Aranzamendi *et al.*, 2013).

In the past two decades, significant studies on the immunological responses and pathological effect of encapsulating tissue-dwelling nematode, *T. spiralis* have identified that the parasite stimulates Th2 immune responses for its establishment (Maizels *et al.*, 2004, 2009; Maizels and Yazdanbakhsh, 2008; Jackson *et al.*, 2009). Furthermore, *T. spiralis* larval and adult products have also been documented to confer protection against inflammatory and auto-immune diseases in mice and humans (Finkelman *et al.*, 2004; Khan and Collins, 2005; Del Prete *et al.*, 2008; Wu *et al.*, 2010; Adisakwattana *et al.*, 2013; Aranzamendi *et al.*, 2013; Rodgers *et al.*, 2014). However, this has not been the case with non-encapsulated nematode like *T. zimbabwensis* that is endemic in Southern Africa (Pozio and Zarlenga, 2005; Pozio, 2013). This

*Corresponding Author: Dr. Nyamongo Onkoba. Institute of Primate Research, P.O. Box 24481-00502 Karen, Nairobi, Kenya.
E-mail: bwonkoba@gmail.com

paucity of studies on metabolic and adaptive immune responses that are induced by *T. zimbabwensis* parasite in infected hosts has hampered efforts to improve tools for diagnosis, surveillance, management and control. In order to improve *Trichinella* infection surveillance and management strategies in sub-Saharan Africa, there is need to understand underlying mechanisms utilized by the parasite in metabolism and induction of immuno-inflammatory responses during chronic *T. zimbabwensis* infection. Thus, this study sought to determine metabolic and immuno-inflammatory responses induced in mice infected *T. zimbabwensis* and the relationship between infection, metabolism and Th1/Th17 type immune response.

Materials and Methods

Study animals

Sixty (60) female BALB/c mice aged between 6 to 8 weeks old were sourced from the University of Cape Town, South Africa. The mice were maintained at the Biomedical Resources Unit (BRU) of the University of KwaZulu-Natal (UKZN), Westville campus, under specific pathogen free conditions where 6 mice were placed in an individually ventilated metabolic cages (Labotec products, RSA). Mice were randomly assigned into two groups; control (n = 30) and *T. zimbabwensis* infected (n = 30) and fed daily on heat sterilized pelleted ration (Meadow feeds, RSA) and clean water was *ad libitum*.

Ethical statement

All experimental protocols and procedures of the study were reviewed and approved by Animals Ethics Committee of the University of KwaZulu-Natal (UKZN) (ref no: 114/13/Animal) in accordance with the South African National guidelines on animal care, handling and use for biomedical research. The experiments are reported in accordance with ARRIVE guidelines (Kilkenny *et al*., 2013).

Parasite isolation and infection of study animals

Crocodile-derived *T. zimbabwensis* strain (Code ISS1209) larvae were obtained from whole eviscerated carcasses of stock rats that were digested as described by Kapel and Gamble (2000). At day 0, each animal in the *Trichinella*-infection group was infected with 500 muscle larvae (ML) through oral lavage as described by Mukaratirwa *et al*. (2001). At day 7, 14, 21 28 and 35 post-infection (pi), six mice from each group were sacrificed, blood was collected for serum, intestines for adult worms (AW) and whole mouse carcass was digested to obtain ML.

Measurement of food and water intake and body weight

The trends in food intake per mouse were derived by weighing the food pellets (Meadow Feeds, RSA) before feeding and 24 hours after feeding the animals on daily basis. After 24 hours from dispensing the pellets to the animals the remaining pellets and pellet crumbs were collected and weighed using Boeco balance (Germany) and the difference from the initial weight was calculated as food intake.

The volume of water intake per mouse was obtained by measuring the difference between final water volume and initial water volume after 24 hours using a laboratory measuring cylinder on daily basis.

Individual mouse body weight was also measured daily using Boeco balance (Germany) and average body weights were calculated for the two groups.

Blood glucose and serum insulin levels

To determine the levels of blood glucose, whole blood was collected using a 25 gauge needle by pricking the tail vein and approximately 10 µL of blood were collected on a glucometer test strip window and used to measure blood glucose using a Contour® TS glucometer according to manufacturer's instructions (Bayer, Basel, Switzerland).

To assay for the levels of insulin in serum following infection with *T. zimbabwensis* parasite, sera were collected from 6 mice from each group sacrificed at days 7, 14, 21 28 and 35 pi were used to measure insulin levels using mouse insulin ELISA kit (cat. No. EZRMI-13K, Millipore, Missouri, USA). Briefly, 96 well plates pre-coated with pre-titered mouse monoclonal antibodies were washed three times with 300µL of 50mM Tri Buffered Saline containing Tween 20. Each serum sample and a pre-determined standard were mixed with 10µL Assay buffer (0.05M phosphosaline, PH 7.4, containing 0.025 M EDTA, 0.08% sodium azide and 1% BSA), 10µL matrix solution containing charcoal-stripped pooled mouse serum and 80µL of pre-titered biotinylated anti-insulin detection antibody per well. The plates were incubated at room temperature for 2 hours while being agitated. Plates were washed as before and 100µL of pre-titered streptavidin peroxidase conjugate solution was added per well and incubated for 30 minutes at room temperature while being agitated. The plates were washed 6 times as before and 100µL of 3, 3', 5, 5' tetra-methylbenzidine solution added per well and placed at room temperature for 15 minutes. The reaction was stopped by adding 50 µL of 0.3M HCL stop solution. Samples and standard optical densities were obtained by reading the plates at 450nm and 590nm wavelengths. A 4 parameter logistic equation was used to determine serum insulin concentrations using GraphPad PRISM version 5.04 for windows (Graph Pad Software, San Diego, CA).

Measurement of cytokine concentrations

To determine the levels of circulating Th1/Th17 cytokines in sera, mouse cytokine specific DuoSet ELISA development system kits (R&D systems, USA) were used to measure IFN-γ (DY485-05) and IL-17 (DY421-05) levels in serum according to manufacturer's instructions. Briefly, NUNC Maxisorp® 96-well ELISA plates were coated with either 4.0 µg/

mL of mouse IFN-γ capture antibody or 2.0 µg/mL of mouse IL-17 capture antibody in PBS and incubated overnight at room temperature. Plates were washed three times with 300 µL of PBS containing 0.05% Tween 20 and blocked with 200 µL of 1% BSA in PBS and incubated for 1 hour at room temperature. Further washing was done five times and 100µl of diluted samples and standards were added to the plates. The standards used were serially diluted in incubation buffer and highest concentrations used were 2000pg/ml for IFN-γ and 1000pg/ml for IL-17. The plates were then incubated for 2 hours at room temperature and washed as before. Biotinylated IFN-γ detection antibody was used at a concentration of 600 µg/ml and IL-17 at 400ng/mL and incubated for 2 hours at room temperature. Plates were then washed as before and 50µl of horseradish peroxidase-conjugated streptavidin was used at a dilution of 1:2000 and incubated for 20 minutes at room temperature. The reactions were stopped by adding 50 µL of 2N H_2SO_4 and absorbance obtained at 450nm and 540 nm. Cytokine concentrations were extrapolated from standards using a 4 parameter logistic equation in Graph Pad PRISM version 5.04 for windows (Graph Pad Software, San Diego, CA).

Data analysis

Cytokine, insulin, blood glucose levels, parasite loads and food and water intake measurements were expressed as means ± standard error (SE) and analysed using repeated measure analysis of variance (ANOVA) and the levels of significance were determined by Bonferroni post-test analyses using Graph pad PRISM version 5.04 for windows (Graph pad software, San Diego, CA, USA) and a *p*-value of < 0.05 was considered to be significant.

Results

Parasite establishment

In the intestines, we were able to recover the *T. zimbabwensis* AW up to 21 days post-infection (Fig. 1). Significantly more adult worms were recovered at day 7 pi compared to days to days 14 and 21 pi ($p<0.001$). At days 14 pi and 21pi, there were no muscle larvae obtained but few larvae were recovered (average of 0.12 larvae per gram (lpg) of muscle). The number of larvae significantly increased to 16 lpg on day 28 ($p<0.05$) and peaking (20 lpg) at day 35 ($p<0.01$).

Food and water intake

At day 3 to 6 pi, the infected group consumed less food compared to the control group (Fig. 2). At day 7 and 18 pi, the trend in the food intake by the infected group increased exponentially in comparison with the control group ($p<0.05$). Where at day 14 pi, the infected group consumed an average of 12 grams of food pellets per day compared to the control group which consumed an average of 4 grams of food pellets per day. At days 19

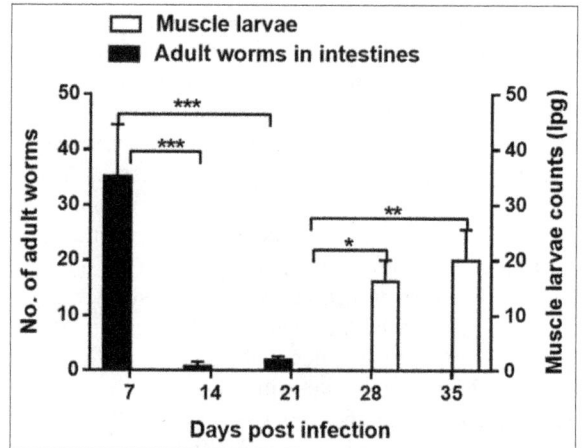

Fig. 1. Mean number of intestinal adult worms (AW) and counts of ML larvae per gram of muscle (lpg) recovered from BALB/c mice infected with *Trichinella zimbabwensis*. Levels of significant differences (* $P<0.05$; ** $P<0.01$, and *** $P<0.001$) were obtained by comparing the parasite loads in the infected and control groups.

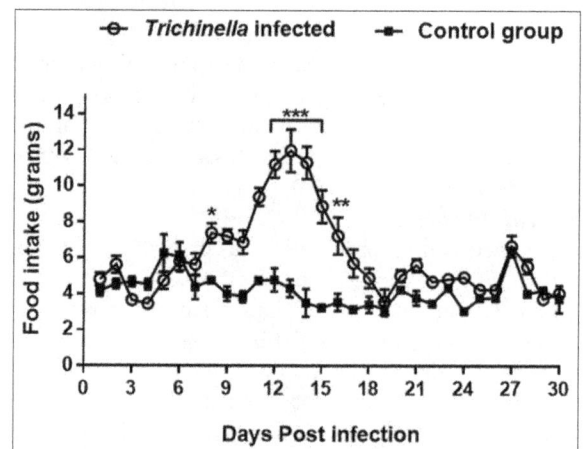

Fig. 2. Graph showing trend of food intake of mice in the infected and control groups during the experimentation period of 30 days. Levels of significant differences (* $P<0.05$; ** $P<0.01$, and *** $P<0.001$) were obtained by comparing the infected and control groups.

to 25 pi, the trend in food intake of the infected group decreased gradually to equal that of the control group. At day 26 through 30 pi, there was no difference in the trend in food intake in both groups. Overall, the infected group had significantly higher food intake compared to the control group ($p<0.001$).

In the two groups, a variations in the trends of water intake was observed although the infected group overally took more water than the control group. The infected group water intake at day 2 pi was higher than the control group ($p<0.01$) (Fig. 3). At days 3 to 11 pi, the water intake by the in mice in the infected group was lower than those in the control group ($p > 0.05$).

Conversely, at days 12 to 17 pi, the control group had a higher water intake than the infected group ($p > 0.05$).

Body weight

Daily measurements of changes in body weight are shown in Fig. 4. We observed at days 3 to 11 pi, the infected group experienced significant weight loss compared to the control group ($p<0.01$). After day 11 pi, the infected group gradually gained weight that at day 15 pi was similar to that of the control group, the upward trend further continued to peak at day 27 pi. During termination of the study (day 30), the body weight change of the infected group was greater ($p<0.01$) than that of the control group.

Insulin and blood glucose levels

The infected group had significantly high insulin levels (0.931 ng/ml) compared to the control group (0.302 ng/ml) at day 7pi. The insulin levels of the

infected group dropped significantly to 0.308 pg/ml (14 dpi), 0.397 pg/ml (21 dpi) and 0.297 pg/ml (35dpi). Comparatively, the insulin levels of mice in the infected group were significantly higher ($p<0.001$) than those in the control group (Fig. 5).

Lower blood glucose levels (101.88 mg/dL) we observed in the infected group in comparison to the control group (116.46 mg/dL). However, the differences were not significant ($p > 0.05$) (data not shown).

Th1/Th17 cytokines

The infected group had elevated levels of IFN-γ cytokine (404.22 pg/ml) ($p<0.001$) at day 7 which slightly decreased at day 14pi (295.46 pg/ml) ($p<0.05$) and at day 21pi (118.21 pg/ml) (Fig. 6). The IFN-γ levels of the control group remained at baseline levels of 77.02 pg/ml throughout the experimental period.

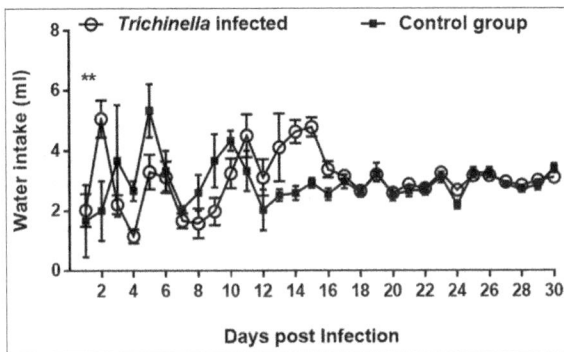

Fig. 3. Graph showing trends of water intake of mice in the infected and control groups during the experimentation period of 30 days. Levels of significant differences (* $P<0.05$; ** $P<0.01$, and *** $P<0.001$) were obtained by comparing the infected and control groups.

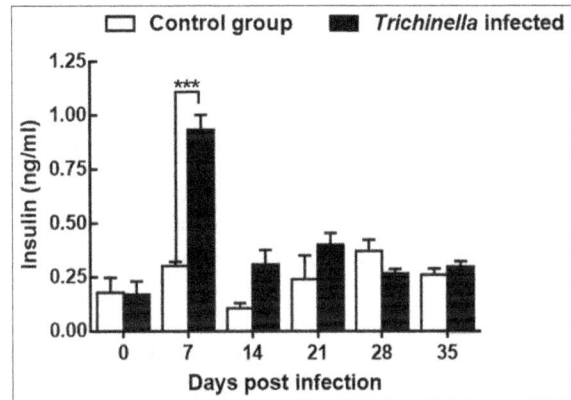

Fig. 5. Levels of insulin in mice during the course of *Trichinella zimbabwensis* infection. Levels of significant differences (* $P<0.05$; ** $P<0.01$, and *** $P<0.001$) were obtained by comparing the infected and control groups.

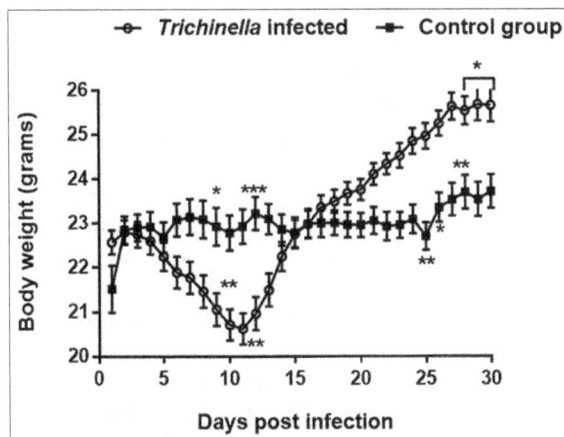

Fig. 4. Graph showing changes in mice body weight during the course of *Trichinella zimbabwensis* infection. Levels of significant differences (* $P<0.05$; ** $P<0.01$, and *** $P<0.001$) were obtained by comparing the infected and control groups.

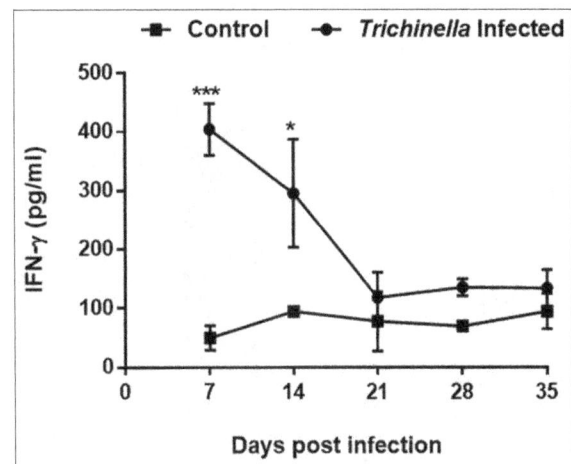

Fig. 6. Levels of Interferon gamma (IFN-γ) cytokine concentration during the course of *Trichinella zimbabwensis* infection. Levels of significant differences (* $P<0.05$; ** $P<0.01$, and *** $P<0.001$) were obtained by comparing the infected and control groups.

Overall trend in IFN-γ levels in the *Trichinella* infection group were significantly higher than that of the control group ($p<0.001$). The IL-17 levels of the infected group were significantly higher (893 pg/ml) compared to the control group (17.60 pg/ml) ($p<0.001$) at day 14 pi (Fig. 7).

Discussion

The results showed that *T. zimbabwensis* adult worms persisted in the small intestines for up to 21 days post-infection and few numbers of *T. zimbabwensis* ML were recovered at day 21. This suggests that the bulk of the larval migrations is mainly at or after day 21pi. Also an indication that ML start to arrive at their site of predilection. In addition, we established that during the enteric phase of *T. zimbabwensis* infection, the infected mice showed a reduced trend in food and water intake. This suggests that inflammatory reactions mediated due to NBL penetration may be playing part in hypophagic response that was accompanied with weight loss. The actual mechanism behind this phenomenon is not clear. However, it has been established by Worthington *et al.* (2013) that in *T. spiralis*-infected mice, hypophagia is due to upregulation of hormone cholecystokinin (CCK). However, the role of the intestines in limiting food ingestion, satiety and delay gastric emptying (Rigaud *et al.*, 1994; Schonhoff *et al.*, 2004) cannot be ruled out as factors influencing the hypophagic response observed.

We also observed that levels of blood glucose and serum insulin in *Trichinella*-infected mice were elevated compared with non-infected control mice. This may indicate that *T. zimbabwensis* ML influence glucose metabolism. However, the alteration in the metabolic responses we observed was short lived until 14 dpi when

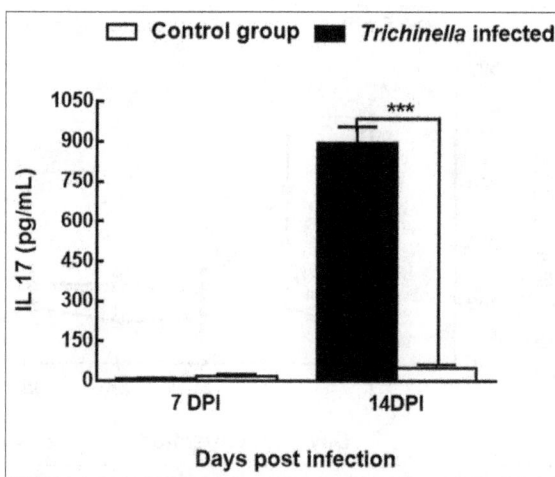

Fig. 7. Levels of Interleukin-17 (IL-17) cytokine concentration during the course of *Trichinella zimbabwensis* infection. Levels of significant differences (* $P<0.05$; ** $P<0.01$, and *** $P<0.001$) were obtained by comparing the infected and control groups.

the levels of insulin returned to normal suggesting that as enteritis resolved and pancreatobiliary secretomotor functions were restored. The migrating larvae may be favouring muscle glucose uptake by inhibiting glucose metabolism, glycogenolysis and controlling feeding behavior and energy expenditure (Szanto and Kahn, 2000). This may be a probable cause of fat mass accumulation and eventual body weight gain. In literature, it has been documented that accumulated fat mass deposits influence secretion of TGF-β, TNF-α and IL-6 cytokines that favour parasite establishment (Trayhurn and Beattie, 2001; Nehete *et al.*, 2014) and IL-17 differentiation (Bettelli *et al.*, 2006; Pappu *et al.*, 2011). In the present study, we observed that there were elevated levels of pro-inflammatory cytokines, IFN-γ and IL-17 which confirms that the known tissue-mediated innate immunity against adult *T. zimbabwensis* infection is initiated and inflammation is due to penetration. After 14 dpi, the levels of IFN-γ were declining and IL-17 were undetectable showing that Th2 immune polarization limit pro-inflammatory cytokine secretion thus worm expulsion (Wakelin *et al.*, 1994; Wu *et al.*, 2010). This is in agreement with our previous study where we observed a decline in the levels of TNF-α and elevated levels of anti-*Trichinella*-specific antibodies (IgG1) and Th2 cytokine (IL-4) and T-regulatory cytokine (IL-10) (Onkoba *et al.*, 2015). This may imply that the parasite may be immuno-modulating host immune system to initiate Th2 polarisation that down regulate production of pro-inflammatory cytokines (Harnett, 2014).

However, the present study could not provide extensive evidence on actual mechanisms involved in glucose metabolism, Th17 secretion and regulation during *T. zimbabwensis* infection. Therefore, further studies are to be undertaken taking into consideration that *T. zimbabwensis* NBL migrates through various body cavities and tissues with diverse immunological responses that are short-lived. Immunological compartmentalization complicates the understanding of tissue-dwelling host-parasite interactions during infection.

In conclusion, *T. zimbabwensis* infection alters host feeding behavior similar to *T. spiralis*. Furthermore, we show for the first time that non-encapsulated *T. zimbabwensis* parasite induces Th1/Th17 type immune response during chronic infection. The data generated contributes to new knowledge on the understanding of how tissue-dwelling helminths manipulate and adapt to host metabolic and immune systems to establish parasitism. Further studies are needed to determine immune responses evoked during *T. zimbabwensis* NBL migratory patterns.

Acknowledgements

Our outmost gratitude goes to Mr. David Buti, Dr. Linda Bester and Dr. Sanil Singh for providing care and housing for study animals at BRU.

Financial support
This study received financial support from the College of Health Sciences of the University of KwaZulu-Natal through PhD studentship bursary awarded to Onkoba W.N.

Conflict of interest
The authors declare that there is no conflict of interest.

References

Adisakwattana, P., Nuamtanong, S., Kusolsuk, T., Chairoj, M., Yenchitsomanas, P.T. and Chaisri, U. 2013. Non-encapsulated *Trichinella* spp., *T. papuae*, diminishes severity of DSS-induced colitis in mice. Asian Pac. J. Allergy Immunol. 31, 106-114.

Appleton, J.A., Kennedy, M. and Harnett, W. 2001. New insights into the intestinal niche of *Trichinella spiralis*, in: Parasitic Nematodes: Molecular Biology, Biochemistry and Immunology. pp: 103-120.

Aranzamendi, C., de Bruin, A., Kuiper, R., Boog, C.J.P., van Eden, W., Rutten, V. and Pinelli, E. 2013. Protection against allergic airway inflammation during the chronic and acute phases of *Trichinella spiralis* infection. Clin. Exp. Allergy 43, 103-115.

Bettelli, E., Carrier, Y., Gao, W., Korn, T., Strom, T.B., Oukka, M., Weiner, H.L. and Kuchroo, V.K. 2006. Reciprocal developmental pathways for the generation of pathogenic effector TH17 and regulatory T cells. Nature 441, 235-238.

Bruschi, F. and Chiumiento, L. 2011. *Trichinella* inflammatory myopathy: Host or parasite strategy? Parasit. Vectors 4, 42. http://doi.org/10.1186/1756-3305-4-42.

Del Prete, G., Chiumiento, L., Amedei, A., Piazza, M., D'Elios, M.M., Codolo, G., de Bernard, M., Masetti, M., Bruschi, F., 2008. Immunosuppression of TH2 responses in *Trichinella spiralis* infection by *Helicobacter pylori* neutrophil-activating protein. J. Allergy Clin. Immunol. 122(5), 908-913. e5.

Despommier, D.D., 1998. How does *Trichinella spiralis* make itself at home? Parasitol. Today 14, 318-323.

Finkelman, F.D., Shea-Donohue, T., Morris, S.C., Gildea, L., Strait, R., Madden, K.B., Schopf, L. and Urban, J.F. 2004. Interleukin-4- and interleukin-13-mediated host protection against intestinal nematode parasites. Immunol. Rev. 201, 139-155.

Gagliardo, L.F., McVay, C.S. and Appleton, J.A. 2002. Molting, Ecdysis, and Reproduction of *Trichinella spiralis* Are Supported *In Vitro* by Intestinal Epithelial Cells. Infect. Immun. 70, 1853-1859.

Gottstein, B., Pozio, E. and Nöckler, K. 2009. Epidemiology, diagnosis, treatment, and control of trichinellosis. Clin. Microbiol. Rev. 22, 127-145.

Harnett, W., 2014. Secretory products of helminth parasites as immunomodulators. Mol. Biochem.

Parasitol. 195(2), 130-136.

Jackson, J.A., Friberg, I.M., Little, S. and Bradley, J.E. 2009. Review series on helminths, immune modulation and the hygiene hypothesis: Immunity against helminths and immunological phenomena in modern human populations: Coevolutionary legacies?. Immunology 126, 18-27.

Kapel, C.M.O. and Gamble, H.R. 2000. Infectivity, persistence, and antibody response to domestic and sylvatic *Trichinella* spp. in experimentally infected pigs. Int. J. Parasitol. 30, 215-221.

Khan, W.I. and Collins, S.M. 2005. Immune-mediated alteration in gut physiology and its role in host defence in nematode infection. Parasite Immunol. 26, 319-326.

Kilkenny, C., Browne, W.J., Cuthill, I.C., Emerson, M. and Altman, D.G. 2013. Improving bioscience research reporting: The arrive guidelines for reporting animal research. Animals 4, 35-44.

La Grange, L.J., Marucci, G. and Pozio, E. 2009. *Trichinella zimbabwensis* in wild Nile crocodiles *(Crocodylus niloticus)* of South Africa. Vet. Parasitol. 161, 88-91.

La Grange, L.J., Marucci, G. and Pozio, E. 2010. *Trichinella zimbabwensis* in a naturally infected mammal. J. Helminthol. 84, 35-38.

Maizels, R.M., Balic, A., Gomez-Escobar, N., Nair, M., Taylor, M.D. and Allen, J.E. 2004. Helminth parasites-masters of regulation. Immunol. Rev. 201, 89-116.

Maizels, R.M., Pearce, E.J., Artis, D., Yazdanbakhsh, M. and Wynn, T.A. 2009. Regulation of pathogenesis and immunity in helminth infections. J. Exp. Med. 206, 2059-2066.

Maizels, R.M. and Yazdanbakhsh, M. 2008. T-cell regulation in helminth parasite infections: Implications for inflammatory diseases. Chem. Immunol. Allergy 94, 112-123.

Mukaratirwa, S., Dzoma, B.M., Matenga, E., Ruziwa, S.D., Sacchi, L. and Pozio, E. 2008. Experimental infections of baboons *(Papio spp.)* and vervet monkeys *(Cercopithecus aethiops)* with *Trichinella zimbabwensis* and successful treatment with ivermectin. Onderstepoort J. Vet. Res. 75, 173-180.

Mukaratirwa, S. and Foggin, C.M. 1999. Infectivity of *Trichinella* sp. isolated from *Crocodylus niloticus* to the indigenous Zimbabwean pig (Mukota). Int. J. Parasitol. 29, 1129-1131.

Mukaratirwa, S., La Grange, L. and Pfukenyi, D.M. 2013. *Trichinella* infections in animals and humans in sub-Saharan Africa: A review. Acta Trop. 125, 82-89.

Mukaratirwa, S., Magwedere, K., Matenga, E. and Foggin, C.M. 2001. Transmission studies on *Trichinella* species isolated from *Crocodylus niloticus* and efficacy of Fenbendazole and

Levamisole against muscle L 1 stages in BALB/ mice. Onderstepoort J. Vet. Res. 68, 21-25.

Murrell, K.D., Dorny, P., Flisser, A., Nash, T. and Pawlowski, Z. 2005. WHO/FAO/OIE Guidelines for the surveillance, prevention and control of taeniosis/cysticercosis.

Nehete, P., Magden, E.R., Nehete, B., Hanley, P.W. and Abee, C.R., 2014. Obesity related alterations in plasma cytokines and metabolic hormones in chimpanzees. Int. J. Inflam. 2014, Article ID 856749. http://dx.doi.org/10.1155/2014/856749.

Nöckler, K., Pozio, E., Voigt, W.P. and Heidrich, J. 2000. Detection of Trichinella infection in food animals. Vet. Parasitol. 93, 335-350.

Onkoba, W.N., Chimbari, M.J., Kamau, J.M. and Mukaratirwa, S. 2015. Differential immune responses in mice infected with the tissue-dwelling nematode *Trichinella zimbabwensis*. J. Helminthol. 90(5), 547-554.

Pappu, R., Ramirez-Carrozzi, V. and Sambandam, A. 2011. The interleukin-17 cytokine family: Critical players in host defence and inflammatory diseases. Immunology 134, 8-16.

Pozio, E. 2013. The opportunistic nature of *Trichinella*-Exploitation of new geographies and habitats. Vet. Parasitol. 194, 128-132.

Pozio, E., Foggin, C.M., Marucci, G., La Rosa, G., Sacchi, L., Corona, S., Rossi, P. and Mukaratirwa, S. 2002. *Trichinella zimbabwensis* n.sp. (Nematoda), a new non-encapsulated species from crocodiles *(Crocodylus niloticus)* in Zimbabwe also infecting mammals. Int. J. Parasitol. 32, 1787-1799.

Pozio, E., Marucci, G., Casulli, A., Sacchi, L., Mukaratirwa, S., Foggin, C.M. and La Rosa, G. 2004. *Trichinella papuae* and *Trichinella zimbabwensis* induce infection in experimentally infected varans, caimans, pythons and turtles. Parasitology 128, 333–342.

Pozio, E. and Zarlenga, D.S. 2005. Recent advances on the taxonomy, systematics and epidemiology of *Trichinella*. Int. J. Parasitol. 35, 1191-1204.

Rigaud, D., Angel, L.A., Cerf, M., Carduner, M.J., Melchior, J.C., Sautier, C., René, E., Apfelbaum, M. and Mignon, M. 1994. Mechanisms of decreased food intake during weight loss in adult Crohn's disease patients without obvious malabsorption. Am. J. Clin. Nutr. 60, 775-781.

Rodgers, D.T., Pineda, M.A, McGrath, M.A, Al-Riyami, L., Harnett, W. and Harnett, M.M. 2014. Protection against collagen-induced arthritis in mice afforded by the parasitic worm product, ES-62, is associated with restoration of the levels of interleukin-10-producing B cells and reduced plasma cell infiltration of the joints. Immunology 141, 457-466.

Schonhoff, S.E., Giel-Moloney, M. and Leiter, A.B. 2004. Minireview: Development and differentiation of gut endocrine cells. Endocrinology 145, 2639-2644.

Szanto, I. and Kahn, C.R. 2000. Selective interaction between leptin and insulin signaling pathways in a hepatic cell line. Proc. Natl. Acad. Sci. U. S. A. 97, 2355-2360.

Trayhurn, P. and Beattie, J.H. 2001. Physiological role of adipose tissue: White adipose tissue as an endocrine and secretory organ. Proc. Nutr. Soc. 60, 329-339.

Wakelin, D., Goyal, P.K., Dehlawi, M.S. and Hermanek, J. 1994. Immune responses to *Trichinella spiralis* and *T. pseudospiralis* in mice. Immunology 81, 475-479.

Worthington, J.J., Samuelson, L.C., Grencis, R.K. and McLaughlin, J.T. 2013. Adaptive Immunity Alters Distinct Host Feeding Pathways during Nematode Induced Inflammation, a Novel Mechanism in Parasite Expulsion. PLoS Pathog. 9(1), e1003122. doi:10.1371/journal.ppat.1003122.

Wu, Z., Nagano, I., Asano, K. and Takahashi, Y. 2010. Infection of non-encapsulated species of *Trichinella* ameliorates experimental autoimmune encephalomyelitis involving suppression of Th17 and Th1 response. Parasitol. Res. 107, 1173-1188.

6

Antimicrobial susceptibility and minimal inhibitory concentration of *Pseudomonas aeruginosa* isolated from septic ocular surface disease in different animal species

L. Leigue[1,2,*], F. Montiani-Ferreira[1] and B.A. Moore[3]

[1]*Department of Veterinary Medicine, Universidade Federal do Paraná; Curitiba, PR, Brazil*
[2]*Department of Microbiology, Institute of Biomedical Sciences, Universidade de São Paulo; São Paulo, SP, Brazil*
[3]*Veterinary Specialty Hospital of San Diego, 10435 Sorrento Valley Road, San Diego, CA 92121, USA*

Abstract

The purpose of this study was to evaluate the antibiotic susceptibility profile of *Pseudomonas aeruginosa* isolated from different animal species with septic ocular surface disease. Sixteen strains of *P. aeruginosa* were isolated from different species of animals (dog, cat, horse, penguin and brown bear) with ocular surface diseases such as conjunctivitis, keratocojnuctivits sicca and ulcerative keratitis. These isolates were tested against 11 different antimicrobials agents using the Kirby-Bauer disk-diffusion method. Minimum inhibitory concentrations (MICs) were determined using E-tests for two antibiotics (tobramycin and ciprofloxacin) commonly used in veterinary ophthalmology practice. Imipenem was the most effective antibiotic, with 100% of the strains being susceptible, followed by amikacin (87.5%), gentamicin, norfloxacin, gatifloxacin and polymyxin (both with 81.5%of susceptibility). MIC_{90} of ciprofloxacin was 2 µg/ml and the values found ranged from 0.094 µg/ml to 32 µg/ml. For tobramycin, MIC_{90} was 32 µg/ml and ranged from 0.25 µg/ml to 256 µg/ml. The most effective *in vitro* antibiotic tested against *P. aeruginosa* in this study was imipenem, followed by amikacin. The 3 mg/ml eye drops commercially available ciprofloxacin presentations were *in vitro* effective against all strains tested in this study if applied up to 4 hours after instillation. Whereas for tobramycin the 3 mg/ml eye drops commercial presentations were not *in vitro* effective against some strains isolated in this study. Thus for ocular infections with *P. aeruginosa* when using tobramycin the ideal recommendation would be to either use eye drops with higher concentrations or decrease the frequency intervals from four to a minimum of every two hours.

Keywords: Antibiotic, Antimicrobial profile, Bacteria, Ocular infections.

Introduction

The eye is typically resistant to primary infection due to the numerous cellular and molecular elements that protect the corneal surface against microorganisms. These elements include tears, corneal nerves, the epithelium, keratocytes, polymorphonuclear cells, and cytokines (Akpek and Gottsch, 2003). The presence of tears is of particular importance since, besides preventing the cornea from drying, it also helps flush foreign particles from the ocular surface and transports antimicrobial proteins (lactoferrin, lysozyme, lipocalin, and beta-lysin) and immunoglobulins to the ocular surface to prevent infections (Mannis and Smolin, 1996). As a consequence of all these factors, with the exception of the herpesviruses and infection with *Moraxella bovis*, microorganisms cannot initiate primary keratitis in animals (Maggs, 2008).

Considering, septic ocular surface disease typically requires an initial injury, such as mechanical or chemical trauma, before a microorganism can infect the cornea (Mayo *et al.*, 1986). Specifically, bacterial infections of ocular surfaces are commonly the result of a predisposing factor or disease that allows the overgrowth of a bacterium that is or is not a part of the ocular surface microbiota (Quinn *et al.*, 1994; Moore *et al.* 1995; Ledbetter *et al.*, 2009).

Pseudomonas aeruginosa, a gram-negative bacillus that is widely distributed in nature, is commonly considered a transitional opportunistic agent and part of the normal ocular surface microbiota (Quinn *et al.*, 1994). However, *P. aeruginosa* is also frequently isolated from ocular surface infections, especially from ocular septic keratitis (Ledbetter *et al.*, 2009). This microorganism is considered one of the most destructive bacteria associated with eye infections in any species (Gutierrez, 1972), having a variety of mechanisms and virulence factors which allow efficient colonization and subsequently compromised ocular tissues and most corneal layers. Examples of such factors include bacterial proteases, and an exotoxin that can destroy epithelial and endothelial cells within 24 hours.

Hemolysins also contribute to *P. aeruginosa's* invasiveness, tissue destruction and efficient

*Corresponding Author: Lucianne Leigue. Department of Veterinary Medicine, Universidade Federal do Paraná; Curitiba, PR, Brazil. Email: lucianne.leigue@usp.br

colonization of ocular tissues (Gutierrez, 1972; Moore et al., 1995; Carter, 1999). Finally, the pigment pyocyanin may also contribute to tissue damage by inhibiting cellular oxygen uptake (Moore et al., 1995). Treatment of ocular surface infections where P. aeruginosa is isolated requires aggressive topical antibiotic therapy (Moore and Naisse, 2000).

However, over time it can be expected that ocular infections become less responsive to antibiotics due to the emergence of resistant bacterial strains. Therefore, it becomes important to implement a strategy for monitoring the emergence and spread of resistance. Antimicrobial susceptibility tests are an indispensable method to determine the most effective antibiotics for the treatment of eye infections.

The Kirby–Bauer disk diffusion test is the routine laboratory test used to determine antimicrobial susceptibility and it is crucial for veterinary ophthalmologists to provide an appropriate antimicrobial therapy (Moore et al., 1995).

Minimum inhibitory concentration (MIC) is the lowest concentration of an antimicrobial drug that will inhibit visible growth of a microorganism after incubation. Since it is a quantitative way to measure the susceptibility of an organism to an antimicrobial, MIC is considered an important tool for confirming resistance of microorganisms to a given antimicrobial agent (Andrews, 2001; CDC, 2002). This is particularly true for ocular surface infections, where a drug can be delivered directly to the site of infection at a high concentration   compared to that of systemic intravenous administration (Levison and Levison, 2009).

Due to the aggressive nature of P. aeruginosa infections and the devastating consequences they can have on the eye, the lag time between diagnosis and antimicrobial susceptibility test results might enable significant and irreversible damage to be done to the eye   prior   to   initiation   of   proper   therapy. Epidemiological data of general susceptibility patterns may be helpful in certain situations such as when empiric rational therapy is indicated. The purpose of the present study was twofold: 1) investigate in vitro antibiotic susceptibilities by disc-diffusion of a panel of 11 antibiotics, and 2) investigate the minimal inhibitory concentrations of tobramycin and ciprofloxacin (two of the most commonly used topical antibiotics used for ocular surface infection) against naturally occurring P. aeruginosa ocular surface infections of dogs, cats, horses as well as two never before reported species, the Magellanic penguin and the brown bear.

Materials and Methods

Specimen collection

This study included sixteen (n=16) clinical isolates of P. aeruginosa from various species of animals presenting to the Comparative Ophthalmology Service at The Federal University of Paraná, Brazil with ocular surface   infections   (conjunctival,   corneal   or conjunctival and corneal). All the procedures using animals were conducted in accordance with the humane principles   set   forth   in   the   ARVO   Statement (Association   for   Research   in   Vision   and Ophthalmology) for the Use of Animals in Ophthalmic and Vision Research and in accordance with UFPR´s (Universidade   Federal   do   Paraná)   Animal   Use Committee.

All animals were first examined for signs of ophthalmic or general clinical disease. A complete ocular examination, including slit lamp biomicroscopy (Hawk Eye;   Dioptrix,   L'Union,   France),   indirect ophthalmoscopy   (Heine   EN20-01   indirect ophthalmoscope; Heine Optotechnik, Herrsching, Germany), rebound tonometry (TonoVet tonometer; ICare Finland Oy, Helsinki, Finland), fluorescein staining (Drogavet; Curitiba-PR, Brazil), and Schirmer tear testing (Drogavet; Curitiba-PR, Brazil) was performed on each animal. Only animals presenting with signs of ocular surface infections without signs of uveitis, glaucoma, or systemic disease and with no history of having received systemic or topical ophthalmic antimicrobials in the preceding 30 days were included in the study.

Bacterial identification

A sterile cotton swab was used to gently sample the corneal and conjunctival surfaces of each infected eye. Swabs were then removed while taking care to avoid contact with eyelashes or skin of the eyelids. The swabs were kept in Stuart´s transport medium, placed on ice and transported within 24 hours for microbiology culture. Swabs were plunged in BHI broth (brain heart infusion), an enrichment medium, for 24 hours at 37°C. The enrichment cultures were then streaked onto 5% Sheep Blood agar (Newprov®, Curitiba, Brazil).

Animals with signs of ocular surface infections in which P. aeruginosa was isolated were deemed to met all the inclusion criteria. Positive bacterial colonies were replicated in selective and differential media for Gram-negative bacteria (MacConkey agar and Brilliant Green agar). P. aeruginosa strains were confirmed by their Gram stain reaction, characteristic colonial morphology,   oxidase   production,   motility   and pyocyanin production (Quinn et al., 1994; Carter, 1999).

Subsequently, only the cases of ocular surface infections where P. aeruginosa was isolated were included. Different animal species that fit this criterion were: dogs (Canis familiaris) (n=10), horses (Equus caballus) (n=3), cat (Felis catus) (n=1), brown bear (Ursus arctos) (n=1) and a Magellanic penguin (Spnenicus megellanucus) (n=1). Ocular surface diseases diagnosed in these animals were: Corneal ulcers   (n=7);   Keratoconjunctivitis   sicca   (n=5);

Blepharoconjunctivits (n=4). Table 1 summarizes and further details the ocular surface diseases diagnosed in each animal species studied.

Table 1. List of animal species and ocular diseases from which *P. aeruginosa* was isolated.

Sample identification	Animal species	Ocular diagnosis
1	Dog	Corneal ulcer
2	Dog	Oronasal fistula + conjunctivitis
3	Dog	KCS*
4	Dog	Corneal ulcer
5	Dog	Corneal ulcer
6	Dog	KCS*
7	Dog	KCS*
8	Dog	Oronasal fistula + conjunctivitis
9	Dog	KCS*
10	Dog	KCS*
11	Cat	Corneal ulcer
12	Horse	Corneal ulcer
13	Horse	Corneal ulcer
14	Penguim[1]	Conjunctivitis
15	Brown Bear[2]	Conjunctivitis
16	Horse	Corneal ulcer

*keratoconjunctivitis sicca.
[1]*Spnenicus megellanucus.*
[2]*Ursus arctos.*

Susceptibility tests

Antimicrobial sensitivity of the isolated *P. aeruginosa* strains was determined by the disk-diffusion technique (also known as Kirby-Bauer method, one of the oldest approaches to antimicrobial susceptibility testing, in which is used Mueller-Hinton agar plates and it is used the direct colony suspension method to make a suspension of the organism in saline to the density of a McFarland 0.5 turbidity standard), in compliance with the National Committee for Clinical and Laboratory Standards (CLSI) (2013) criteria or European Committee on Antimicrobial Susceptibility Testing (EUCAST, 2013). Isolates whose antibiogram yielded intermediate results were considered resistant. Eleven (11) available antimicrobial discs (Newprov®, Curitiba, Brazil) were used: enrofloxacin (10µg), ciprofloxacin (5µg), norfloxacin (10µg), gatifloxacin (10µg), tobramycin (10µg), gentamicin (10µg), amikacin (30µg), streptomycin (10µg), neomycin (30µg), imipenem (10gµ), polymyxin B (300U).

All the strains were tested to the minimal inhibitory concentration (MIC) test for tobramycin (antibiotic strip impregnated with the antibiotic and in which the concentration ranged from 0.016-128 µg/ml) and ciprofloxacin (antibiotic strip impregnated with the antibiotic and in which the concentration tested ranged from 0.002 – 32 µg/ml), using a commercially available strip antibiotic test (E-test, AB Biodisk®, Sweden). Etest® is a rapid and well-established method for antimicrobial resistance testing.

It consists of a predefined gradient of antibiotic concentrations on a plastic strip that carries a continuous concentration gradient of stabilized and dried drug. The intersection of the inhibitory zone with the strip is the MIC. The zone of inhibition was interpreted and classified as sensible, resistant and intermediate according to the manufacturer's manual (E-test, AB Biodisk®, Sweden). It was used Mueller-Hinton agar plates and used the direct colony suspension method to make a suspension of the organism in a saline solution to the density of a McFarland 0.5 turbidity standard. The MIC breakpoints were determined according to CLSI (2013) guidelines: CIP, ciprofloxacin (S≤1; I 2; R≥4); TOB, tobramycin (S≤4; I 8; R≥16); intermediate results were considered resistant. *P. aeruginosa* ATCC 27853 was used as quality control.

Results

Typical signs encountered in the animals with septic ocular surface disease included blepharospasm, ocular discharge, conjunctival venous congestion and hyperemia, chemosis, low Schirmer tear test results, and corneal malacia, opacification, edema, neovascularization and ulceration. Imipenen was the only drug to which 100% of *P. aeruginosa* strains showed *in vitro* susceptibility in this study. A high susceptibility rate (87.5%) was demonstrated to amikacin, followed by gentamicin, norfloxacin, gatifloxacin and polymyxin (81.5%) and a low susceptibility rate to enrofloxacin (25%). Results for all antibiotics tested are summarized in Table 2 and the breakpoints used to definy the strains as susceptiple or resistant were according CLSI (2013) guidelines.

Four strains of *P. aeruginosa* were resistant to ciprofloxacin: An isolate from a dog with corneal ulcer and oronasal fistula (sample 1), another isolate from a dog with keratoconjunctivitis sicca (sample 6), an isolate from cat with a corneal ulcer (sample 11), and an isolate from a horse with a deep corneal ulcer (sample 16). Five strains were resistant to tobramycin: The sample from a dog with corneal ulcer and oronasal fistula (sample 1), one from a dog with keratoconjunctivitis sicca (sample 6) three two from horses with corneal ulcers (sample 12 and 16 respectively), and one from a cat with corneal ulcer (case 11).

Table 2. Antimicrobial susceptibility patterns of *P. aeruginosa* isolated from eyes of different species of animals.

Drugs[a]/sample	1[b]	2[b]	3[b]	4[b]	5[b]	6[b]	7[b]	8[b]	9[b]	10[b]	11[c]	12[d]	13[d]	14[e]	15[f]	16[d]	S %	R%
ENO	S	R	R	S	S	R	R	R	R	R	R	R	S	R	R	R	25	75
CIP	R	S	S	S	S	R	S	S	S	S	R	S	S	S	S	R	75	25
NOR	S	S	S	S	S	R	S	S	S	S	S	R	S	S	S	R	81.25	18.75
GAT	S	S	S	S	S	R	S	S	S	S	S	R	S	S	S	R	81.25	18.75
TOB	R	S	S	S	S	R	S	S	S	S	R	R	S	S	S	R	68.75	31.25
GEN	S	S	S	S	S	R	S	S	S	S	S	R	S	S	S	R	81.25	18.75
AMI	S	S	S	S	S	R	S	S	S	S	S	S	S	S	S	R	87.5	12.5
EST	S	S	S	R	S	R	S	R	S	S	S	R	S	S	R	R	62.5	37.5
NEO	S	R	R	S	S	R	R	R	S	S	S	R	S	S	S	R	56.25	43.75
POL	R	S	S	S	S	R	S	S	S	R	S	S	S	S	S	S	81.25	18.75
IMI	S	S	S	S	S	S	S	S	S	S	S	S	S	S	S	S	100	0

a. Drugs: ENO: enrofloxacin; CIP: ciprofloxacin; NOR: norfloxacin; GAT: gatifloxacin; TOB: tobramycin; GEN: gentamicin; AMI: amikacin; EST: streptomycin; NEO: neomycin; POL: polymyxin B; IMI: imipenem. Susceptibilities: (S): susceptible; (R): resistant.
(b): Strain isolated from dog.
(c): Strain isolated from cat.
(d): Strain isolated from horse.
(e): Strain isolated from penguin.
(f): Strain isolated from black bear.

Table 3. Minimum inhibitory concentration (MIC) of 16 strains of *P. aeruginosa* recovered from eyes of different species of animals.

Sample	CIP (µg/mL)[a]	Sus.	TOB (µg/mL)[a]	Sus.
1[b]	4.00	R	8.00	R
2[b]	0.19	S	2.00	S
3[b]	0.13	S	2.00	S
4[b]	0.094	S	1.50	S
5[b]	0.25	S	0.25	S
6[b]	12.00	R	≤256	R
7[b]	0.19	S	3.00	S
8[b]	0.38	S	4.00	S
9[b]	0.094	S	1.00	S
10[b]	0.094	S	1.00	S
11[c]	2.00	R	32.00	R
12[d]	0.094	S	1.50	S
13[d]	0.094	S	1.00	S
14[e]	0.094	S	1.50	S
15[f]	0.094	S	1.00	S
16[d]	≤32	R	≤256	R

a. Drugs: CIP, ciprofloxacin (S≤1; I 2; R≥4); TOB, tobramycin (S≤4; I 8; R≥16). Sus. Susceptibilities; S: susceptible; R: resistant.
(b): Strain isolated from dog.
(c): Strain isolated from cat.
(d): Strain isolated from horse.
(e): Strain isolated from penguin.
(f): Strain isolated from black bear.

Table 3 summarizes the MIC (µg/ml) results to ciprofloxacin and tobramycin of all 16 strains of *P. aeruginosa*. According to the CLSI (2013) MIC breakpoints, four isolates presented MIC values that demonstrated resistance to ciprofloxacin. Four isolates were resistant to tobramycin (same were resistant to ciprofloxacin). The four resistant strains were recovered from a dog (corneal ulcer; case 1), dog (KCS; case 6), a cat (corneal ulcer, case 11) and a horse (corneal ulcer, case 16).

In general MIC values for tobramycin were higher than for ciprofloxacin for all strains of *P. aeruginosa* evaluated. MIC values for ciprofloxacin varied from 0.13µg/ml to 32 µg/ml and the average MIC value was 3.24 ± µg/ml. MIC_{90} of ciprofloxacin was 3 µg/ml and MIC_{50} was 0.94 µg/ml. MIC values for tobramycin varied from 0.25 µg/ml to 256 µg/ml. The average MIC value was 35.76 µg/ml. The MIC_{90} was 48 µg/ml and the MIC_{50} was 1.50 µg/ml.

Discussion

Animals, especially dogs, are well known naturally-occurring *P. aeruginosa* ulcerative keratitis models. The infection is considered appropriate for comparative investigations since this bacterial agent in canine infections is congruent with the classic genotype-phenotype pattern reported for human corneal isolates (Ledbetter *et al.*, 2009).

P. aeruginosa strains isolated from ocular infections have a particularly important role when prior ocular surface disease provides an opportunity for colonization and stabilization of an eye infection.

These conditions include keratoconjunctivitis sicca, corneal ulcers, chronic conjunctivitis and dental problems combined with infraorbital fistulas (Moore *et al*., 1995; Ledbetter *et al*., 2009; Wada *et al*., 2010). The majority of these primary conditions were observed in the eyes of subjects in the present study (Table 1). Treatment with antibiotics effective against Gram-negative bacteria is usually successful. However, in some cases emergence of strains resistant to available antibiotics makes treatment difficult and poses as a real threat to an eye (Wada *et al*., 2010).

A low *in vitro* susceptibility rate (25%) was observed for enrofloxacin against *P. aeruginosa* isolated from ocular tissues. This result was also observed by other authors while researching strains of *P. aeruginosa* from cases of keratitis in cats and dogs (Lin and Petersen-Jones, 2007, 2008). Conversely, the *in vitro* action of norfloxacin against *P. aeruginosa* was considered good since only three strains were resistant, one from a dog and two from horses. Another study investigating strains from dogs with septic keratitis also found good susceptibility rates for this drug, since only one strain (1/27) was resistant (Lin and Petersen-Jones, 2007). Ciprofloxacin demonstrated a satisfactory degree of *in vitro* activity against *P. aeruginosa* (75% susceptible strains) and four resistant strains were detected. Lin and Petersen-Jones (2007) encountered high *in vitro* susceptibility of this drug against *P. aeruginosa*, where 95% of the isolates from dogs with corneal ulcers were susceptible. In another investigation (Lin and Petersen-Jones, 2008), *P. aeruginosa* isolates from ulcerative keratitis of cats showed an even better result, with 100% of the strains being susceptible to ciprofloxacin. The fourth-generation fluorquinolone tested here, gatifloxacin, also showed a good *in vitro* susceptibility against *P. aeruginosa*, since three strains demonstrated resistance (81.5%). Another report (Ledbetter *et al*., 2007) found 100% of strains from ulcerative keratitis in dogs susceptible for gatifloxacin. Compared with earlier generations, fourth-generation fluoroquinolones have an expanded spectrum of activity against Gram-positive bacteria, anaerobic bacteria, mycobacteria, and species of *Chlamydia, Chlamydophila, Mycoplasma*, and *Ureaplasma* (Moore *et al*., 1995; Kowalski *et al*, 2003; Ledbetter *et al*., 2007). Gram-negative bacterial spectrum of the third- and fourth-generation fluoroquinolones is preserved. However, compared with earlier generations (especially ciprofloxacin), they are less active *in vitro* against many Gram-negative bacteria, including *P. aeruginosa* (Kowalski *et al*, 2003; Ledbetter *et al*., 2007). Therefore, even though there is a mass marketing pressure for clinicians to prescribe newer antibiotic drugs it is noteworthy that according to the literature (Jensen *et al*., 2005) and the results presented in this study, there was no difference between the *in vitro* activity of gatifloxacin (fourth

generation) and ciprofloxacin (second generation fluoroquinolone) against strains of *P. aeruginosa*; all strains that were resistant to ciprofloxacin, were also resistant to gatifloxacin.

Four pseudomonas strains isolated in this study demonstrated resistance to at least one of the aminoglycosides tested here. A total of 87.5% were susceptible to amikacin, 81.5% to gentamicin and 68.7% to tobramycin. Hariharan *et al*. (1995) found that 100% of pseudomonas strains from dogs were susceptible to tobramycin and amikacin, and 95% to gentamicin. Lin and Petersen-Jones (2008) found high susceptibility *in vitro* rates for amikacin (100%), tobramycin (80%) and gentamicin (75%) isolated from dogs with keratitis. Our results corroborate previous investigations of *P. aeruginosa* isolates indicating that these drugs are still effective. Aminoglycosides are an important antibiotic group available in veterinary ophthalmic formulations. When compared with another bacterial genera frequently isolated from animal eyes, e.g. *Staphylococcus*, gentimicin and tobramycin are not very effective (47.5% of the strains were resistant to gentamicin and 65% were resistant to tobramycin) (Varges *et al*., 2009). This confirms the importance of identifying the specific pathogen in a given bacterial ocular surface disease and determining its respective sensitivity pattern. The use of topical amikacin has been suggested as a better empiric alternative to gentamicin or tobramycin (Hariharan *et al*., 1995). In our results, two strains that were resistant to tobramycin were susceptible for amikacin (cases n° 11 and 12) and two strains were resistant to all aminoglycosides tested (cases n° 6 and 16). The appearance of strains resistant to amikacin is of some concern since this drug is one of the most useful agents for treatment of severe *P. aeruginosa* infections (Hariharan *et al*., 1995).

In this investigation, 56.5% of the strains were susceptible to neomycin, similar to the susceptibility reported in another study of *P. aeruginosa* isolates from feline ulcerative keratitis (63%) (Lin and Petersen-Jones, 2008). Neomycin is commonly prescribed in combination with bacitracin and polymyxin B for topical therapy of eye infections in triple antibiotic formulations. Triple antibiotic formulations maximize the spectrum of antibacterial activity against both Gram-positive and Gram-negative bacteria. *Pseudomonas* spp. is often resistant to neomycin, but polymixin B is rapidly bactericidal against Gram-negative bacteria, including *P. aeruginosa* (Lima Filho and Batistuzzo, 2006). In our study, 81% of *P. aeruginosa* were susceptible *in vitro* to polymixin B. However, previous studies have conflicting results, ranging from 100% susceptibility of veterinary isolates (Hariharan *et al*., 1995) to susceptibility rates as low as 40% (Ledbetter *et al*., 2009). We also observed that nearly all strains that were resistant neomycin were susceptible to polymixin B, or vice-versa. Thus, our *in vitro* results corroborate the clinical recommendation for this triple antibiotic combination to be used as a first choice option for treatment of ocular surface *P. aeruginosa* infections (Maggs, 2008).

No isolates tested in this study were resistant to imipenem. The carbapenems antibiotics are commonly used in human multi-resistant pseudomonas infections. The lack of apparent resistance of *P. aeruginosa* strains to imipenem should be highlighted, especially when compared to those findings obtained from cases of human *P. aeruginosa* isolates, in which the *in vitro* resistance can reach 4% (Mohammadpour *et al.*, 2011) to 40% (Fernandes *et al.*, 2015). Although this drug is rarely used in veterinary medicine and is not approved for use in animals by the Food and Drug Administration, veterinarians can legally prescribe imipenem as an extra-label drug for ocular infections consisting of multi-resistant strains of *P. aeruginosa*. Although use of intravenous imipenem preparations topically on the eye has been suggested for ocular infections with multi-resistant *P. aeruginosa* strains, the high price, instability of imipenem solutions [it should be used within 48 hours and kept under refrigeration (Lima Filho and Batistuzzo, 2006)], and debate about reservation for human use make it a rare treatment choice.

Based on this study, the best *in vitro* activities against *P. aeruginosa* isolated from animal's eyes could be ranked as 1: imipenem, 2: amikacin, 3: gatifloxacin, norfloxacin, gentamicin or polymyxin. Imipenem and amikacin eye drops are only available in extemporaneous compounding formulations. Gatifloxacin, norfloxacin, gentamicin and polymyxin are commercially available in the form of eye drops in most countries.

Even with a small sample size of 16 positive *P. aeruginosa* cultures, this work presents interesting data. Notice that diagnoses include conjunctivitis and keratoconjunctivitis sicca, which are normally not primarily caused by *Pseudomonas*, but high resistant strains were isolated, could complicate or delay the disease resolution.

This investigation also determined the MIC values of two important antibiotics commercially available in the form of eye drops and commonly used in veterinary and medical ophthalmology: ciprofloxacin and tobramycin. *In vitro* resistance breakpoints are based on antibiotic concentrations in the blood (CLSI, 2013). However, because ocular antibiotics can reach higher concentrations, this breakpoint does not truly represent bacterial resistance in the eye. Ocular antibiotics will most likely have a higher resistance breakpoint value than systemic antibiotics. For example, a 1% drop with a concentration of 10 µg/mL results in a concentration of 10.000 µg/mL on the eye. Alternatively, in the serum, tissues, or blood, the level may only be 10 µg/mL when the same drug is administered orally (Mah, 2003). Therefore, bacteria identified as resistant elsewhere in the body (e.g. lung) may respond differently if located in the eye and are exposed to topical antibiotic. Studies conducted by Kaye *et al.* (2009) showed that topical administration of an antimicrobial to the cornea may achieve a different concentration and bioavailability in the tissue than the serum levels. In the treatment of bacterial keratitis, the MIC values are an important measure for evaluating the potential effectiveness of topically applied antimicrobials (Sueke *et al.*, 2010).

Both tobramycin and ciprofloxacin formulated as eye drops have a concentration of 3mg/mL in commercially available solutions (Peiffer and Stowe, 1981; Viana, 2007). If one drop (approximately 0.05 mL as commercially droppers delivery a 25 a 50 µL/ drop of solution or suspension), is instilled into the eye, the solution maintains a good antibiotic concentration (0.15 mg). Knowing that the conjunctival fornix of the eye will hold only one drop (Peiffer and Stowe, 1981) (which means 0.05mL) and only 10 to 25 µL of drug are retained in the conjunctival fornix and tear film (Peiffer and Stowe, 1981; Viana, 2007), the concentration of the drugs still will be at 75 µg.

The MIC values found for ciprofloxacin in this study ranged from 0.094 to 32 µ/mL, so, for this drug, the amount present in the conjunctival fornix, exceed the MIC of the strains tested. For tobramycin, the MIC ranged from 0.25 to 256 µg/mL. One MIC isolate tested was 48 µg/mL (case n°11) and two others (cases n° 6 and 16) exceed the MIC (256 µg / mL) of this antibiotic, and for this isolate, the use of eye drops might not be medically effective. A study conducted in ophthalmology centers in the United Kingdom demonstrated the MICs for *P. aeruginosa* isolated from human keratitis ranged from 0.016 to 6.000 mg/L (Sueke *et al.*, 2010).

The average concentration of antibiotics in tears may vary. For ciprofloxacin (0.3% ophthalmic solution) 4 hours after instillation, tear concentration becomes 16 µg/mL in human beigns (Limberg and Buggé, 1994) and 36.25 µ/mL for horses (Hendrix *et al.*, 2007). Considering that the MIC of the strains tested in this study did not exceed 12 µg/mL, the concentration of this drug in tears within four hours is still most likely higher, so instillation of one drop of ciprofloxacin is effective if repeated every four hours.

One study (Tang-Liu *et al.*, 1994) showed that 4 hours after instillation, tobramycin has an average concentration of 8µg/mL in human tears. Therefore, this concentration would still be effective against most strains tested in this study, since most strains had an MIC of 1.00 µg/mL. However, four strains obtained higher MICs (8 µg/mL, 48 µg/mL and two isolated with

256 µg/mL). These MICs suggest poor response to treatment *in vivo* with tobramycin considering the possible MICs that can be achieved in the most common eye drop treatment protocols. Therefore, it is recommended to increase the frequency of administering tobramycin from every four to approximately every two hours.

MIC at the site of a *P. aeruginosa* ocular surface infection must reach high concentrations in order to be effective. The evaluation of *P. aeruginosa* susceptibility by microbiology laboratories is typically made with reference to concentrations in human serum. However, concentrations of antibiotics obtained from the ocular surface by local application of eye drops or ointments are higher, and it is important to determine the MIC to better assess the antibiotic susceptibility of specific bacterial strains isolated from ocular surface infections.

Our study revealed that the antimicrobials with the best *in vitro* actions against *P. aeruginosa* isolated from the eyes of selected animals from Brazil were 1: imipenem, 2: amikacin, 3: gatifloxacin, norfloxacin, gentamicin or polymyxin. This study also showed that commercially available concentrations of ciprofloxacin eye drops used for local treatment (3 mg/ml) was effective against all strains tested in this study if applied up to 4 hours after instillation. For tobramycin eye drops as commercially presentation the concentrations of 3mg/ml, however, cannot reach an ideal MIC for some resistant strains with. Thus for ocular surface infections with *P. aeruginosa* when using tobramycin the ideal recommendation would be to either to use eye drops with higher concentrations or decrease the frequency intervals from four hours to a minimum of every two hours.

Conflict of interest

No competing financial interests exist.

References

Akpek, E.K. and Gottsch, J.D. 2003. Immune defense at the ocular surface. Eye (Lond). 17, 949-956.

Andrews, J.M. 2001. Determination of minimum inhibitory concentrations. J. Antimicro. Chemoth. 48, 5-16.

Carter, G.R. 1999. Pseudomonas. In Carter, G.R.: Fundamentos em Bacteriologia e Micologia Veterinária, 1ed, Ed Roca, São Paulo.

CDC. 2002. Addressing the problem of antimicrobial resistance. National Center for Infectious Disease. Target Area Booklet CDC.

Clinical and Laboratory Standards Institute (CLSI). 2013. Performance Standards for Antimicrobial Susceptibility Testing: Twenty-third Informational Supplement M100-S23. LSI, Wayne, PA, USA.

European Committee on Antimicrobial Susceptibility Testing (EUCAST). 2013. EUCAST guidelines for detection of resistance mechanisms and specific resistances of clinical and/or epidemiological importance. EUCAST, Basel, Switzerland: http://www.eucast.org/clinical_breakpoints.

Fernandes, M., Vira, D., Medikonda, R. and Kumar, N. 2015. Extensively and pan-drug resistant *Pseudomonas aeruginosa* keratitis: clinical features, risk factors, and outcome. Graefes. Arch. Clin. Exp. Ophthalmol. 254, 315-322.

Gutierrez, E.H. 1972. Bacterial infections of the eye. In: D.Locatcher-Khorazo and B.C. Seegal. (ed), Microbiology of the eye. The C.V. Mosby Co., St. Louis, pp: 69-70.

Hariharan, H., Mcphee, L., Heaney, S. and Bryenton, J. 1995. Antimicrobial drug susceptibility of clinical isolates of *Pseudomonas aeruginosa*. Can. Vet. J. 36, 166-168.

Hendrix, D.V.H., Stuffle, J.L. and Cox, S.K. 2007. Pharmacokinetics of topically applied ciprofloxacin in equine tears. Vet. Ophthtalmol. 10, 344-347.

Jensen, H., Zerouala, C., Carrier, M. and Short, B. 2005. Comparison of ophthalmic gatifloxacin 0.3% and ciprofloxacin 0.3% in healing of corneal ulcers associated with *Pseudomonas aeruginosa*-induced ulcerative keratitis in rabbits. J. Ocul. Pharmacol. Ther. 21, 36-43.

Kaye, S.B., Neal, T., Nicholson, S., Szkurlat, J., Bamber, S., Baddon, A.C., Anderson, S., Seddon, K., Dwyer, N., Lovering, A.M. and Smith, G. 2009. Concentration and bioavailability of ciprofloxacin and teicoplanin in the cornea. Invest. Ophthalmol. Vis. Sci. 50, 3176-3184.

Kowalski, R.P., Dhaliwal, D.K., Karenchak, L.M., Romanowski, E.G., Mah, F.S., Ritterband, D.C. and Gordon, Y.J.2003. Gatifloxacin and moxifloxacin: an in vitro susceptibility comparison to levofloxacin, ciprofloxacin, and ofloxacin using bacterial keratitis isolates. Am. J. Ophthalmol. 136, 500-505.

Ledbetter, E.C., Hendricks, L.M., Riis, R.C. and Scarlett, J. 2007. In vitro fluoroquinolone susceptibility of *Pseudomonas aeruginosa* isolates from dogs with ulcerative keratitis. Am. J. Vet. Res. 68, 638-642.

Ledbetter, E.G., Mun, J.J., Kowbel, D. and Fleiszig, S.M.J. 2009. Pathogenic phenotype and genotype of *Pseudomonas aeruginosa* isolates from spontaneous canine ocular infections. Investig. Ophthalmol. Visual. Sci. 50, 729-736.

Levison, M.E. and Levison, J.H. 2009. Pharmacokinetics and Pharmacodynamics of Antibacterial Agents. Infect. Dis. Clin. North Am. 23, 791-815.

Lima Filho, A.A.S. and Batistuzzo, J.A.O. 2006. Formulações Magistrais em oftalmologia, Cultura Médica, Rio de Janeiro, Brasil.

Limberg, M. and Buggé, C. 1994. Tear concentrations of topically applied ciprofloxacin. Cornea 13, 496-499.

Lin, C.T. and Petersen-Jones, S.M. 2007. Antibiotic susceptibility of bacterial isolates from corneal ulcers of dogs in Taiwan. J. Small Anim. Pract. 48, 271-274.

Lin, C.T. and Petersen-Jones, S.M. 2008. Antibiotic susceptibility of bacteria isolated from cats with ulcerative keratitis in Taiwan. J. Small Anim. Pract. 49, 80-83.

Maggs, D.J. 2008. Cornea and sclera. In: Maggs, D.J., Miller, P.E. and Ofri, R. Slatter's Fundamentals of Veterinary Ophthalmology 4th Ed. Saunders Elsevier, St Louis. pp: 175-202.

Mah, F.S. 2003. New antibiotics for bacterial infections. Ophthalmol. Clin. North Am. 16, 11-27.

Mannis, M.J. and Smolin, G. 1996. Natural defense mechanisms of the ocular surface. In: Pepose, J.S., Holland, G.N. and Wilhelmeus, K.R. (eds). Ocular Infection and Immunity. Mosby: St Louis, MO, pp: 185-190.

Mayo, M.S., Cook, W.L., Schlitzer, R.L., Ward, M.A., Wilson, L.A. and Ahearn, D.G. 1986. Antibiograms, serotypes, and plasmid profile of *Pseudomonas aeruginosa* associated with corneal ulcers and contact lens wear. J. Clinic. Microbiol. 24, 372-376.

Mohammadpour, M., Mohajernezhadfard, Z., Khodabande, A. and Vahedi, P. 2011. Antibiotic Susceptibility Patterns of Pseudomonas Corneal Ulcers in Contact Lens Wearers. Middle East African J. Ophthalmol. 18, 228-231.

Moore, C.P., Collins, B.K. and Fales, W.H. 1995. Antibacterial susceptibility patterns for microbial isolates associated with infectious keratitis in horses: 63 cases (1986-1994). J. Am. Vet. Med. Assoc. 207, 928-933.

Moore, C.P. and Naisse, M.P. 2000. Clinical Microbiology. In: Gellat, K.N. Veterinary Ophthalmology. 3rd Ed, pp: 259-289.

Peiffer, R.L. and Stowe, C.M. 1981. Veterinary ophthalmic pharmacology. In: Gelatt, K.N. ed. Veterinary Ophthalmology. 2nd ed. Philadelphia: Lea & Febiger, pp: 160-205.

Quinn, P.J., Carter, M.E., Markey, B. and Marter, G.R. 1994. *Pseudomonas* species. In: Ibid. (Eds), Clinical Veterinary Microbiology. Wolfe, London, pp: 237-242.

Sueke, H., Kaye, S. and Neal, T. 2010. Minimum inhibitory concentrations of standard and novel antimicrobials for isolates from bacterial keratitis," Invest. Ophthalmol. Vis. Sci. 51, 2519-2524.

Tang-Liu, D.D.S., Schob, D.L., Usansky, J. and Gordon, Y.J. 1994. Comparative tear concentrations over time of ofloxacin and tobramycin in human eyes. Clin. Pharmacol. Therapeutics 55, 284-293.

Varges, R., Penna, B., Martins, G., Martins, R. and Lilenbaum, W. 2009. Antimicrobial susceptibility of *Staphylococcus* isolated from naturally occurring canine external ocular diseases. Vet. Ophthalmol. 12, 216-220.

Viana, F.A.B. 2007. Guia terapêutico veterinário. 2ed., Editora CEM, Lagoa Santa.

Wada, S., Hobo, S. and Niwa, H. 2010. Ulcerative keratitis in thoroughbred racehorses in Japan from 1997 to 2008. Vet. Ophthalmol. 13, 99-105.

7

Developmental ossification sequences of the appendicular and axial skeleton in Kuttanad duck embryos (*Anas platyrhynchos domesticus*)

A.D. Firdous[1,*], S. Maya[2], K. Massarat[1] and M.A. Baba[1]

[1]*Division of Veterinary Anatomy and Histology, FVSC & AH Shuhama Alusteng Jammu and Kashmir, India*
[2]*Department of Veterinary Anatomy and Histology, CV& AS, Mannuthy, Kerala, India*

Abstract

The processes of ossification sequences are poorly investigated for birds in general, even for domestic and experimental species and when it comes to the waterfowl it is almost negligible. Such sequences constitute a rich source of data on character evolution, and may even provide phylogenetic information. A pre-hatch developmental study on ossification sequences of axial and appendicular skeletal system in Kuttanad duck embryos was undertaken using 78 viable embryos. From day 3 to day 7 of incubation no ossification densities were seen both by alizarin red staining and computerized radiography. The first indication of ossification as small ossification centers in skull bones, clavicle, scapula, humerus, radius and ulna in forelimb and ilium, pubis femur and fibula in hind limb were observed on the 9th day of incubation. The ossification of the body of the ribs started at the 11th day of incubation towards the proximal extremity. On day 13th the ossification process of vertebrae was started from cervical end. The variation in appearance of the ossification centers in different bones at different stages of incubation period suggests relative importance of phylogeny to the sequences.

Keywords: Alizarin red, Duck, Ossification, Radiography.

Introduction

It is poorly understood or still in infancy, what factors influence ossification sequences and what the relative importance of phylogeny is to the sequences. Galliformes are among domestic birds that could be considered as a good model to examine these variables. Waterfowl comes second to the Galliformes and will substitute the domestic fowl in many ways as an experimental valuable model for studying the vertebrate skeletal defects. These birds are osteologically conservative, have precocial young, but have a broad spectrum of body sizes and incubation periods. Birds are said to show the least embryonic variation of all groups of vertebrates (Kerr, 1919; Richardson *et al.*, 1997). It has been argued that specific differences between birds arise largely through modifications at later stages of development (Ricklefs and Starck, 1998). Patterns of early embryonic development have traditionally been viewed as invariant within vertebrate taxa. The passive components of avian skeletal system i.e. bone development and health is an important subject in avian research, because of its significance in the poultry industry. Many of the pathological skeletal deformities are still common and do not appear to be linked to define causes e.g. varus and valgus deformation of the long bones are examples. Although there are dissimilarities between human and avian bone development, the avian is considered as a valuable model for human skeletal defects (Cook, 2000). Though a lot of work has been done on the developmental aspects of the skeletal system

in birds; research on skeletal system development waterfowl is scanty. Hence the aim of this study was to investigate the developmental way of the passive part of the skeletal system of Kuttanad duck embryos that will add the knowledge in the anatomical literature and will help the allied subjects on comparative basis.

Materials and Methods

The material of this study consisted of 78 Kuttanad duck's viable embryos, collected from 3rd to 28th day of incubation procured from the University Poultry and Duck Farm, Mannuthy, Thrissur Kerala, India. The number of viable embryos collected in a given period of incubation is shown in Table 1 (6 embryos at each time point). The eggs were incubated at 37-38.9°C with humidity of 30-35%. The eggs were rotated at least three times a day, half turn each rotation. Starting from 3rd day of incubation, six eggs with viable embryos were collected. At day 25th the incubation temperature was decreased to 36-37°C and the humidity was increased to 70%.

Techniques to access the sequence of ossification
Toluidine Blue-Alizarin Red S Staining of Cartilage and Bone protocol (Burdi, 1965)
Cartilage and bone were differentiated in whole-mount preparations with toluidine blue-alizarin red S staining after formalin, acetic acid and alcohol (FAA) fixation. Specimens were fixed in FAA solution having the ratio of three components as 1:1:8 for approximately 40 minutes. Then they were stained in 0.06% toluidine blue made in 70% ethyl alcohol for 48 hours at room temperature.

*Corresponding Author: Firdous Ahmad Dar. Division of Veterinary Anatomy and Histology, FVSC & AH Shuhama Alusteng Jammu and Kashmir, India. E-mail: drromey@gmail.com

Table 1. Number of viable embryos collected at different days of incubation.

Incubation period (days)	3rd	5th	7th	9th	11th	13th	15th	17th	19th	21st	23rd	25th	27th
Number of embryos collected	6	6	6	6	6	6	6	6	6	6	6	6	6

Twenty volumes of stain solution to the estimated volume of the specimen were used. Soft tissues were destained in 35% ethyl alcohol for 20 hours; 5% for 28 hours and 70% for 8 hours respectively. The specimens were counterstained in a freshly prepared 1% aqueous solution of KOH to which 2-3 drops of 0.1% alizarin red S per 100 ml of solution was added. The specimens were transferred into the fresh 1% KOH-alizarin mixture daily for 3 days, or until the bones had reached the desired intensity of red and soft tissues. The specimens were rinsed in water, placed in a 1:1 mixture of glycerol and ethyl alcohol for 1-2 hours and then transferred into fresh glycerol-alcohol for final clearing and storage.

Radiography

Ex ovo radiographs of the skeletal system were taken at different ages to reach the extent of ossification and development of various components of this system. Radiographs were taken by computerized digital radiography equipment, which was provided by Department of Veterinary Surgery and Radiology, College of Veterinary and Animal sciences, Mannuthy.

Stereozoom microscopy

The embryos were viewed by stereozoom microscope, which was provided by Department of Veterinary Physiology and Department of Veterinary Parasitology.

Results

No ossification centers were seen from the 3rd to the 7th day of incubation. Both alizarin red staining and computerized radiography could not detect any ossification densities (Fig. 1). The degree of ossification during different stages of incubation period in Kuttanad duck was efficiently visualized by computerized radiography (Fig. 2, 3 and 4). For convenience of description, the skeleton was divided into four parts, *viz.*, skull, vertebrae, ribs and sternum and forelimb and hind limb. In earlier stages of the embryonic life in Kuttanad ducks most elements of the skull were still separated. By 27 days of incubation facial bones were largely fused but the skull was still opened dorsally. The bones of the skull from 3rd day of incubation till 7th day did not stain with alizarin red. The first indication of ossification in skull bones as a small ossification centers were observed in squamosal bone on 9th day of incubation (Fig. 5 and 6). The process of ossification was followed by palatine, pterygoid, prefrontal, and the bones forming the beak such as maxilla, jugal, quadratojugal, splenial, angular, supraangular and premaxilla. The last bones to be ossified were the frontal and nasal bones and by 13th day all skull bones appeared and were maximally ossified (Fig. 7). The red regions of each skull bone were enlarged with the advancement of incubation period.

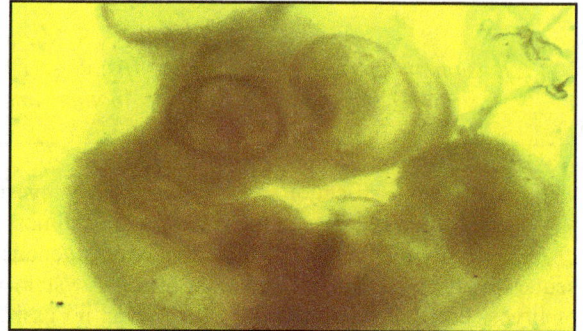

Fig. 1. 5th day of incubation of Kuttanad duck embryo without any signs of ossification. Alizarin red staining.

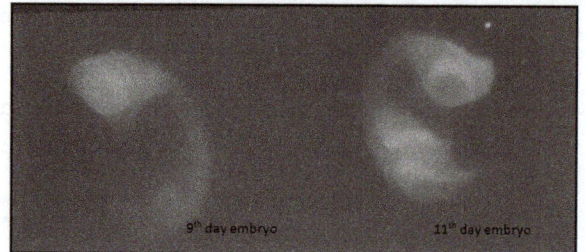

Fig. 2. Digital radiograph of Kuttanad duck embryos.

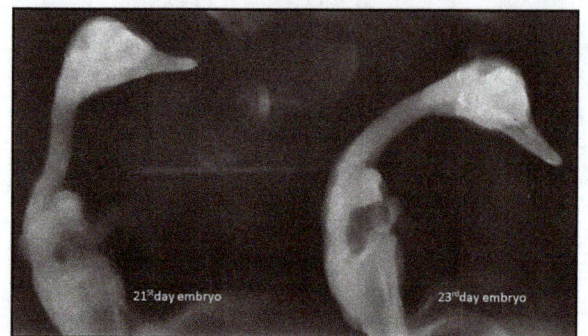

Fig. 3. Digital radiograph of Kuttanad duck embryos showing ossification centers in different bones.

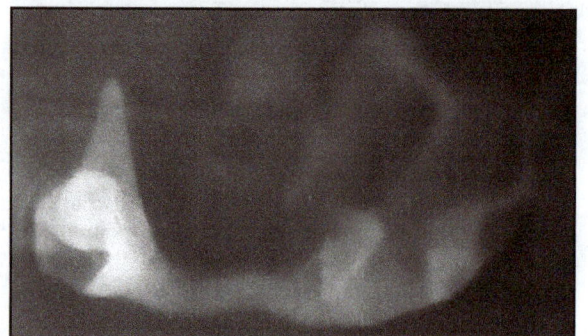

Fig. 4. Digital radiograph of 25th day old Kuttanad duck embryo showing ossification centers.

The long bones in the post cranial part of the skeleton in the Kuttanad duck were the first to show the process of mineralization. The fore and hind limbs showed endochondral calcification and the ossification process started at the center of the diaphysis and extended towards the epiphysis. On the 9th day of incubation small ossification centers were observed in clavicle, scapula, humerus, radius and ulna in forelimb and ilium, pubis femur and fibula in hind limb (Fig. 8). By day 11 of incubation the size of the ossification centers got increased. On day 13th of incubation new ossification centers were observed on radius, ulna, carpometacarpal joint, ulnar carpal, metatarsus, tibiotarsus, first phalanx of digit ii and second phalanx of digit iii. Day 15 marked the ossification centers on digit ii, iii, iv of forelimb and additional ossification centers were observed in 1st, 2nd, 3rd phalanx of digit iii and 4th phalanx of digit ii of pelvic limb. Between days 17 and 19 of incubation there were prominent and clear increase of ossification centers in both limbs (Fig. 9). Right and left clavicles showed the process of ossification on the 9th day but were not fused. Both clavicles were joined on 23rd day of incubation but not properly fused. On 28th day of developmental process the growth plates of long bones were still open. On 17th day of incubation the vertebral arches of all the cervical, thoracic, lumbar and sacral vertebrates showed ossification (Fig. 10 and 11). On day 21st of incubation ossification was seen on pygostyle. The calcification of

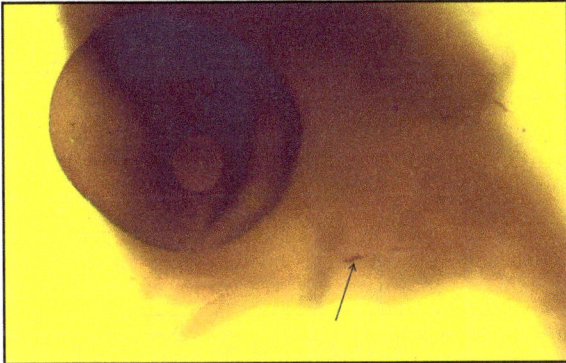

Fig. 5. First indication of ossification in skull at 9th day of incubation (arrow). Alizarin red staining.

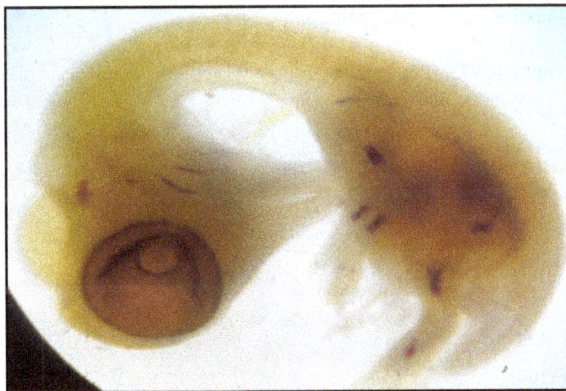

Fig. 6. Ossification centers in skull bones at 11th day of incubation in Kuttanad duck embryo. Alizarin red staining.

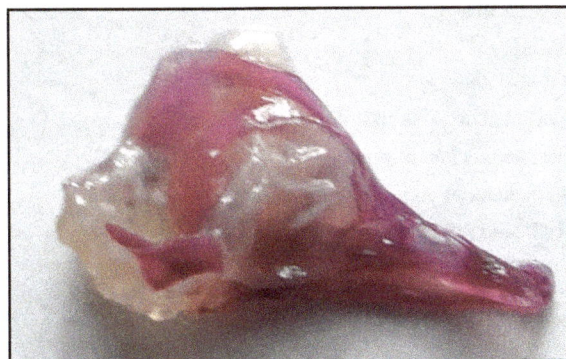

Fig. 7. Maximally ossified 13th day incubated skull bones of Kuttanad duck embryo. Alizarin red staining.

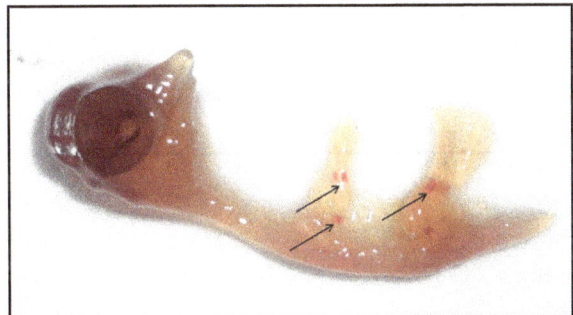

Fig. 8. Ossification centers (arrows) appeared in long bones on 9th day of incubation. Alizarin red staining.

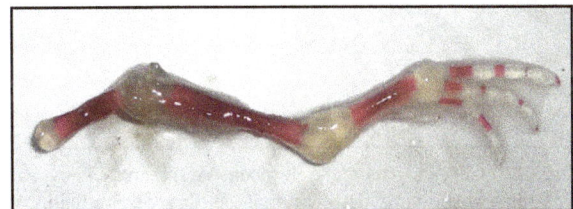

Fig. 9. Prominent ossification centers at 19th day of incubation in hind limb. Alizarin red staining.

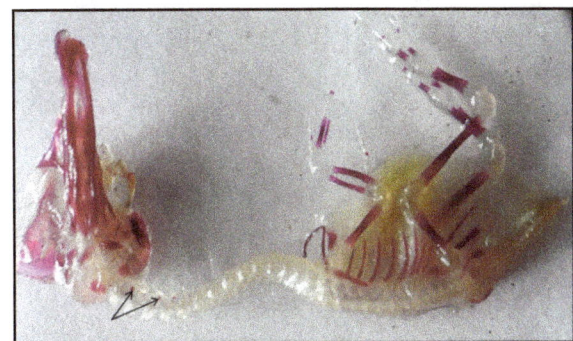

Fig. 10. Ossification centers of vertebrae at cervical end (arrows). Alizarin red staining.

the body of the ribs started at the 11th day of incubation towards the proximal extremity (Fig. 12). In both vertebral and sternal ribs, ossification first occurred at the middle region and then progressed towards the proximal and distal regions. As the ossification extended in both ways an area towards the vertebra remained cartilaginous till hatching. The uncinate process of the rib first appeared as cartilage then it was calcified. In Kuttanad ducks the keel bone began to ossify firstly towards the caudal side and then cranially. The ossification of the Axial and Appendicular bones in a given incubation period is shown in Table 2.

Discussion

A detailed description of skeletogenesis and ossification sequence for the chicken and Japanese quail has been provided by many researchers (Rogulska, 1962; Hogg, 1980; Nakane and Tsudzuki, 1999). The ossification sequence of the Kuttanad duck variety has not previously been described. This study besides describing the process of ossification in Kuttanad duck may also reveal the relative importance of egg size and incubation period to ossification sequence in this species. The relative sequence of ossification was the same whether enzymatic clearing and staining or histological sections are used, and so studies using different methodologies are also comparable (Clark and Smith, 1993). In this regard, a pre-hatch developmental study of ossification sequences of axial and appendicular skeletal system in Kuttanad duck embryos was undertaken using 78 viable embryos.

The first indication of ossification in skull bones of Kuttanad duck embryos was seen as a small ossification centers and observed in squamosal bone on the 9th day of incubation. In contradictory to quail as reported by Jollie (1957) the skull bones appeared on 11th day of incubation. The wing ossified earlier as compared to the foot. Vasiliauskas *et al.* (2003) reported the same in hind limb of chicks but in disagreement to Zukiene *et al.* (2003) in mice. The ossification process of the forelimbs is in agreement

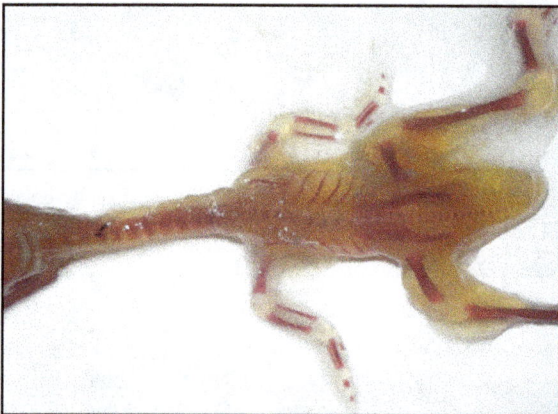

Fig. 11. Cervical, thoracic, lumbar, sacral and coccygeal vertebrates showing ossification (25th day of incubation). Alizarin red staining.

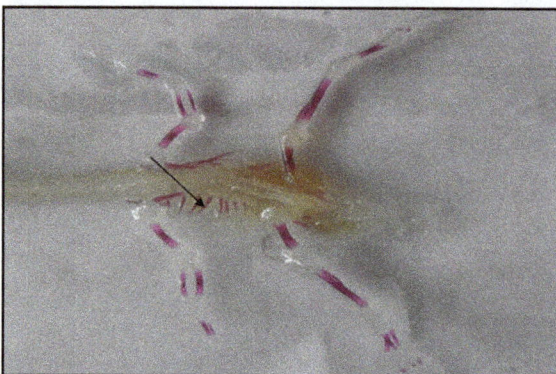

Fig. 12. Ossification of ribs (13th day old embryo). Alizarin red staining.

Table 2. The ossification of bones of Axial and Appendicular skeleton in Kuttanad duck embryos in given incubation period.

Structures ossified	Time of ossification (days)
Squamosal bone of skull	9
Palatine, pterygoid, prefrontal	13
Maxilla, Jugal, Quadratojugal, Splenial, Angular, Supraangular, Premaxilla	13
Clavicle	9
Scapula	9
Humerus	9
Radius	9-13
Ulna	9-13
Ilium	9-11
Pubis	9-11
Femur	9-11
Fibula	9
Carpometacarpal joint	13
Ulnar carpal	13
Metatarsus	13
Tibiotarsus	13
First phalanx of digit ii	13
Second phalanx of digit iii	13
4th phalanx of digit ii of pelvic limb	15
Right and left clavicles	9
Vertebral arches of all the cervical, thoracic, lumbar and sacral vertebrates	17
Pygostyle	21
Ribs	11

to the studies of Saunder (1998) in forelimbs of chicks. Both clavicles were joined on 23rd day of incubation but not properly fused. Ruchon *et al.* (1998) reported in mice the vertebrates ossified at the 16th day, however, Lecanda *et al.* (2000) reported the process of vertebral ossification on the 15th day of incubation. The ossification of the cervical vertebrate body in chick embryo started at the 12th-13th day of incubation while as sacral vertebrae get ossified on day 19th of incubation (Shapiro, 1992).

Sawad *et al.* (2009) said that in Gallus the primary calcification of the rib body at the proximal extremity at the 10th day of incubation. In case of chicken as reported by Hamburger and Hamilton (1951) the uncinate process calcifies directly. Nakane and Tsudzuki (1999) reported in quail that sternum ossification occurred in the laterocaudal process at the 14th day of incubation and in the laterocranial process at the 15th day of incubation.

Conclusion

In the present study, embryonic ossification sequences of skeletal system in Kuttanad duck were revealed. In this paper it is presumed that the stages of ossification of various elements of the body presented will be useful as a normal control in the fields of general embryology, developmental engineering, and teratological studies. The difference in the sequence of ossification of various skeletal elements in Kuttanad duck may be due to the appearance of ossification centers at different stages of incubation. Besides there was also a difference on comparative basis possibly due to the difference in the incubation period among different birds.

Acknowledgments

The authors highly acknowledge the Dean of faculty for providing the necessary facilities to carry out this work. The authors are grateful to the Department of Veterinary Physiology, Department of Veterinary Parasitology and Department of Veterinary Surgery and Radiology for providing the facilities.

References

Burdi, A.R. 1965. Toluidine Blue-Alizarin Red S Staining of Cartilage and Bone in Whole-Mount Skeletons in Vitro. Stain Technol. 40, 45-48.

Clark, C.T. and Smith, K.K. 1993. Cranial osteogenesis in Monodelphis domestica (Didelphidae) and Macropus eugenii (Macropodidae). J. Morphol. 215, 119-149.

Cook, M.E. 2000. Skeletal deformities and their causes: Introduction. Poult. Sci. 79, 982-984.

Hamburger, V. and Hamilton, H.L. 1951. A series of normal stages in the development of the chick embryo. J. Morphol. 88, 49-92.

Hogg, D.A. 1980. A reinvestigation of the centers of ossification in the avian skeleton at and after hatching. J. Anat. 130, 725-743.

Jollie, M.T. 1957. The head skeleton of the chicken and remarks on the anatomy of this region in other birds. J. Morphol. 100, 389-436.

Kerr, J.G. 1919. Textbook of Embryology. Vol 2. MacMillan. London.

Lecanda, F., Warlow, P.M., Sheikh, S., Furlan, F., Steinberg, T.H. and Civitelli, R. 2000. Connexin43 deficiency causes delayed ossification, craniofacial abnormalities, and osteoblast disfunction. J. Cell Biol. 151, 931-944.

Nakane, Y. and Tsudzuki, M. 1999. Development of the skeleton in Japanese quail embryos. Dev. Growth Differ. 41, 523-534.

Richardson, M.K., Hanken, J., Gooneratne, M.L., Pieau, C., Raynaud, A., Selwood L. and Wright, G.M. 1997. There is no highly conserved embryonic stage in vertebrates: implications for current theories of evolution and development. Anat. Embryol. 196, 91-106.

Ricklefs, R.E. and Starck, J.M. 1998. Embryonic growth and development. In: Avian Growth and Development. Evolution within the Altricial-Precocial. Academic Press, Oxford, pp: 31-58.

Rogulska, T. 1962. Differences in the process of ossification during the embryonic development of the chick (*Gallus domesticus*), rook (*Corvus frugilegus*) and black-headed gull (*Larusridi bundus*). Zool. Pol. 12, 223-236.

Ruchon, A.F., Marcinkiewicz, M., Siegfried, G., Tenenhouse, H.S., DesGroseillers, L., Crine, P. and Boileau, G. 1998. Pex mRNA is localized in developing mouse osteoblasts and odontoblasts. J. Histchem. Cytochem. 46, 459-468.

Saunder, J.W.Jr. 1998. The proximo-distal sequence of the origin of the parts of chick wing and the role of the ectoderm. J. Exp. Zool. 282, 628-668.

Sawad, A.A., Hana, B.A. and Al-Silawi, A.N. 2009. Morphological Study of the Skeleton Development in Chick Embryo (*Gallus domesticus*). Int. J. Poul. Sci. 8(7), 710-714.

Shapiro, F. 1992. Vertebral development of chick embryo during days 3-19 of incubation. J. Morphol. 213, 317-333.

Vasiliauskas, D., Laufer, E. and Stern, C.D. 2003. A role for hairy 1 in regulating chick Limb bud growth. Dev. Biol. 262, 94-106.

Zukiene, J., Zalgeviciene, V. and Rizgeliene, R. 2003. The influence of azathioprine on the osteogenesis of the limbs. Medicina 39, 584-588.

8

Haemangiosarcoma in a captive Asiatic lion (*Panthera leo persica*)

F. Vercammen[1,*], J. Brandt[1], L. Van Brantegem[2], L. Bosseler[2] and R. Ducatelle[2]

[1]Centre for Research and Conservation, Royal Zoological Society of Antwerp, K. Astridplein 26, B-2018 Antwerp, Belgium

[2]Department of Pathology, Bacteriology and Avian Medicine, Faculty of Veterinary Medicine, University of Ghent, Salisburylaan 133, B-9820 Merelbeke, Belgium

Abstract

A 2.7-year-old male captive Asiatic lion (*Panthera leo persica*) died unexpectedly without preceding symptoms. Gross necropsy revealed liver and lung tumours, which proved to be haemangiosarcomas by histopathology. Some of the liver tumours were ruptured, leading to massive intra-abdominal haemorrhage and death. Haemangiosarcomas are rare in domestic and exotic felids, occurring in skin, thoracic-abdominal cavity and bones. Although these tumours mainly appear to be occurring in older cats, they are sometimes observed in younger animals, as in the present case. This is the first description of haemangiosarcoma in a young Asiatic lion.

Keywords: Asiatic lion, Haemangiosarcoma, Histopathology, Neoplasia, *Panthera leo persica*.

Introduction

Asiatic lions (*Panthera leo persica*) are large felids once found throughout most of southwest Asia and genetically distinct from African lions (*Panthera leo*). Now, they are confined to India and the International Union for the Conservation of Nature lists these animals as endangered, with an estimated population of only 250 animals inside and 100 animals outside the Gir Forest protected area in the State of Gujarat (Breitenmoser *et al.*, 2008). The major threats for this population are unpredictable events, such as epidemics or large forest fires, poaching and drowning incidents (Breitenmoser *et al.*, 2008). Today, the Zoological Information Management System (ZIMS) by the International Species Information System (ISIS) lists 325 captive animals in 57 institutions in Asia, Europe and the United States of America.

Searching the international literature, the authors could find few reports on infectious diseases (Ramanathan *et al.*, 2007; Pawar *et al.*, 2012) and only three reports on neoplasms in Asiatic lions, i.e. one case of ocular squamous cell carcinoma, one case of lymphocytic leukaemia, and one report describing two cases of visceral haemangiosarcoma (Hruban *et al.*, 1992; Kelawala *et al.*, 2001; Amaravathi *et al.*, 2012). There are two case reports of visceral haemangiosarcoma in other exotic felids: a cheetah (*Acinonyx jubatus*) and a Bengal tiger (*Panthera tigris*) (Ervin *et al.*, 1988; Kang *et al.*, 1996). Although haemangiosarcomas are also rarely observed in domestic cats, several such reports exist (Liu *et al.*, 1974; Quigley and Leedale, 1983; Scavelli *et al.*, 1985; Schultheiss, 2004; Johannes *et al.*, 2007; Wobeser *et al.*, 2007; Culp *et al.*, 2008).

The present report describes the gross necropsy and histopathology of a fatal haemangiosarcoma in a young captive Asiatic lion. This case is not only noteworthy because of the rarity of this tumour in large felids, but also the young age at which this animal developed the neoplasm is remarkable.

Case Details

At the Wild Animal Park Planckendael of the Royal Zoological Society of Antwerp, an adult, male Asiatic lion, 2.7 years old, was found dead in his inside enclosure without preceding clinical abnormalities. Gross post-mortem examination revealed a normal body condition with a body weight of 140 kg and the following salient findings: anaemic mucosae; 10 litres of blood in the abdominal cavity; pale-coloured pancreas and spleen; multiple nodular lung masses (a few mm to 10 cm diameter, filled with blood clots) (Fig. 1); multiple (2 mm – 8 mm diameter) kidney cysts (filled with clear transparent liquid); multiple liver nodules (a few mm to 10 cm diameter, filled with blood clots, some with grapelike appearance, others were ruptured) (Fig. 2). An additional macroscopic finding, i.e. an extensive proximal diaphyseal new bone formation on the right humerus, was identified later after the preparation of the skeleton at the Royal Belgian Institute of Natural Sciences in Brussels. No anomalies were detected in any other organ.

A set of tissue samples (liver, lung, spleen, kidney, bronchial lymph node) was collected and fixed in 10% neutral buffered formalin, embedded in paraffin, sectioned at 4 μm, and stained with haematoxylin and eosin and Prussian blue for histologic examination. Immunohistochemistry was performed on 4-μm sections using Factor VIII-related antigen or von

*Corresponding Author: Dr. Francis Vercammen. Centre for Research and Conservation, Royal Zoological Society of Antwerp, K. Astridplein 26, B-2018 Antwerp, Belgium. E-mail: *francis.vercammen@kmda.org*

Willebrand factor (vWf) (polyclonal rabbit antibody, reference A0082, Dako, Glostrop, Denmark) and the platelet-endothelial cell adhesion molecule or cluster of differentiation 31 (CD31) (monoclonal mouse antibody, Clone JC70A, reference M0823, Dako, Glostrup, Denmark). External positive controls for the immunohistochemical stainings were spleen from a pig for vWf and mesenteric blood vessels from a dog for CD31. Internal controls consisted of normal endothelial cells in the examined tissues. No non-specific staining was observed in any of the slides.

In the liver, there were multifocal areas where the normal architecture was lost and most of the parenchyma had been replaced by non-encapsulated, poorly demarcated, infiltrative and moderately cellular masses. The masses were composed of loosely arranged streams and poorly defined capillary-like channels, supported by a moderate amount of eosinophilic stroma and occasionally large vascular channels, filled with variable amounts of blood (Fig. 3a). Neoplastic cells were mainly polygonal to spindle shaped, with indistinct cell borders, moderate amounts of eosinophilic cytoplasm with a round to oval, centrally placed nucleus with a finely stippled chromatin pattern and 1 nucleolus. There was moderate anisokaryosis and anisocytosis. Mitotic figures ranged from 1 to 4 per high power field. There were larger areas of haemorrhage and necrosis. The neoplastic cells

labelled strongly positive for vWf and CD31 (Fig. 3b). In the lung similar neoplastic foci were observed, which also labelled positive for vWf and CD31. There was mild fibrosis of the renal capsule. There were no neoplastic lesions in the kidney. The capsule of the spleen showed focal mesothelial cell proliferation without signs of neoplastic masses in the spleen. In the bronchial lymph node, and especially in its subcapsular sinuses, there was a multifocal mild infiltration of macrophages. Many of those macrophages had an intracytoplasmic accumulation of a yellowish-brown granular pigment. Prussian blue staining confirmed the pigment as haemosiderin. Other macrophages showed erythrophagocytosis. The lesion in the humerus, detected during the preparation of the skeleton, was not examined histopathologically.

Tissue impression smears of bronchial lymph node, liver, lung and also of the abdominal blood were made for bacteriological examinations. Giemsa stain, Gram stain and Ziehl-Neelsen stain were all negative. Cultivation on tryptone-soya-agar and blood agar demonstrated no growth of bacteria.

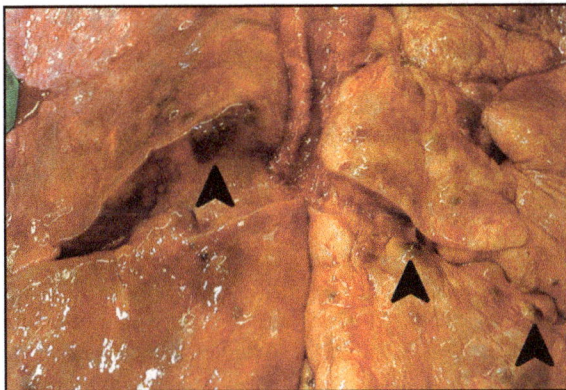

Fig. 1. Gross necropsy: lung tumours in an Asiatic lion with haemangiosarcoma.

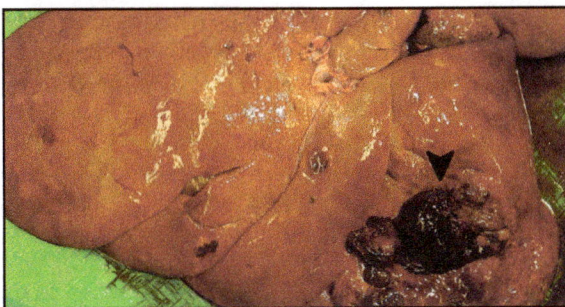

Fig. 2. Gross necropsy: liver tumours in an Asiatic lion with haemangiosarcoma.

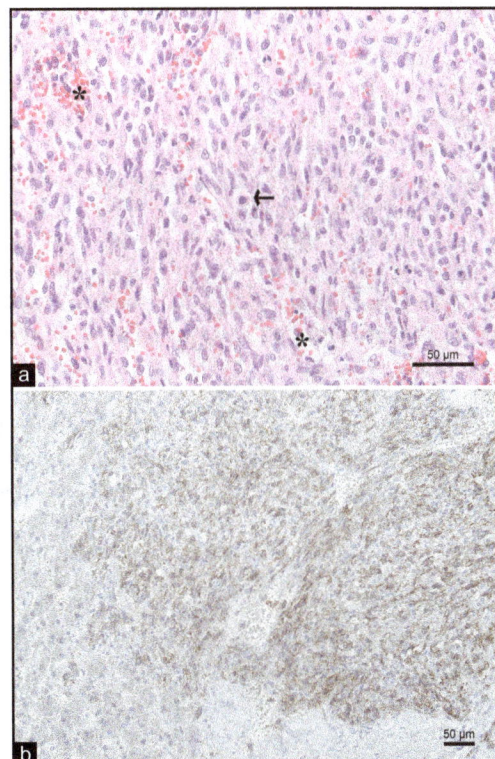

Fig. 3. Histopathology of liver haemangiosarcoma in an Asiatic lion. (a) The masses are composed of streams and capillary-like channels (asterisk) formed by polygonal to spindle shaped neoplastic cells. A mitotic figure is indicated (arrow). Mitoses range from 1 to 4 per high power field (Haematoxylin and eosin - H&E). (b) Cluster of differentiation 31 (CD31) positive immunohistochemistry. On the left side of the image CD31 negative hepatocytes are seen.

Discussion

Haemangiosarcomas are very rare in domestic cats as well as in large captive cats. In a retrospective study covering 6 years and 1912 domestic animals, only 72 cats (3-17 years old) were diagnosed with haemangiosarcoma, of which 59 involved the skin, 2 the bones and 11 the viscera (Schultheiss, 2004). Johannes et al. (2007) found 10 cats with visceral haemangiosarcoma out of 53 domestic cats with haemangiosarcoma over a period of 10 years. In a large survey totalling 3145 domestic cats, a haemangiosarcoma prevalence of 0.6% was observed (Patnaik and Liu, 1977). In a retrospective evaluation of surgical cases involving 31 domestic cats between 4 and 15 years old, 15 abdominal haemangiosarcomas, 2 thoracic, 13 subcutaneous and 1 haemangiosarcoma of the nasal cavity were found (Scavelli et al., 1985). One report considered only amputated feline digits and found 5 domestic cats (2-13 years old) out of 63 with haemangiosarcomas (Wobeser et al., 2007).

Visceral haemangiosarcoma involving the liver has been described only twice in the Asiatic lion and remains a very rare tumour in non-domestic felids (Amaravathi et al., 2012). The prevalence of this tumour is very low even in domestic cats, where the mean age of occurrence is 9.5 years (range between 2-18 years) (Quigley and Leedale, 1983; Scavelli et al., 1985; Schultheiss, 2004; Wobeser et al., 2007). The age of the young Asiatic lion in the present case (2.7 years) falls within the age range reported for domestic cats, but deviates from the mean age (9.5 years) and is in very sharp contrast with the very old age of 22 and 24 years in the only two reported cases in Asiatic lions (Amaravathi et al., 2012). Moreover, these two animals had been suffering from progressive weakness and debilitation for several months as opposed to our clinically healthy young animal (Amaravathi et al., 2012). Probably these symptoms are the result of the progressive increase in abdominal serosanguinous fluid, contrary to the abrupt liver haemorrhages in the present case. Furthermore, the old lions presented with masses in their liver and spleen, whereas our lion had liver and lung tumours. Unfortunately, all our observations did not allow us to determine the primary neoplastic site. Clinicians should be aware that neoplasia is a potential differential diagnosis in a sick Asiatic lion and that pathological surveillance of all captive animals in all age categories is of great value to the breeding and conservation effort.

In domestic cats, bone involvement is rare, but two out of 58 bone neoplasms (one in the humerus and one in the tibia) were diagnosed as haemangiosarcoma, both in older animals, 17 and 18 years respectively (Quigley and Leedale, 1983). Another report described only one domestic cat with a soft tissue haemangiosarcoma with bone involvement out of 29 cats with soft tissue tumours involving bone (Liu et al., 1974). The extensive new bone formation on the humerus was not examined in histopathology because it was discovered after the preparation of the skeleton for the museum. Yet, this lesion is probably not a result of a metastasising haemangiosarcoma, which normally provokes extensive osteolysis rather than new bone formation (Quigley and Leedale, 1983).

In conclusion, this is the first description of haemangiosarcoma in a young captive Asiatic lion that died suddenly due to massive liver haemorrhages.

Acknowledgments

The authors wish to thank Mr. W. Wouters of the Royal Belgian Institute of Natural Sciences in Brussels for the preparation of the skeleton and the Flemish Government for structural support to the Centre for Research and Conservation.

References

Amaravathi, P., Srilatha, C., Sujatha, K. and Sailaja, N. 2012. Histopathological and immunohistochemical study of hemangiosarcoma in lions. Indian J. Vet. Pathol. 36, 120-121.

Breitenmoser, U., Mallon, D.P., Khan, J.A. and Driscoll, C. 2008. *Panthera leo ssp. persica*. IUCN 2013. IUCN Red List of Threatened Species. http://www.iucnredlist.org.

Culp, W.T., Drobatz, K.J., Glassman, M.M., Baez, J.L. and Aronson, L.R. 2008. Feline visceral hemangiosarcoma. J. Vet. Intern. Med. 22, 148-152.

Ervin, A.M., Junge, R.E., Miller, R.E. and Thornburg, L.P. 1988. Hemangiosarcoma in a cheetah (*Acinonyx jubatus*). J. Zoo Wildl. Med. 19, 143-145.

Hruban, Z., Vardiman, J., Meehan, T., Frye, F. and Carter, W.E. 1992. Haematopoietic malignancies in zoo animals. J. Comp. Pathol. 106, 15-24.

Johannes, C.M., Henry, C.J., Turnquist, S.E., Hamilton, T.A., Smith, A.N., Chun, R. and Tyler, J.W. 2007. Hemangiosarcoma in cats: 53 cases (1992-2002). J. Am. Vet. Med. Assoc. 231, 1851-1856.

Kang, B., Kim, D., Shin, N. and Kwon, S. 1996. Spontaneous hemangiosarcoma in a Bengal tiger (*Panthera tigris*). Korean J. Vet. Res. 36, 143-150.

Kelawala, N.H., Parsiana, R.R., Sabapara, R.H. and Prajapati, K.S. 2001. Ocular neoplasm in an Asiatic lion (*Panthera leo persica*) - a case report. Intas Polivet 2, 222-223.

Liu, S.K., Dorfman, H.D. and Patnaik, A.K. 1974. Primary and secondary bone tumours in the cat. J. Small Anim. Pract. 15, 141-156.

Patnaik, A.K. and Liu, S.K. 1977. Angiosarcoma in cats. J. Small Anim. Pract. 18, 191-198.

Pawar, R.M., Lakshmikantan, U., Hasan, S., Poornachandar, A. and Shivaji, S. 2012. Detection and molecular characterization of ascarid nematode infection (*Toxascaris leonina* and *Toxocara cati*) in captive Asiatic lions (*Panthera leo persica*). Acta Parasitol. 57, 67-73.

Quigley, P.J. and Leedale, A.H. 1983. Tumors involving bone in the domestic cat: a review of fifty-eight cases. Vet. Pathol. 20, 670-686.

Ramanathan, A., Malik, P.K. and Prasad, G. 2007. Seroepizootiological survey for selected viral infections in captive Asiatic lions (*Panthera leo persica*) from western India. J. Zoo Wildl. Med. 38, 400-408.

Scavelli, T.D., Patnaik, A.K., Mehlhaff, C.J. and Hayes, A.A. 1985. Hemangiosarcoma in the cat: retrospective evaluation of 31 surgical cases. J. Am. Vet. Med. Assoc. 187, 817-819.

Schultheiss, P.C. 2004. A retrospective study of visceral and nonvisceral hemangiosarcoma and hemangiomas in domestic animals. J. Vet. Diagn. Invest. 16, 522-526.

Wobeser, B.K., Kidney, B.A., Powers, B.E., Withrow, S.J., Mayer, M.N., Spinato, M.T. and Allen, A.L. 2007. Diagnoses and clinical outcomes associated with surgically amputated feline digits submitted to multiple veterinary diagnostic laboratories. Vet. Pathol. 44, 362-365.

9

The pulsed light inactivation of veterinary relevant microbial biofilms and the use of a RTPCR assay to detect parasite species within biofilm structures

M. Garvey[1,*], G. Coughlan[2,3], N. Murphy[2] and N. Rowan[3]

[1]*Department of Life Sciences, Institute of Technology Sligo, Sligo, Ireland*
[2]*Department of Parasitology, National University of Ireland Maynooth, Maynooth, Ireland*
[3]*Bioscience Research Institute, Athlone Institute of Technology, Athlone, Ireland*

Abstract

The presence of pathogenic organisms namely parasite species and bacteria in biofilms in veterinary settings, is a public health concern in relation to human and animal exposure. Veterinary clinics represent a significant risk factor for the transfer of pathogens from housed animals to humans, especially in cases of wound infection and the shedding of faecal matter. This study aims to provide a means of detecting veterinary relevant parasite species in bacterial biofilms, and to provide a means of disinfecting these biofilms. A real time PCR assay was utilized to detect parasite DNA in *Bacillus cereus* biofilms on stainless steel and PVC surfaces. Results show that both *Cryptosporidium* and *Giardia* attach to biofilms in large numbers (100-1000 oo/cysts) in as little as 72 hours. Pulsed light successfully inactivated all test species (*Listeria, Salmonella, Bacillus, Escherichia*) in planktonic and biofilm form with an increase in inactivation for every increase in UV dose.

Keywords: Biofilms, *Cryptosporidium*, *Giardia*, PCR, Veterinary.

Introduction

The prevention and control of veterinary related infections is an important aspect of public health and safety due to the occurrence of zoonotic infections. The spread of pathogenic species within veterinary practices can lead to infection of both the housed animals and veterinary staff. Veterinary clinics are a focus for human and animal interaction, often in situations dealing with infected wounds or faecal matter. This is a significant concern for immunocompromised individuals who are animal owners. Animal associated pathogens of concern to immunocompromised persons include *Cryptosporidium, Salmonella, Listeria, Bacillus, Escherichia coli, Campylobacter* and *Giardia* (Grant and Olsen, 1999). Furthermore, many research studies have highlighted the connection between the spread of pathogenic organisms from surfaces to patients (Gebel *et al.*, 2013). Consequently, the use of surface disinfectants for the control of pathogens in clinical and veterinary settings has become important due to the increase in antibiotic resistant microbial species and zoonotic infections. However, issues have arisen where some pathogens have shown resistance to commonly used chemical based disinfectants. Such pathogens include the parasites Cryptosporidium and Giardia, bacterial endospores and bacterial biofilm structures (Betancourt and Rose, 2004). Planktonic microbial cells are able to attach to and colonise environmental surfaces by producing an extracellular polymeric substance (EPS), these adherent (sessile) cells are referred to as biofilms. The descriptive terms sessile and planktonic are used to describe surface adherent and free floating bacterial cells respectively. Veterinary important species such as *Listeria, Escherichia, Bacillus* and *Salmonella* are capable of producing these biofilm structures allowing them to gain resistance to standard chemical disinfection methods. Biofilms communities spread largely by breaking of in clumps from the primary structure, these detached biofilm clumps may contain enough bacteria to give an infective dose to housed animals making them a potential health risk. Indeed, biofilms or sessile communities are believed to be the causative agent in diseases such as pneumonia, liver abscesses, enteritis, wound infections and mastitis infections in animals (Clutterbuck *et al.*, 2007). Ingestion of a biofilm bacterial clump present in the surrounding environment could play an important role in the transmission of disease. In addition, in hosts with functioning innate and adaptive immune responses, biofilm-based infections are often very persistent and remain unresolved. In fact, surrounding tissues often undergo extensive damage by immune complexes and invading neutrophils when trying to eradicate the infection (Stewart and Costerton, 2001).

The prevention of biofilm formation on surfaces located in areas of animal housing would provide the best control measures for these robust structures; however, there is no agent available that will prevent cell adhesion and biofilm formation. Current methods rely on the use of disinfection agents and regular cleaning of surfaces exposed to possible pathogens. Research has indicated that sessile communities can be

*Corresponding Author: Dr. Mary Garvey. Department of Life Sciences, Institute of Technology Sligo, Ash Lane, Sligo, Ireland. E-mail: garvey.mary@itsligo.ie

up to 1000 times more resistant to chemotherapeutics such as chlorhexidine than their planktonic counterparts (Garvey et al., 2014a). Furthermore, resistant bacteria originated in sessile communities can spread from animal to animal through veterinary staff, veterinary surfaces and equipment or farm equipment such as feeders and water dispensers (Aguilar-Romero et al., 2010) resulting in extended infection problems. Biofilm structures are also capable of trapping or incorporating other pathogenic species including enteric noroviruses (Wingender and Flemming, 2011) and parasites such as Giardia and Cryptosporidium (DiCesare et al., 2012). Harbouring of such species shields them from cleaning and disinfection techniques, increasing their already high resistance to such treatments. Studies have shown that aquatic biofilms represent a significant, long-term reservoir for pathogens such as Cryptosporidium and Giardia, which can be released back into water (Wingender and Flemming, 2011). Thus, explaining the presence of parasites in water networks long after disinfection protocols are completed following an outbreak. Ultraviolet (UV) light is well known for its antimicrobial activity, due to its bacteriostatic properties affecting the DNA of the organism, breaking DNA bonds, causing the formation of DNA adducts thus preventing bacterial cell replication (Ochoa-Velasco et al., 2014). Additionally, research focusing on the use of a pulsed light (PL) system for the inactivation of parasite species and bacterial endospores has shown this system to be highly efficient (Garvey et al., 2014a). PL technologies differ from standard UV lamps in their mode of delivery, penetration depth and wavelength range (Garvey et al., 2014a) making them a more potent disinfection system. Here we report on the use of a PL system for the disinfection of veterinary relevant biofilms on polyvinylchloride (PVC) and stainless steel surfaces. The use of polymerase chain reaction (PCR) methods provides a rapid species specific means of identifying species type and cell numbers present. Indeed, PCR methods have been used extensively to detect and quantify bacterial cells in food products and in biofilms (Pan and Breidt, 2007). Therefore, the present study also utilised a real time PCR assay to determine the extent at which Bacillus biofilm structures incorporated parasite species into their matrix, subsequently providing shelter from disinfection techniques.

Materials and Methods

Microbial test species

For this study a range of veterinary relevant biofilm forming microbial species Listeria monocytogenes (ATCC 11994), Bacillus cereus (ATCC 11778), Salmonella typhimurium (ATCC 13311) and Escherichia coli (ATCC 11775) were chosen for biofilm formation and PL inactivation studies. All strains were cultured and maintained in nutrient agar and nutrient broth (Cruinn Diagnostics Ltd, Ireland) at 37°C. Giardia lamblia cysts and Cryptosporidium parvum oocysts were purchased from Waterborne Inc USA. Oocysts and cysts were stored in sterile PBS (0.01 M phosphate buffer, containing 0.0027 M KCL and 0.137 M NaCl at a pH of 7.4) with 100 U of penicillin/ml, 100 µg of streptomycin/ml and 100 µg of gentamicin/ml at 4°C. Prior to use parasite identity was confirmed by a dye staining method comprising of propidium iodide (PI) 1 mg/ml in 0.1 M sterile PBS and 4', 6'-Diamidino-2-Phenylindole (DAPI) 2 mg/ml in methanol and a fluorescein-labelled mouse-derived monoclonal antibody Giardi-a-Glo™ or Crypt-a-Glo™ (Waterborne Inc, New Orleans, USA). Oo/cysts were counted using a haemocytometer and inverted microscope (Olympus, CKX41) with camera (Olympus, IX2-SLP) attached.

Growth of sessile communities using Centers for Disease Control (CDC) biofilm reactor

The CDC biofilm reactor (Biosurface Technologies Corp, Bozeman, Montana, USA) was used for the growth of biofilm structures as per the recommended procedure of the American Society for Testing and Materials (ASTM, 2012). Furthermore, the CDC reactor is a recognised method for the growth of biofilms under high shear and continuous flow (Coenye and Nelis, 2010) and is of sufficient capacity to provide numerous samples of biofilms for disinfection studies. In order to establish a dose response relationship for biofilm inactivation with UV light it is necessary to first obtain biofilm communities which were dense, reproducible and also treatable. For this study both PVC and stainless steel coupons were chosen as biofilm growth surfaces as both materials are commonly used in veterinary settings and are excellent matrixes for biofilm adhesion and proliferation.

For the growth of microbial biofilms methods were followed as per the recommended procedure for continuous fluid shear flow biofilm formation (ASTM E2562-12 2012) and Garvey et al., 2014b. The reactor was prepared containing 350 mL of tryptone soy broth (TSB) and 2% glucose as this concentration was previously found to promote biofilm adhesion and proliferation (Senevirantne et al., 2013). Once satisfied that the coupons were completely submerged the apparatus was sterilised by autoclaving. 1 mL of a 12 hour microbial culture was added to the reactor chamber to ensure that cells were in the log phase of reproduction. For each test strain the reactor was incubated at 37°C for 72 and 96 hours under rotatory conditions at 125 rpm. To allow for the enumeration of colony forming units (cfu) per microbial biofilm, all coupons were removed aseptically from each reactor rod and rinsed with sterile phosphate-buffered saline (PBS) to remove any planktonic cells. Biofilms were removed from each coupon by scraping the coupon using a sterile cell scraper into 10 mL of sterile PBS. The standard plate count technique was used to determine the cfu/mL bacterial population in the biofilm as per the recommended procedure (ASTM E2562-12 2012). To allow for the entrapment of parasite test species within the biofilm matrix 1×10^6 oo/cysts per mL was added to the reactor chamber and incubated for 72 hours. For biofilms containing parasite test species, 1 mL from the 10 mL PBS containing the scrapped biofilm was stained with parasite specific dyes as previously described to confirm identity and numbers present.

Pulsed Ultraviolet (PUV) light

The PUV machine used throughout this study was sourced through Samtech Ltd, Strathclyde, Scotland, UK. The bacteriostatic effects of PL are caused by the rich and broad-spectrum UV content, the short duration, and the high peak power of the pulse. The system was used as per Garvey et al. (2010) and is therefore not described in further detail herein.

Pulsed light inactivation of planktonic microbial species

E. coli, S. typhimurium, L. monocytogenes and B. cereus cultures were grown and maintained as previously described. For PUV studies a single colony of the test strain was aseptically transferred to 100 mL of sterile nutrient broth followed by incubation at 37°C for 12 hours at 125 rpm. For surface treatment 100 µL of an appropriate dilution was spread onto agar surfaces. Test plates were then exposed to pulses of UV light at 16.2 J at varying doses (obtained by varying the pulse number) at a rate of 1 pulse per second as per Garvey et al. (2014). PUV studies were also conducted on samples diluted from the 12 hour broth in 20 mL final volumes of sterile PBS at 8 cm from the light source, after which 100 µL of treated liquid was transferred to suitable agar and incubated at 37°C for 24 hours.

Pulsed light inactivation of sessile communities

Coupons were aseptically removed from the reactor, rinsed with sterile PBS and transferred to a sterile petri dish. Samples were exposed to pulses of UV light at 16.2J at 8 cm from the light source at varying UV doses which were obtained by increasing the pulse number. Once treated, coupons were submerged in 10 mL of sterile PBS and surface scraped using a sterile cell scraper to remove the treated biofilms and to allow for the determination of inactivated rates. The liquid was then transferred to a sterile 20 mL container and centrifuged at 800 g for 10 minutes to pellet the cells. The sample was then re-suspended and agitated manually to ensure biofilm dispersion. Serial dilutions were made from the biofilms suspension and 100 µL spread on triplicate agar plates to determine the cfu/mL of treated samples. This process was repeated for coupons at varying UV doses ($< 8 \mu J/cm^2$) to determine the Log_{10} reduction obtained with increasing UV dose. Plates were incubated for 24 hours at 37°C to allow for the growth of bacterial colonies, which were subsequently gram stained and identify confirmed to ensure no contamination of the rector system had occurred.

Parasite entrapment and DNA extraction from biofilm structures

Biofilms of B. cereus were allowed to form while in the presence of 1×10^6 oo/cysts per mL in the biofilm reactor, to allow for the entrapment of parasite species within the biofilm matrix. This species was chosen due to its enteric pathogenic nature and it greater resistance to PUV inactivation. Following 72 hours incubation, coupons were aseptically removed from the bioreactor to sterile petri dish. Coupons were then aseptically scrapped in to 10 mL volumes of PBS, which was subsequently centrifuged at 800g for 10 minutes to pellet the cells, followed by re-suspension in 200 µl of sterile PCR grade water. Target DNA extraction for B. cereus, G. lamblia and C. parvum was conducted as per kit instructions for B. cereus biofilm suspensions using a Roche DNA extraction kit and HP PCR template preparation kit (Roche Diagnostics, Roche, Ireland). All steps were performed as per manufacturer's instructions with treated and untreated microbial pellets which were suspended in 200 µL of sterile PBS.

Real time PCR

All primers and probes were sourced from Tib Molbiol, Berlin, Germany. For B. cereus the forward primer ACACACGTGCTACAATGGATG and reverse primer AGTTGCAGCCTACAATCCGAA with the taqman probe sequence F-ACAAAGGGCTGCAAGACCGCG—Q coding for the phaC gene was used as per Nayak et al. (2013). Primers coding for β-giardin of G. lamblia were used as per method of Bertrand et al. (2009) with the forward primer 5'-AAGCCCGACGACCTCACCCGCAGTGC-3' and reverse primer 5'-GAGGCCGCCCTGGATCTTCGAGACGAC-3'. The Taqman probe with the following sequence: 5'-FAM TCACCCAGACGATGGA CAAGCCCTAMRA-3 was utilised for this study. For Cryptosporidium parvum the 18Si reverse primer 5'- CCTGCTTTAAGCACTTAATTTTC and 18Si forward primer 5'- ATGGACAAGAAATAACAATACAGG as first described by Morgan et al. (1997) were utilised as per Garvey et al. (2010). The Taqman probe had the following sequence: 5-'-(6-FAM) ACCAGACTTGCCCTCC (TAMRA) as per Keegan et al. (2003). Amplification reactions (20 µL) contained 5 µL of sample DNA (0.5 µM of each primer, 0.2 µM of probe) and 15 µL of reaction buffer (Roche Diagnostic, West Sussex, England). Both positive and negative controls were included in RT-PCR to validate the results. DNase–RNase free water was used as negative control throughout. Cycling parameters were initial denaturation for 10 min at 95°C followed by 65 cycles of denaturation for 10 s at 95°C, annealing for 40 s at 40 °C, extension for 1 s at 70°C and cooling for 30 s at 40°C on a Nanocycler® device (Roche Diagnostics). These cycling parameters were the same for all samples. Additionally, large numbers of cycles were used to ensure detection of low levels of infection. On completion of each RT-PCR run amplification curves were analysed by Nanocycler software (Roche Diagnostics) and a standard curve (Fig. 1) of cell DNA concentration determined. DNA standards were prepared from fresh cells or oo/cysts ranging in concentration from 10 to 10^8 oocysts or cysts/mL by dilution in PBS following standard viable count determinations.

Statistics

All experimental data is an average of 3 experimental replicates with 3 internal replicates. Bacterial inactivation is expressed as $\log_{10}$ reduction of the untreated control. Student's t-tests and ANOVA one-way model (MINITAB software release 16; Mintab Inc., State College, PA) were used to compare the relationship between UV treatments and bacterial inactivation at 95% level of confidence. Student t-tests were used to determine the relationship between the sensitivity of biofilms from different strains to PL treatment.

Results

Sessile communities and parasite detection

All bacterial strains under study formed densely populated sessile communities on both PVC and stainless steel surfaces after 72 hours. Findings also demonstrate (data not shown) that with longer incubation times, exceeding 72 hours (96 hours), there was no increase in cell number of the biofilms as detected by plate counts. Following 72 hours, a ca. 5 and 6.6 $\log_{10}$ biofilm formed for *B. cereus* and *S. typhimurium* respectively, and a 6 $\log_{10}$ for *E. coli* and 6.5 $\log_{10}$ for *L. monocytogenes* on PVC surfaces. A similar level of cell density was detected on stainless steel surfaces, where a ca. 5 $\log_{10}$ to 6.6 $\log_{10}$ biofilm formed for *B. cereus, L. monocytogenes, S. typhimurium* and *E. coli*. The determination of cell number for *B. cereus* biofilms via PCR was slightly higher than the standard cell count method. A Ct value of 18.39, corresponding to a cell count of ca. 7 $\log_{10}$ cfu/ml (Fig. 1) for both materials was determined by analysis of the standard curve. An important fact to note is that PCR detects the presence of target DNA, but cannot differentiate between live and dead cells. In contrast, the standard cell count technique reports viable cell numbers only via the enumeration of colonies grown on nutrient agar. The lack of an increase in biofilm cell density after a 72 hours period suggests the presence of a stationary phase or steady state of biofilm growth. PCR analyses showed the presence of total cells (non-viable and viable) at 72 hours, when viable cell counts as determined by the spread plate technique are subtracted from this, a value for non-viable cells

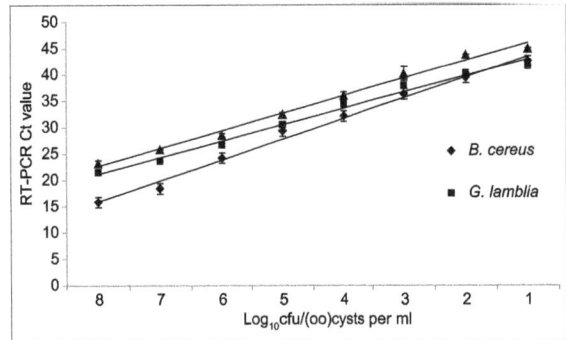

Fig. 1. Linear regression analysis of DNA standard curve as determined by real time PCR analysis for planktonic *Bacillus cereus* ($\log_{10}$ cfu/ml) and the parasite species *Cryptosporidium parvum* ($\log_{10}$ oocysts/ml) and *Giardia lamblia* ($\log_{10}$ cfu/(oo) cysts per ml) (+/-S.D) using species specific primers.

can be determined. In this case a biofilm viable cell density of 5 $\log_{10}$ was formed, indicating that approximately 2 $\log_{10}$ of non-viable cells were also present in the biofilm matrix as detected by PCR. The presence of these non-viable cells further confirms that incubation for 72 hours provided an optimal period of time for biofilm formation, after which cell death occurs to some extent. These findings correspond to that of Senevirantne *et al.* (2013), who concluded that 72 hours was also the optimal incubation time for the growth of *Enterococcus faecalis* biofilms. Therefore, the findings of this study suggest that 72 hour duration of incubation is sufficient to reproducibly produce a robust, densely populated biofilm of *B. cereus, E. coli, L. monocytogenes* and *S. typhimurium* using a CDC reactor. Consequently, 72 hour biofilms were used for inactivation studies for all test species.

Both parasites species were detected in the *B. cereus* biofilms at a concentration of between 2 and 3 $\log_{10}$ for PVC and stainless steel surfaces by PCR (Fig. 2). Additionally, PCR proved a more efficient reliable method of detecting *Cryptosporidium* and *Giardia* than the use of specific dyes. Fluorescent dye staining of biofilms containing oo/cysts greatly underestimated the number of organisms present. A maximal oo/cyst count of 10 (+/-2) was measured for *C. parvum* and 14 for *G. lamblia* (+/-4) via fluorescent staining. Issues arose in relation to non-specific binding of dyes to biofilm constitutes believed to be EPS components resulting in unreliable counting of parasite numbers.

The impact of PL on microbial species was assessed for surface treated organisms, organisms in suspension and sessile communities. All test strains proved to be susceptible to the pulsed light treatment, albeit with varying levels of sensitivity as shown in (Figs. 3 and 4) *E. coli* showed the greatest level of inactivation on agar surfaces (Fig. 3a) with complete inactivation of an initial concentration of ca. 9 $\log_{10}$ with as little as 5 μJ/cm^2 of pulsed light. The order of decreasing sensitivity for test strains was *E. coli*, *L. monocytogenes*, *B. cereus* and *S. typhimurium* on surfaces. When treated in suspension this sensitivity changed with *L. monocytogenes* showing the highest resistance to PL treatment and

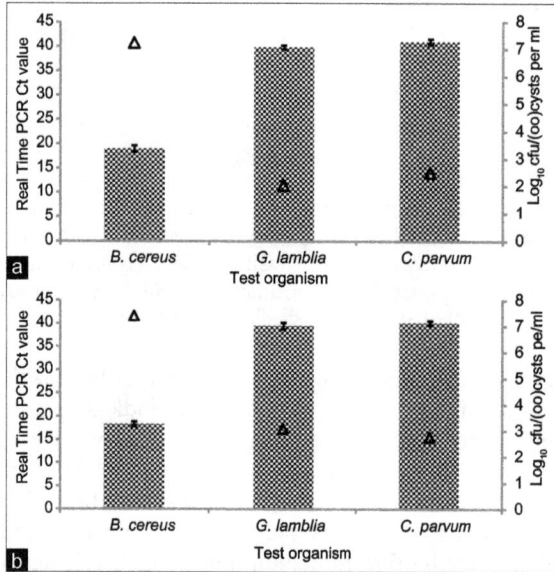

Fig. 2. Real time PCR Ct value (column graph) for microbial test species and corresponding cell count in $\log_{10}$ cfu/(oo)cysts per ml (Δ) as determined by using the equation of the line of the standard curves, results show both parasite test species as detected in *B. cereus* biofilms on (a) PVC and (b) stainless steel surfaces (+/- S.D).

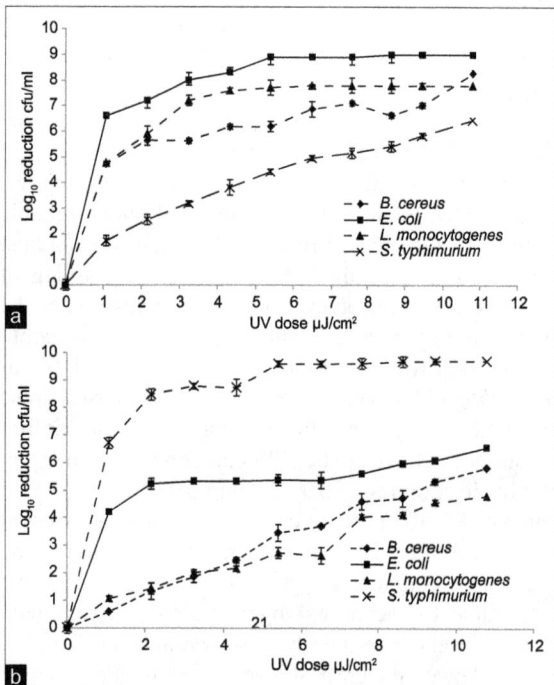

Fig. 3. Pulsed light inactivation of a range of Gram negative and Gram positive test species on (a) agar surfaces and (b) in suspension (+/- S.D).

S. typhimurium showing the greatest sensitivity to pulsed light (Fig. 3b) for all treatment doses (p<0.05). Indeed a maximal 9.6 $\log_{10}$ inactivation of *S. typhimurium* was achieved with 5.39 μJ/cm² compared to a 2.73 $\log_{10}$ for *L. monocytogenes*. This same dose resulted in a 3.45 and 5.38 $\log_{10}$ inactivation of *B. cereus* and *E. coli* respectively, highlighting the significant difference in susceptibility to pulsed light. These findings are in conjunction with Cheigh *et al.* (2012) where *E. coli* also proved more sensitive to PL than *L. monocytogenes* when treated in suspension. High levels of biofilm inactivation were also achieved for all test strains present on both surface materials (Fig. 4). For the Gram negative species *E. coli* and *S. typhimurium* a 4.04 and 5.11 $\log_{10}$ reduction in viable cell counts was obtained on PVC surfaces with 5.39 μJ/cm² (Fig. 4a). This same dose resulted in a significantly (p<0.05) greater level of inactivation of the same species on stainless steel surfaces, with a maximal 4.2 and 6.6 $\log_{10}$ reduction obtained for *E. coli* and *S. typhimurium* respectively (Fig. 4b). Both Gram positive species tested showed increased sensitivity on stainless steel surfaces compared to PVC. A dose of 5.39 μJ/cm² resulted in a 3.23 and a 4.34 $\log_{10}$ inactivation on PVC and 5.95 and 4.6 $\log_{10}$ inactivation on stainless steel for *B. cereus* and *L. monocytogenes* respectively. A PL dose of 7.56 μJ/cm² resulted in complete inactivation of *L. monocytogenes* and *S. typhimurium* of ca. 6.51 $\log_{10}$ (Fig. 4a) on PVC surfaces.

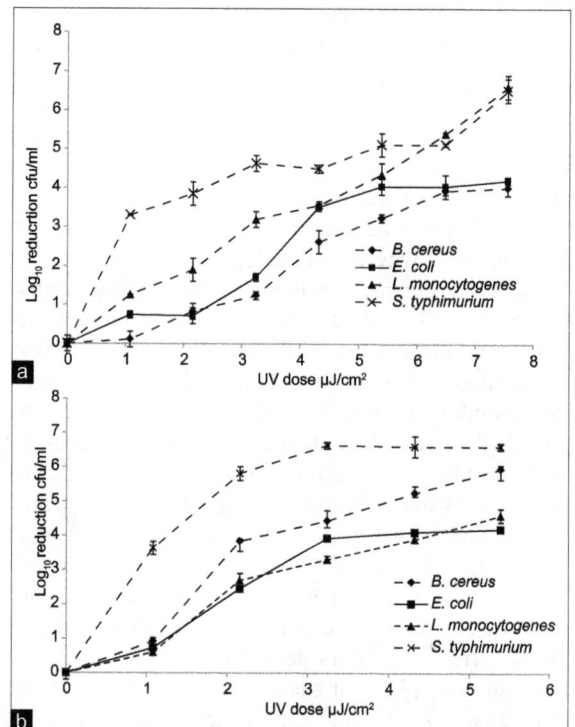

Fig. 4. Pulsed light inactivation of bacterial biofilms of varying test species on (a) PVC surfaces and (b) stainless steel surfaces (+/- S.D).

Discussion

The change from a planktonic free floating cell to that of a biofilm sessile cell induces physiological changes in bacteria, occurring via a series of gene expression alterations including gene repression and induction (Donlan and Costerton, 2002). It is the induction of genes, relating to antibiotic resistance that leads to the increased pathogenicity of sessile bacteria over their planktonic counterparts (O'Leary et al., 2015). Consequently, this causes the increased resistance to antibiotics and disinfectants such as chlorine commonly observed with these complex structures (Aguilar-Romero et al., 2010). For this reason, it is of the upmost importance to establish alternative ways of eradicating these problematic often pathogenic structures from veterinary surfaces. The pulsed light system used in this study proved successful at disinfecting densely populated biofilms of veterinary relevant microorganisms. Indeed, complete inactivation of a 6.5 $\log_{10}$ biofilm of L. monocytogenes and S. typhimurium was achieved with 7.56 $\mu J/cm^2$. However, there was a significant difference ($p<0.05$) in the susceptibility of biofilm communities on PVC and stainless steel surfaces. S. typhimurium and B. cereus proved more sensitive to pulsed light inactivation on stainless steel surfaces compared to PVC. Stainless steel is the predominant material used in veterinary practices as clinical surfaces and animal housing due to their easy to clean nature. Consequently, the higher susceptibility of microbial biofilms on stainless steel surfaces further establishes this materials benefit for use in such environments.

Traditionally, the sensitivity of planktonic cells to disinfection has been used as an indication of biofilm sensitivity and resistance (Buckingham-Meyer et al., 2007). However, disinfection studies such as those described herein based on actual biofilm communities is much more representative of the environmental situation. Additionally, high levels of planktonic cell inactivation (4 – 9 $\log_{10}$ cfu/ml) were also achieved following pulsed UV exposure for both surface treated and microbial suspensions. Therefore, pulsed light as a disinfectant has the ability to reduce biofilm formation at the planktonic stage of attachment, which can be assisted by choosing surface materials that are more readily disinfected by this approach such as stainless steel.

The findings of this study confirm that both parasite species studied can quickly attach or become entrapped in bacterial biofilms. This is in keeping with the findings of recently published literate outlining the presence of parasite species in biofilm structures (DiCesare et al., 2012; Koh et al., 2013). The findings of Koh et al. (2013) conclude that biofilm communities accumulate Cryptosporidium species over time as determined by qPCR detection. The detection of these pathogens within biofilm structures has important public health implications in relation to animal and human exposure. The infectious dose for Cryptosporidium has been established to be less than 20 oocysts (Zambriski et al., 2013) with prolonged infection occurring with little success following medical intervention. The robust, chemical disinfection resistant nature of biofilms and these parasites increases the probability that the survival and detachment of biofilm-associated viable parasites may occur at concentrations exceeding that required for infection. This possibility needs to be considered in risk assessments relating to the cleaning of veterinary environments particularly where animals are housed.

Previous studies by this research group reported a ca. 5 $\log_{10}$ inactivation of Cryptosporidium parvum (Garvey et al., 2013) and ca. 1 $\log_{10}$ inactivation of Giardia lamblia (Garvey et al., 2014b) with a PL dose of 7.38 $\mu J/cm^2$. Nevertheless, further studies are warranted to determine the exact dose required to inactivate parasites within biofilm matrixes, which will undoubtedly shield parasites to some extent. However, issues are expected to arise in relation to viability determination post treatment and cell culture infectivity. Specifically, issues relating to the sterility of the parasites following extraction from biofilms and subsequent exposure to mammalian cell lines. Nonetheless, PL shows potential for use as a disinfectant for veterinary environments given its highly effective bacteriostatic properties towards bacterial biofilms and parasite species. Regardless of microbial exposure to PL in suspension or on surfaces findings demonstrate that cell inactivation increased significantly ($p<0.05$) with increasing UV dose or treatment time.

In conclusion, the findings reported here contribute to existing literature in many ways:

Firstly, all veterinary relevant strains produced densely populated biofilms structures on both surface materials used.

Secondly, PL repeatedly inactivated the range of test species on surfaces and in suspension. Additionally, it provided high levels of biofilm inactivation on PVC and stainless steel surfaces.

Thirdly, a real time PCR assay proved successful for determining the level of C. parvum and G. lamblia present in the biofilms of B. cereus where fluorescent staining greatly underestimated the numbers present.

Finally, pulsed light doses (7.38 $\mu J/cm^2$) which have been previously shown to inactivate both parasite species (Cryptosporidium and Giardia), have also provided complete inactivation of all biofilms tested.

Acknowledgments

All research studies were conducted in the Bioscience Research Institute, Athlone Institute of Technology, Ireland.

Conflict of interest

The authors declare that there is no conflict of interest.

References

Aguilar-Romero, F., Perez-Romero, A.N., Diaz-Aparicio, E. and Hernandez-Castro, R. 2010. Bacterial biofilms: Importance in animal diseases. Current Research, Technology and Education topics in Applied Microbiology and Microbial Biotechnology. A Mendez Vilas Edition, pp: 700-703.

ASTM. 2012. ASTM E2562 - 12: Standard Test Method for Quantification of Pseudomonas aeruginosa Biofilm Grown with High Shear and Continuous Flow Using CDC Biofilm Reactor. In Annual Book of ASTM Standards; ASTM International: West Conshohocken, PA, USA.

Bertrand, I., Maux, M., Helmi, K., Hoffmann, L., Schwartzbrod, J. and Cauchie, H.M. 2009. Quantification of Giardia transcripts during in vitro excystation: Interest for the estimation of cyst viability. Water Res. 43, 2728-2738.

Betancourt, W.Q. and Rose, J.B. 2004. Drinking water treatment processes for removal of Cryptosporidium and Giardia. Vet. Parasitol. 126(1-2), 219-234.

Buckingham-Meyer, K., Goeres, D.M. and Hamilton, M.A. 2007. Comparative evaluation of biofilm disinfectant efficacy tests. J. Microbiol. Methods 70, 236-244.

Cheigh, C.I., Park, M.H., Chung, M.S., Shin, J.K. and Park, Y.S. 2012. Comparison of intense pulsed light- and ultraviolet (UVC)-induced cell damage in Listeria monocytogenes and Escherichia coli O157:H7. Food Control 25(2), 654-659.

Clutterbuck, A.L., Woods, E.J., Knottenbelt, D.C., Clegg, P.D., Cochrane, C.A. and Percival, S.L. 2007. Biofilms and their relevance to veterinary medicine. Vet. Microbiol. 121, 1-17.

Coenye, T. and Nelis J.J. 2010. In vitro and in vivo model systems to study microbial biofilm formation. J. Microbiol. Methods 83, 89-105.

DiCesare,E.A.,Hargreaves,B.R.andJellison,K.L.2012. Biofilm roughness determines Cryptosporidium parvum retention in environmental biofilms. Appl. Environ. Microbiol. 78(12), 4187-4193.

Donlan, R.M. and Costerton, J.W. 2002. Biofilms: survival Mechanisms of Clinically Relevant Microorganisms. Clin. Microbiol. Rev. 15(2), 167-193.

Garvey, M., Rabbit, D., Stocca, A. and Rowan, N. 2014a. Pulsed Ultraviolet light inactivation of Pseudomonas aeruginosa biofilms. Water Environ. J. 29, 36-42. DOI: 10.1111/wej.12088.

Garvey, M., Stocca, A. and Rowan, N. 2014b. Development of a combined in vitro cell culture - quantitative PCR assay for evaluating the disinfection performance of pulsed light for treating the waterborne enteroparasite Giardia lamblia. Exp. Parasitol. 144, 6-13.

Garvey, M., Clifford, E., O'Reilly, E. and Rowan, N. 2013. Efficacy of using harmless Bacillus endospores to estimate the inactivation of Cryptosporidium parvum oocysts in water. J. Parasitol. 99(3), 448-452.

Garvey, M., Farrell, H., Cormican, M. and Rowan, N. 2010. Investigations of the relationship between use of in vitro cell culture-quantitative PCR and a mouse-based bioassay for evaluating critical factors affecting the disinfection performance of pulsed UV light for treating Cryptosporidium parvum oocysts in saline. J. Microbiol. Methods 80(3), 267-273.

Gebel, J., Exner, M., French, G., Chartier, Y., Christiansen, B., Gemein, S., Goroncy-Bermes, P., Harteman, P., Heudorf, U., Kramer, A., Maillard, J.Y., Oltmanns, P., Rotter, M. and Sonntag, G.H. 2013. The role of surface disinfection in infection prevention. GMS Hyg. Infect. Control 8(1): Doc10. doi:10.3205/dgkh000210.

Grant, S. and Olsen, C.W. 1999. Preventing Zoonotic Diseases in Immunocompromised Persons: The Role of Physicians and Veterinarians. Emerg. Infect. Dis. 5(1), 159-163.

Keegan, A.R., Fanok, S., Monis, P.T. and Saint, C.P. 2003. Cell culture-Taqman PCR assay for evaluation of Cryptosporidium parvum disinfection. Appl. Environ. Microbiol. 69, 2505-2511.

Koh, W., Clode, P.L., Monis, P. and Thompson, R.C. 2013. Multiplication of the waterborne pathogen Cryptosporidium parvum in an aquatic biofilm system. Parasit. Vectors. doi: 10.1186/1756-3305-6-270.

Morgan, U.M., Constantine, C.C., Forbes, D.A. and Thompson, R.C. 1997. Differentiation between human and animal isolates of Cryptosporidium parvum using rDNA sequencing and direct PCR analysis. J. Parasitol. 83(5), 825-830.

Nayak, P.K., KumarMohanty, A., Gaonkar, T., Kumar, A., Bhosle, S.N. and Garg, S. 2013. Rapid Identification of Polyhydroxyalkanoate Accumulating Members of Bacillales Using Internal Primers for phaC Gene of Bacillus megaterium. ISRN Bacteriol. 1-12: doi:10.1155/2013/562014.

Ochoa-Velasco, C.E., Cruz-Gonzalez, M. and Guerrero-Beltran, J.A. 2014. Ultraviolet-C light inactivation of Escherichia coli And Salmonella typhimuriumin coconut (Cocos nucifera L.) milk. Innovative Food Sci. Emerg. Technol. 26, 199-204.

O'Leary, D., McCabe, E.M., McCusker, M.P., Martins, M., Fanning, S. and Duffy, G. 2015. Acid environments affect biofilm formation and gene expression in isolates of Salmonella enterica Typhimurium DT104. Int. J. Food Microbiol. 206, 7-16.

Pan, Y. and Breidt, F. 2007. Enumeration of Viable Listeria monocytogenes Cells by Real-Time PCR with Propidium Monoazide and Ethidium

Monoazide in the Presence of Dead Cells. Appl. Environ. Microbiol. 73(24), 8028-8031.

Senevirantne, C.J., Yip, J.W., Chang, J.W., Zhang, C.F. and Samaranayake, L.P. 2013. Effect of culture media and nutrients on biofilm growth kinetics of laboratory and clinical strains of Enterococcus faecalis. Arch. Oral Biol. 58, 1327-1334.

Stewart, P.S. and Costerton, J.W. 2001. Antibiotic resistance of bacteria in biofilms. Lancet 358(9276), 135-138.

Wingender, J. and Flemming, H.C. 2011. Biofilms in drinking water and their role as reservoir for pathogens. Int. J. Hyg. Environ. Health 214(6), 417-423.

Zambriski, J.A., Nydam, D.V., Wilcox, Z.J., Bowman, D.D., Mohammed, H.O. and Littoa, J.L. 2013. *Cryptosporidium parvum*: Determination of ID50 and the dose–response relationship in experimentally challenged dairy calves. Vet. Parasitol. 197, 104-112.

10

Unusual haemodynamics in two dogs and two cats with portosystemic shunt - implications for distinguishing between congenital and acquired conditions

Mario Ricciardi*

"Pingry" Veterinary Hospital, via Medaglie d'Oro 5, Bari, Italy

Abstract

Extrahepatic porto-systemic shunt (PSS) in small animals can be congenital (CPSS) or acquired (APSS) as a consequence of portal hypertension (PH), and are distinguished on the bases of their anatomical pattern. A precise morphologic imaging assessment, along with clinical and histopathologic findings, is important for distinguishing patients with PH from those with congenital PSSs, which require different therapeutic approach. Expected findings in patients with PH are presence of ascites, multiple APSS, and a confirmed cause of portal flow obstruction. On the other hand, a single PSS, absence of ascites and no evidence of portal vein, caudal vena cava or hepatic disorders are typical findings of CPSS patients. This paper describes four cases of PSSs in which the combination of the computed tomographic imaging findings did not match the standards for APSS nor for CPSS: one dog had chronic hepatitis causing PH and ascites and a splenoazygos PSS, to date considered a CPSS pattern. One dog showed a left splenogonadal PSS and porto-caval varices, to date considered an APSS pattern, without ascites, portal vein obstruction, primary structural hepatic disorders nor evidence of PH. Two cats, with and without diffuse hepatic structural disorders respectively, had a single left splenogonadal PSS without ascites. Possible interpretation of such unusual haemodynamic conditions and clinical repercussion, especially for orientation of treatment choice, are discussed.

Keywords: Cat, Computed tomography, Dog, Portal hypertension, Portosystemic shunt.

Introduction

Abnormal venous porto-caval connections are widely described in small animal veterinary literature, with majority of cases reported in dogs (Lamb, 1996; Bertolini *et al.*, 2006; Bertolini, 2010a, 2010b; Bruehschwein *et al.*, 2010; Nelson and Nelson, 2011; Fukushima *et al.*, 2014). These vascular anomalies are divided in two main categories according to their origin: congenital PSS (CPSS) deriving from embryogenetic errors in the development of vitelline and cardinal venous systems (Ferrell *et al.*, 2003), and acquired PSS (APSS) deriving from recanalization of pre-existing, vestigial embryonic vascular connections between portal and caval systems as a consequence of portal hypertension (PH) (Fossum, 2002; Szatmari *et al.*, 2004; Bertolini, 2010a).

Ultrasound and computed tomography (CT) are reliable imaging techniques for the non-invasive diagnosis of PSSs and for distinction between acquired and congenital shunts (Szatmari and Rothuizen, 2002; Szatmari *et al.*, 2004; Ricciardi, 2016). Such imaging distinction is essential for differentiating hypertensive patients, which need further investigations in order to diagnose the cause of the underlying PH, from those that need surgical closure of a congenital vascular malformation. The most useful imaging findings which are taken into account for discriminating APSS and CPSS are: the anatomical pattern of vascular anomalies (distinct vascular patterns have been observed within each category without any overlapping of anatomical pathway between APPS and CPPS), their number (more than one porto-caval shunt are typically found in dogs with PH and MAPSS) and presence/absence of ascites (which is typically absent in dogs with CPSS) (Ricciardi, 2016).

This paper describes four cases of PSSs in two dogs and two cats in which the combination of the computed tomographic imaging findings did not match the standards for APSS nor for CPSS. Possible interpretation and clinical repercussion, especially for orientation of treatment options, of such unusual haemodynamic conditions are discussed.

Case details

Dog 1

A 12-year-old intact male Yorkshire terrier dog was evaluated for a 2-week history of inappetence and abdominal distension. Clinical examination findings included thinnes (Body Condition Score: 3/9) (Baldwin *et al.*, 2010) and free fluid in the abdomen. No clinical evidence of heart disease was present.

Complete blood count revealed neutrophilia with right shift (segmented neutrophils 7946/μl, reference interval [RI] 3601–6056) and monocytosis (702/μl, RI 172–462). Serum chemistry revealed marked increase in liver enzyme activity (aspartate aminotransferase 530 IU/l, RI 20–31; alanine aminotransferase 638 IU/l, RI 22–78), hypoalbuminemia (2.1 g/dl, RI 2.7–3.6) and increase in C-reactive protein (1.36 mg/dl, RI 0.01–0.09), and urinalysis revealed marked increase in urinary bile acids levels (249 mmol/l, RI 2.9– 9.5). Abdominal fluid was consistent with pure transudate.

B-mode ultrasound abdominal examination (Esaote MyLab 30 Gold, Esaote SpA, Genoa, Italy) revealed abundant anechoic peritoneal effusion, with normoechoic and diffusely inhomogeneous hepatic parenchyma. Because of abundant ascites and overlying gastrointestinal content the portal vein was visualized with difficulty.

In order to clarify any possible abdominal or thoracic vascular disease that could explain the portal hypertension, thoracic and abdominal CT scan was performed immediately after the ultrasound examination using a 16-slice MDCT scanner (*Somatom Emotion*, *Siemens*, Forchheim, *Germany*). Computed tomography images were acquired before and after the intravenous injection of iodinate contrast medium (640 mg I/kg; *Iopamigita® Insight Agents GmbHR, Heildeberg, Germany*). Scanning and reconstruction parameters were as follows: helical modality, 0.6 sec/gantry rotation, 1 mm slice thickness; 180 kV, 110 mAs; soft tissue reconstruction algorithm.

Three-dimensional (3D) multiplanar reformatted and volume-rendered images were obtained using a dedicated 3D software (Pixmeo, OsiriX; OsiriX DICOM-viewer; Pixmeo, Geneva, Switzerland). Computed tomography scans showed a large amount of free fluid in the abdomen, and a large, single tortuous vessel connecting the splenic vein with the azygos vein. The liver appeared slightly reduced in volume, with irregular margins and without macroscopic parenchymal abnormalities or attenuation changes. No compressions/thrombosis of the portal vein or caudal vena cava were present (Fig. 1).

Based on the imaging findings a diffuse microscopic hepatic disorder with secondary portal hypertension, associated with a spleno-azygos portosystemic shunt, was suspected.

Specimens of liver biopsy samples were sent for histopathologic evaluation in a certified veterinary laboratory (*San Marco Veterinary Laboratory, Padova, Italy*). Histopathologic evaluation of a liver biopsy sample revealed cytoplasmic expansion of hepatocytes with infiltration of lymphocytes, plasma cells and macrophages between hepatocyte layers. Sinusoidal congestion, dilation of centrilobular veins and surrounding lymphatic vessels and stromal expansion with centro-central bridging surrounded by inflammatory cells were evident in centrilobular tracts. These findings were consistent with subacute-cronic centrolobular and midzonal hepatitis.

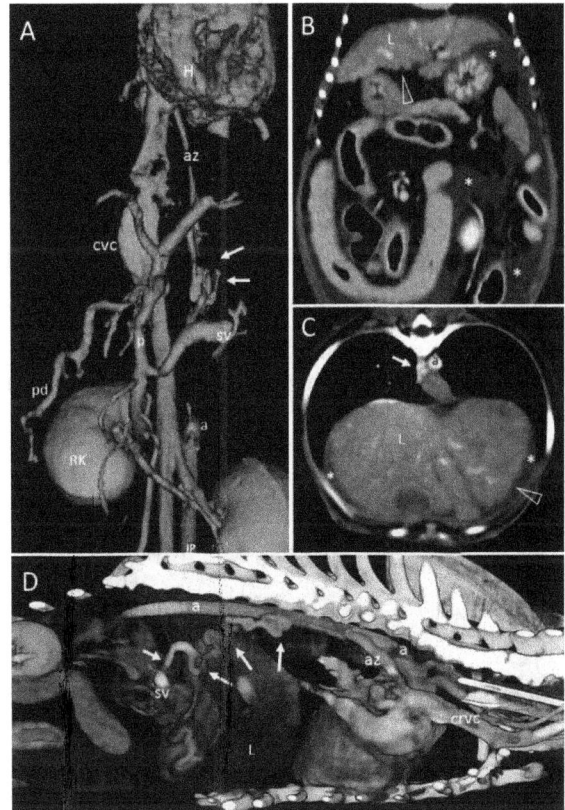

Fig. 1. Dog 1. (A): Ventral three-dimensional volume-rendered CT angiography of portal system, caudal vena cava, heart and azygos vein showing a splenoazygos PSS (arrows) connecting splenic vein (sv) and azygos vein (az). (B) Dorsal and (C) transverse multiplanar reformatted contrast-enhanced CT images of abdomen. The liver (L) appears slightly reduced in volume, with irregular margins (arrowheads) and without macroscopic parenchymal abnormalities or attenuation changes. A large amount of fluid (ascites) is evident in the background (asterisks). The section of the splenoazygos PSS is evident adjacent to Aorta (a), on the right (C-arrow). (D): Oblique right lateral thick-slab multiplanar reformatted contrast-enhanced CT image of abdomen and thorax showing in detail the tortuous splenoazygos PSS (arrows) and its connection with azygos vein (az). H: heart; p: portal vein; cvc: caudal vena cava; pd: pancreaticoduodenal vein; RK: right kidney; crvc: cranial vena cava.

In order to avoid worsening of portal hypertension surgical closure of the spleno-azygos PSS was not considered. A supportive therapy with spironolactone (2mg/kg q12h), amoxicilline-clavulanic acid (20 mg/kg q 12 h) and a commercial therapeutic diet for hepatic health (Prescription Diet l/d Canine, Hill's Pet Nutrition Inc, Topeka, Kan) were started. Three months later the dog was still alive.

Dog 2

An 8-year-old intact male mongrel dog was evaluated for a 1-month history of waxing and waning abnormal mentation and sporadic episodes of vomiting. At time of clinical examination the dog was normal. Complete blood count was unremarkable. Serum chemistry revealed increase in liver enzyme activity (aspartate aminotransferase 95 IU/l, RI 16–38; alanine aminotransferase 463 IU/l, RI 16–123) and hypoalbuminemia (2.2 g/dl, RI 2.7–3.6), and urinalysis revealed increase in urinary bile acids levels (87 mmol/l, RI 2.9– 9.5). Abdominal ultrasound and CT of thoracic and abdominal region were performed as described for dog 1. Imaging evaluation revealed microhepatia without macroscopic structural abnormalities of liver parenchyma, a large tortuous vessel connecting splenic vein and left gonadic vein and a network of small and tortuous vessels (varices) cranio-medially to the left kidney connecting left phrenicoabdominal vein and portal vein (Fig. 2).

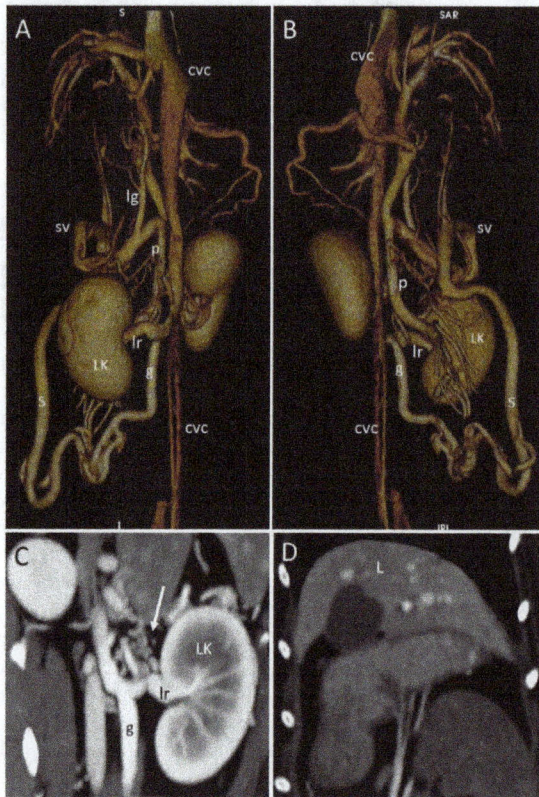

Fig. 2. Dog 2. (A) Left dorso-lateral and (B) right ventro-lateral three-dimensional volume-rendered CT angiography of portal system and caudal vena cava showing a large left splenogonadal PSS (s) connecting splenic vein (sv) and left gonadic vein (g) and entering the left renal vein (lr). (C): Dorsal maximum intensity projection (MIP) reformatted contrast-enhanced CT image of abdomen at level of kidneys. Porto-caval varices (arrow) are visible medially to the left kidney (LK). The enlarged left gonadal vein (g), which constitutes part of the left splenogonadal PSS, is visible at level of left renal vein (lr). (D): Dorsal multiplanar reformatted contrast-enhanced CT image of abdomen. The liver (L) appears slightly reduced in volume without macroscopic structural parenchymal abnormalities. P: portal vein; cvc: caudal vena cava; lg: left gastric vein.

Based on the imaging findings a diffuse microscopic hepatic disorder with secondary non-ascitic portal hypertension and MAPSS was suspected. In order to evaluate the presence and quantify eventual underlying portal hypertension, invasive portal pressure was measured during laparotomy for liver biopsy sampling. According to the described technique (Bojrab et al., 2014) a 22-Gauge intravenous catheter was placed into a jejunal vein and was attached to an extension set, a 3-way stopcock, a syringe and a water manometer with a zero point at the level of the right atrium. A value of 11.5 cm H_2O (reference interval: 8-13 cm H_2O) was recorded.

Histopathologic evaluation of a liver biopsy sample revealed diffuse lobular hypoplasia, portal venous hypoplasia, arteriolar and biliary hyperplasia, non-specific hepatocellular degeneration and multifocal lipogranulomes. These findings were suggestive of parenchymal damage caused by portal hypoperfusion. Supportive therapy with lactulose (10 mg PO q8h), metronidazole (7.5 mg/kg q12h) and a commercial therapeutic diet for hepatic health (Prescription Diet l/d Canine, Hill's Pet Nutrition Inc, Topeka, Kan) was started.

Four months later the dog was in good clinical condition with significant reduction of neurologic signs.

Cat 1

An 11-year-old spayed female domestic short-hair cat was referred for CT staging of a histopathologically confirmed lumbar cutaneous sarcoma. Clinical examination confirmed a cutaneous mass at level of lumbar region and a palpable firm mass in the cranial abdomen.

Haematology, serum chemistry analyses and urinalysis results were within normal limits. CT of the whole body was performed as described for dog 1. CT findings included: two large irregularly marginated, inhomogeneous, hypervascularized lumbar cutaneous and subcutaneous masses isoattenuating to the soft tissue with inhomogeneous contrast-enhancement; multiple irregularly marginated rounded hepatic masses (maximum dimensions: 3 x 5 x 4 cm), hypoattenuating to soft tissue with irregular contrast-enhancement; multiple, regularly marginated rounded pulmonary nodules (maximum dimensions: 3 x 3 x 3 mm) and a large tortuous vessel connecting splenic vein and left gonadic vein. No free fluid in the abdomen was evident (Fig. 3). An imaging diagnosis of metastatic soft tissue sarcoma with a left splenogonadal PSS was made.

Cat 2

A 13-year-old spayed female domestic short-hair cat was referred for CT staging of a histopathologically confirmed soft tissue sarcoma at the level of right scapular region.

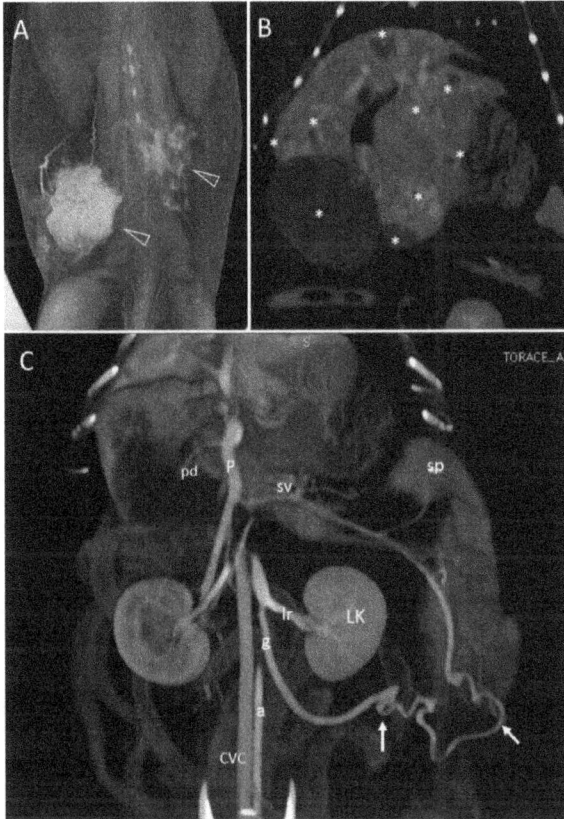

Fig. 3. Cat 1. (A) Dorsal thick-slab multiplanar reformatted contrast-enhanced CT image of lumbar region showing two large irregularly marginated, inhomogeneous, hypervascularized cutaneous and subcutaneous neoplasms (arrowheads). (B) Dorsal multiplanar reformatted contrast-enhanced CT image of abdomen. Multiple, irregularly marginated, rounded hepatic masses, hypoattenuating to soft tissue, with irregular contrast-enhancement, compatible with primary or metastatic diffuse hepatic neoplasia, are evident (asterisks). (C) Dorsal thick-slab multiplanar reformatted contrast-enhanced CT image of abdomen showing a large left splenogonadal PSS (arrows) connecting the splenic vein (sv) with the left gonadic vein (g) and entering the left renal vein (lr). No ascitic fluid is evident in the background (B,C). P, portal vein; a, aorta; cvc, caudal vena cava; pd, pancreaticoduodenal vein; LK, left kidney; sp, spleen.

Clinical examination confirmed a cutaneous mass at the level of right scapular region and did not reveal any other abnormalities. Haematology, serum chemistry analyses and urinalysis results were within normal limits. CT of the whole body was performed as described for dog 1. CT findings included: a large, irregularly marginated, multilobulated, hinomogeneous, hypervascularized cutaneous and subcutaneous masse isoattenuating to the soft tissue with inhomogeneous contrast-enhancement latero-caudal to the right scapula. Mild enlargement of ipsilateral axillary lymph node was present. No volume abnormalities of the liver nor macroscopic structural or attenuation changes were evident. A large tortuous

vessel connecting splenic vein and left gonadic vein was observed with no evidence of free fluid in the abdomen (Fig. 4). An imaging diagnosis of soft tissue sarcoma associated with a left splenogonadal PSS was made. Table (1) shows the main clinical, imaging and histopathologic findings for each patient.

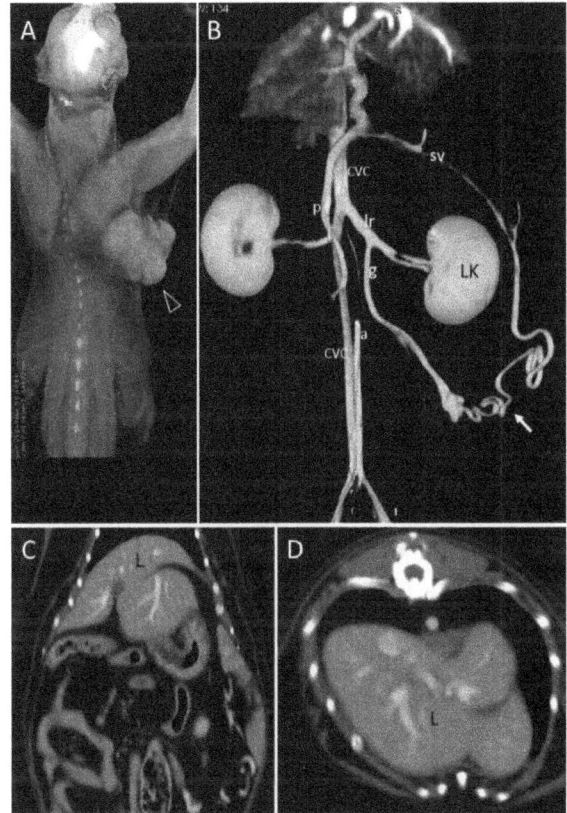

Fig. 4. Cat 2. (A) Dorsal thick-slab multiplanar reformatted contrast-enhanced CT image of thoracic region showing a large, irregularly marginated, multilobulated, hypervascularized cutaneous mass isoattenuating to the soft tissue with inhomogeneous contrast-enhancement latero-caudal to the right scapula (arrowhead). (B) Ventral three-dimensional volume-rendered CT angiography of portal system and caudal vena cava showing a large left splenogonadal PSS (arrow) connecting splenic vein (sv) with left gonadic vein (g) and entering the left renal vein (lr). (C) Dorsal and (D) transverse multiplanar reformatted contrast-enhanced CT images of abdomen at level of liver (L) showing absence of hepatic macroscopic structural abnormalities or attenuation/volume changes. Also note absence of ascites in the background (C). P, portal vein; a, aorta; cvc, caudal vena cava; LK, left kidney; sv, splenic vein.

Discussion

In veterinary medical literature the classical expected clinical and imaging findings in patients with portal hypertension are ascites, multiple APSS (either varices and large shunts) and a confirmed cause of portal flow obstruction at level of extrahepatic portal vein, liver, hepatic veins, posthepatic caudal vena cava, or right atrium (Buob *et al.*, 2011).

Table 1. Major clinical, imaging and histopatologic findings of each patient.

Case	Signalment	Clinical signs/clinical findings	Abdominal effusion	Pattern of porto-caval connections	invasive portal pressure measurement (cm H_2O)	CT appearance of the liver	Histopatologic diagnosis from liver biopsy
Dog 1	12-year-old intact male, Yorkshire Terrier	Inappetence, abdominal distension	Pure transudate	Single splenoazygos PSS	N/A	Mild decrease in liver volume with irregular margins	subacute-cronic centrolobular and midzonal hepatitis
Dog 2	8-year-old intact male mongrel	waxing and waning abnormal mentation; sporadic vomiting	absent	Left splenogonadal PSS; Gastro-phrenic varices;	11,5 (RI in normal dogs: 8-13; RI in dogs with PSS: 0-12)	microhepatia without parenchymal abnormalities	portal hypoperfusion
Cat 1	11-year-old spayed female DSH	lumbar cutaneous neoplasm (sarcoma)	absent	Single left splenogonadal PSS	N/A	multiple hepatic masses of presumptive metastatic origin	N/A
Cat 2	13-year-old spayed female DSH	Scapular cutaneous neoplasm (soft tissue sarcoma)	absent	Single left splenogonadal PSS	N/A	normal appearance	N/A

N/A: Not available; RI: Reference interval.

On the other hand patients with congenital PSS are traditionally described as having a single porto-caval connection without ascites or portal flow obstruction (Szatmari et al., 2004; Bertolini et al., 2006; Nelson and Nelson, 2011; Fukushima et al., 2014). Furthermore, current classification of canine PSS differentiate repeatable and distinct vascular patterns of CPSS and APSS without any overlapping of anatomical pathway between each category (Ricciardi, 2016). These differences in the course of CPSS and APSS allow for their categorization during an angiographic study and help, in addition to other clinical and imaging findings, in the distinction between patients with PH from other with congenital porto-caval connection (Ricciardi, 2016). In the cases reported herein, some overlapping between clinical, histopathologic and imaging findings of PH and CPSS were observed, making the categorization of patients challenging.

In dog 1, a single splenoazygos PSS was observed in a patient with diffuse subacute-cronic hepatitis, which caused PH and ascitis. In major classifications of porto-caval connections in dogs the splenoazygos PSS pattern has been described among CPSS and never in the APSS group (Szatmari et al., 2004; Bertolini et al., 2006; Nelson and Nelson, 2011; Fukushima et al., 2014). In the author's opinion, the presence of such PSS pattern in a dog with PH would corroborate two hypotheses:

1) Pre-existence of CPSS of splenoazygos pattern in a patient which has developed PH in adulthood due to an acquired liver disease. In this case, a CPSS may be not sufficient to alleviate PH caused by primary diffuse intrahepatic parenchymal disease. Consequently, APSS and ascites develop. Interestingly a similar condition has been already reported in two dogs with PH in which a splenophrenic PSS, traditionally described as CPSS, was found in addition to other MAPSS (Ricciardi, 2016). This hypothesis would disavow the theory that the presence of a CPSS, in a dog with portal flow obstruction at level of the liver, would make development of PH unlikely bypassing portal blood in the systemic (caval) circulation, that presents the lowest resistance, (Szatmari, 2003). This eventuality would help refine imaging evaluation of patients with PH and CPSS reconsidering their haemodynamics.

2) The splenoazygos PSS may also be a pattern of APSS until now unreported, which regains patency if PH develops. The portal vein in the normal dog has at least three embryonic connections with the systemic venous system, which usually are not, or only minimally perfused. One of these connects the cardiac branches of the left gastric vein with the oesophageal branches of the azygos vein (Huntington and Mcclure, 1920; Bertolini, 2010a; Moubarak et al., 2012). Such embryonic pathways of porto-caval connection may develop in splenoazygos APSS when PH occurs. Such hypothesis has already been considered for the splenophrenic PSS pattern - traditionally described as CPSS but also found in dogs with PH (Ricciardi, 2016) - since embryonic connections between phrenic vein and small branches of portal vein have also been

described in dogs (Huntington and Mcclure, 1920; Bertolini, 2010a; Moubarak et al., 2012).

Interestingly, in human medical literature, a portoazygos shunt associated with multiple paraesophageal, retroperitoneal, parasplenic and gastric varices has been reported in an adult patient with liver cirrhosis and portal hypertension (Gebrael et al., 2013). In this case, the authors considered the portoazygos PSS an acquired portal collateral developed as a consequence of PH. If splenoazygos and splenophrenic PSS represent pattern shared by both APSS and CPSS, categorization of the vascular anomaly based only on imaging findings (anatomical pathway) may be challenging.

In this case, the distinction between PH with APSS and CPSS may be influenced by the presence or absence of abdominal effusion as a frequent distinctive hallmark between these two conditions. However, as reported in humans (Gines et al., 1987; Sarin and Kapoor, 2002; Sarin et al., 2007) and dogs (Adam et al., 2012; Ricciardi, 2016) ascites may be absent in some PH cases especially if the APSS are completely effective in alleviating portal pressure.

Hence, as previously reported for the splenophrenic PSS pattern (Ricciardi, 2016), in cases of primary microvascular or parenchymal hepatic disorders macroscopically undetectable on imaging evaluation (such as PHPV or hepatitis like in dog 1 of this series), the possible absence of ascites and the presence of a single acquired splenoazygos shunt (without other MAPSS) may disorient the presumptive diagnosis of PH (acquired splenoazygos PSS misinterpreted as CPSS). However, the number of PSSs may be helpful in such distinction since presence of more than one porto-caval connections has been considered a constant imaging finding shared among dogs with PH (Bertolini, 2010a; Ricciardi, 2016).

In dog 2, a large left splenogonadal PSS and varices near to the left kidney, also known as gastrophrenic varices (Bertolini, 2010a; Ricciardi et al., 2014; Ricciardi, 2016), were found without ascites. These patterns of porto-caval connection have been reported as two of the most consistently observed route of APSSs in dogs (Szatmari et al., 2004; Bertolini, 2010a; Ricciardi et al., 2014; Ricciardi, 2016) suggesting non-ascitic PH in this patient. Regarding the portal vein pressure, in normal dogs it is between 8 and 13 cm H_2O, while patients with a PSS, because of the diversion of portal blood flow into the systemic circulation, the portal pressure is usually lower, ranging between 0 and 12 cm H_2O (Johnson et al., 1987; Slatter, 2003). In our patient the portal pressure was 11.5 cm H_2O resulting not very helpful in discriminating between a PH and a normal portal pressure, even if a much lower value could be expected in the presence of such large splenogonadal PSS.

Liver histopathology was suggestive of parenchymal damage caused by portal hypoperfusion, as typically reported in patients with CPSS (Borrows, 2003; Isobe et al., 2008). However, histopathologic liver changes may be identical in case of primary diseases causing PH (idiopathic non-cirrhotic PH (NCPH), portal venous hypoplasia, hepatic microvascular dysplasia and congenital arterioportal fistula) or in the case of reduced portal perfusion (congenital PSS). Thus, differentiation between PH with MAPSS due to primary liver disease and CPSS may not be possible based only on liver histopathologic findings (Van den Ingh et al., 1995a, 1995b; Center, 1996; Bunch et al., 2001). Hence, based on the overall histopathologic and imaging findings in this patient, three diagnostic hypotheses may be reasonably considered:

1) A PH due to primary liver diseases (idiopathic NCPH, portal venous hypoplasia, or hepatic microvascular dysplasia) with completely efficient MAPSS which avoided development of ascites. In this case, surgical closure of the PSS, as therapeutic approach for hepatic encephalopathy of this dog, would not be recommendable.

2) Transient PH developed in adulthood due to a self-limiting hepatic or portal disease (such us portal vein thrombosis or inflammatory liver disease), subsequently regressed, with opening of MAPSS. In this case, the multiple acquired PSS may represent the remnant of a transient episode of PH and, as responsible for the occurrence of hepatic encephalopathy without any other hemodynamic utility, may need surgical closure.

3) Multiple congenital porto-caval connections in a patient without PH. Although considered a rare phenomenon, multiple CPSS have also been described in dogs (Johnson et al., 1987; Wilson et al., 1997; Morandi et al., 2005; Leeman et al., 2013); in all cases however, large porto-caval or porto-azygous vascular connections were reported without varices nor splenogonadal pattern. Hence, this last hypothesis would redefine the classifications of CPSSs including among these even the left splenogonadal PSS and the porto-caval varices close to the left kidney. This implies that the finding of a single left splenogonadal PSS in a non-ascitic patient without macroscopic evidence of liver disease on imaging evaluation would be a diagnostic challenge – for discrimination between underlying PH and CPSS – especially in the case of unspecific liver histopathologic results (as those of dog 2) and doubt/border-line portal pressure values.

Regarding the hypothesis no. 1, NCPH is one of the most reported cause of presinusoidal intrahepatic PH in humans and dogs and, from histopathological point of view, it resembles primary hypoplasia of the portal vasculature (PHPV) so that the latter term is recommended by the World Small Animal Veterinary Association liver study group (Buob *et al.*, 2011). It is unclear, however, if the lesion in NCPH-PHPV patients is in all cases a primary hypoplasia of the intrahepatic portal vasculature or a consequence of a primary congenital or acquired disorder in hepatic perfusion (Buob *et al.*, 2011).

In humans the basic criteria to diagnose NCPH are: 1) presence of unequivocal signs of portal hypertension, 2) absence of diffuse liver diseases that can cause PH and 3) absence of occlusive disorders of the hepatic veins or of the portal vein (Schouten *et al.*, 2015). In our dog, the portal pressure measurement failed to testify an unequivocal condition of PH so that the hypothesis of an underlying NCPH-PHPV and MAPSS seems unlikely and a condition of multiple CPSS, of both large and small calibre, without PH, could not be ruled out.

Moreover, the hypothesis of a congenital origin of the left splenogonadal PSS has been previously reported in veterinary literature (Valentine and Carpenter, 1990).

Interestingly a single left splenogonadal PSS without ascites was found in the two cats described in this series.

In cat 1 the finding of diffuse hepatic structural disorder (suggestive of diffuse hepatic metastases) made it reasonable to consider the splenogonadal PSS as a classical APSS recanalized as a consequence of raised intrahepatic portal pressure. In this cat, as previously described (Ricciardi, 2016), the lack of ascites may be explained by a complete effectiveness of the acquired splenogaonadal PSS in alleviating portal pressure.

On the contrary, in cat 2, the left splenogonadal PSS was found as an incidental finding not associated with attenuation changes, nor volume abnormalities nor macroscopic structural alterations of the liver. Ascites was also absent.

In this case, two hypotheses may be reasonably considered:

1) as discussed in the third hypothesis of dog 2, the left splenogonadal PSS may be considered a congenital porto-caval connection, until now unreported among classification of CPSSs, causing subclinical, unrecognized or misinterpreted clinical signs (this cat had no history of clinical sign attributable to PSS).

2) as discussed in the second hypothesis of dog 2, transient PH developed in adulthood because of a self-limiting hepatic or portal disease with a single remnant APSS.

Unfortunately liver histopathology and ultrasonographic assessment of portal flow direction were not available in this patient.

In a series of 33 cats with single PSS connecting the splenic vein and the left renal vein or the adjacent segment of caudal vena cava, only 14 patients had a hepatopathy with the potential for associated PH. Adult spayed females were significantly overrepresented, as the cats of this report, and the portal blood flow, available in a limited number of patients, resulted to be hepatopetal in the majority of cases.

In this study, the authors concluded that the aetiology of the splenosystemic PSS in cats could not be definitely determined but, as hypothesized for the cat 2 reported herein, it may represent an acquired shunts secondary to past or present portal hypertension or it can be a congenital shunt of unknown clinical significance (Palerme *et al.*, 2013).

In the author's opinion, findings from these cases should prompt to reconsider porto-caval haemodynamic in dogs and cats with PSS, in the light of shunt phenotype and number, presence/absence of ascites, presence of macroscopic liver structural disorders, liver histopathologic results and, when possible, portal pressure measurement.

The splenoazygos PSS pattern, may be considered a classical CPSS pattern (Szatmari *et al.*, 2004; Bertolini *et al.*, 2006; Nelson and Nelson, 2011; Fukushima *et al.*, 2014) or an APSS until now unreported.

The left splenogonadal PSS and porto-caval varices near to the left kidney may be considered, as traditionally described, classical APSSs when found in patients with ascites and a confirmed cause of portal flow obstruction (Ricciardi *et al.*, 2014; Ricciardi, 2016), however, in non-ascitic patients without macroscopic evidence of liver disease, without evidence of hepatofugal portal blood flow or portal pressure measurement suggestive of PH, such PSS patterns may be also considered as CPSSs (encountered either as single CPSS, like in cat 2, or as multiple CPSSs, like in dog 2). In this last circumstance, the univocal presumptive diagnosis of NCPH with MAPSS may be questionable. Hence, as previously described for the splenophrenic PSS pathway (Ricciardi, 2016), acquired and congenital large PSSs may share the same anatomical pathway of porto-caval connection (here described for splenoazygos and left splenogonadal pattern). Such preliminar observations may help in reconsidering the distinction between CPSS and APSS, traditionally based on the shunt phenotype assessed by imaging evaluations (Bertolini *et al.*, 2006; Bertolini, 2010a, 2010b; Nelson and Nelson, 2011; Fukushima *et al.*, 2014; Ricciardi *et al.*, 2014; Ricciardi, 2016) and consequently the distinction between patient with PH from those with congenital PSS(s).

These findings, however, need to be enriched by further data regarding the direction of portal blood flow in patients with and without signs of PH and presence of left splenogonadal or splenoazygos PSS.

Finally, this case series emphasizes the importance of the precise imaging assessment of the PSS pattern, along with clinical and histopathologic findings, during diagnostic workup of patients with and without PH.

Conflict of interests

The Author declare that there is no conflict of interest.

Acknowledgments

The author wish to thank Dr. Ilaria Carrieri, DVM in Taranto (TA), Italy, Dr. Marcello Lanci, DVM in Fano (PU), Italy, Dr. Vito Manfredi, DVM in Triggiano (BA), Italy and the staff of the "Pingry" Veterinary Hospital of Bari (BA), Italy for their assistance with data collection. The author is also grateful to Dr. Swan Specchi and Dr. Simona Morabito (Istituto Veterinario di Novara, Granozzo con Monticello (NO), Italy, for the constructive exchange of ideas on complex and controversial hemodynamic aspects of the vascular disorders described in this paper.

References

Adam, F.H., German, A.J., McConnell, J.F., Trehy, M.R., Whitley, N., Collings, A., Watson, P.J. and Burrow, R.D. 2012. Clinical and clinicopathologic abnormalities in young dogs with acquired and congenital portosystemic shunts: 93 cases (2003-2008). J. Am. Vet. Med. Assoc. 241, 760-765.

Baldwin, K., Bartges, J., Buffington, T., Freeman, L.M., Grabow, M., Legred, J. and Ostwald, D.Jr. 2010. AAHA nutritional assessment guidelines for dogs and cats. J. Am. Anim. Hosp. Assoc. 46(4), 285-296.

Bertolini, G. 2010a. Acquired portal collateral circulation in the dog and cat. Vet. Radiol. Ultrasound. 51, 25-33.

Bertolini, G. 2010b. MDCT for abdominal vascular assessment in dogs: MDCT basics, CT angiography, normal anatomy and congenital anomalies. LAMBERT Academic Publishing, Saarbrucken, Germany.

Bertolini, G., Rolla, E.C., Zotti, A. and Caldin, M. 2006. Three-dimensional multislice helical computed tomography techniques for canine extrahepatic portosystemic shunt assessment. Vet. Radiol. Ultrasound. 47, 439-443.

Bojrab, M.J., Waldron, D.R. and Toombs, J.P. 2014. Current Techniques in Small Animal Surgery. 5th ed. Jackson, W.Y.: Teton New Media, pp: 334.

Borrows, C.F. 2003. Liver disorders. In: Clinical Medicine of the Dog and Cat, 1st ed, (Schaer, M. ed.), Veterinary Press, London, England, pp: 337-349.

Bruehschwein, A., Foltin, I., Flatz, K., Zoellner, M. and Matis, U. 2010. Contrast-enhanced magnetic resonance angiography for diagnosis of portosystemic shunts in 10 dogs. Vet. Radiol. Ultrasound. 51, 116-121.

Bunch, S.E., Johnson, S.E. and Cullen, J.M. 2001. Idiopathic noncirrhotic portal hypertension in dogs: 33 cases (1982-1998). J. Am. Vet. Med. Assoc. 218, 392-399.

Buob, S., Johnston, A.N. and Webster, C.R. 2011. Portal hypertension: pathophysiology, diagnosis, and treatment. J. Vet. Intern. Med. 25, 169-186.

Center, S.A. 1996. Hepatic Vascular Diseases, In: Strombeck's Small Animal Gastroenterology. 3rd ed. W.B. Saunders Company, Philadelphia, pp: 802-846.

Ferrell, E.A., Graham, J.P., Hanel, R.S., Randell, S., Farese, J.P. and Castleman, W.L. 2003. Simultaneous congenital and acquired extrahepatic portosystemic shunts in two dogs. Vet. Radiol. Ultrasound. 44, 38-42.

Fossum, T.W. 2002. Small Animal Surgery, 2nd ed., Mosby, St. Louis, pp: 457-468.

Fukushima, K., Kanemoto, H., Ohno, K.M., Takahashi, R., Fujiwara, R., Nishimura, R. and Tsujimoto, H. 2014. Computed tomographic morphology and clinical features of extrahepatic portosystemic shunts in 172 dogs in Japan. Vet. J. 199(3), 376-381.

Gebrael, J., Yu, H. and Hyslop, W.B. 2013. Spontaneous Portoazygos Shunt in a Patient with Portal Hypertension. J. Radiol. Case Rep. 7(7), 32-36.

Gines, P., Quintero, E., Arroyo, V., Terés, J., Bruguera, M., Rimola, A., Caballería, J., Rodés, J. and Rozman, C. 1987. Compensated cirrhosis: natural history and prognostic factors. Hepatology 7(1), 122-128.

Huntington, G.S. and Mcclure, C.F.W. 1920. The development of the veins in the domestic cat (Felis domestica) with especial reference, (1) to the share taken by the supracardinal veins in the developmentof the postcava and azygos veins and (2) to the interpretation of the variant conditions of the postcava and its tributaries as found in the adult. Anat. Rec. 20, 1-30.

Isobe, K., Matsunaga, S., Nakayama, H. and Uetsuka, K. 2008. Histopathological Characteristics of Hepatic Lipogranulomas with Portosystemic Shunt in Dogs. J. Vet. Med. Sci. 70, 133-138.

Johnson, C.A., Armstrong, P.J. and Hauptman, J.G. 1987. Congenital portosystemic shunts in dogs: 46 cases (1979-1986). J. Am. Vet. Med. Assoc. 191, 1478-1483.

Lamb, C.R. 1996. Ultrasonographic diagnosis of congenital portosystemic shunts in dogs: Results of a prospective study. Vet. Radiol. Ultrasound. 37, 281-288.

Leeman, J.J., Kim, S.E., Reese, D.J., Risselada, M. and Ellison, G.W. 2013. Multiple congenital PSS in a dog: case report and literature review. J. Am. Anim. Hosp. Assoc. 49, 281-285.

Morandi, F., Cole, R.C., Tobias, K.M., Berry, C.R., Avenell, J. and Daniel, G.B. 2005. Use of 99mTCO4(-) trans-splenic portal scintigraphy for diagnosis of portosystemic shunts in 28 dogs. Vet. Radiol. Ultrasound. 46, 153-161.

Moubarak, E., Bouvier, A., Boursier, J., Lebigot, J., Ridereau-Zins, C., Thouveny, F., Willoteaux, S. and Aubé, C. 2012. Portosystemic collateral vessels in liver cirrhosis: a three-dimensional MDCT pictorial review. Abdom Imaging. 37(5), 746-766.

Nelson, N.C. and Nelson, L.L. 2011. Anatomy of extrahepatic portosystemic shunts in dogs as determined by computed tomography angiography. Vet. Radiol. Ultrasound. 52, 498-506.

Palerme, J.S., Brown, J.C., Marks, S.L. and Birkenheuer, A.J. 2013. Splenosystemic shunts in cats: a retrospective of 33 cases (2004-2011). J. Vet. Intern. Med. 27, 1347-1353.

Ricciardi, M. 2016. Splenophrenic portosystemic shunt in dogs with and without portal hypertension: can acquired and congenital porto-caval connections coexist? Open Vet. J. 6, 185-193.

Ricciardi, M., Martino, R. and Assad, E.A. 2014. Imaging diagnosis--celiacomesenteric trunk and portal vein hypoplasia in a pit bull terrier. Vet. Radiol. Ultrasound. 55, 190-194.

Sarin, S.K. and Kapoor, D. 2002. Non-cirrhotic portal fibrosis: current concepts and management. J. Gastroenterol. Hepatol. 17, 526-534.

Sarin, S.K., Kumar, A., Chawla, Y.K., Baijal, S.S., Dhiman, R.K., Jafri, W., Lesmana, L.A., Guha Mazumder, D., Omata, M., Qureshi, H., Raza, R.M., Sahni, P., Sakhuja, P., Salih, M., Santra, A.,

Sharma, B.C., Sharma, P., Shiha, G. and Sollano, J. 2007. Noncirrhotic portal fibrosis/idiopathic portal hypertension: APASL recommendations for diagnosis and treatment. Hepatol. Int. 1(3), 398-413.

Schouten, J.N., Verheij, J. and Seijo, S. 2015. Idiopathic non-cirrhotic portal hypertension: a review. Orphanet. J. Rare Dis. 10, 67.

Slatter, D.H. 2003. Textbook of Small Animal Surgery, 3rd ed. Philadelphia: Saunders, pp: 738.

Szatmari, V. 2003. Simultaneous congenital and acquired extrahepatic portosystemic shunts in two dogs. Vet. Radiol. Ultrasound. 44, 486-487.

Szatmari, V. and Rothuizen, J. 2002. How can you tell with ultrasound that a patient with high blood ammonia has a congenital or acquired portosystemic shunt or no shunt at all? In the Proceedings of the 27th Congress of the World Small Animal Veterinary Association, October 3-6, Granada, Spain, pp: 42.

Szatmari, V., Rothuizen, J., van den Ingh, T.S., van Sluijs, F. and Voorhout, G. 2004. Ultrasonographic findings in dogs with hyperammonemia: 90 cases (2000-2002). J. Am. Vet. Med. Assoc. 224(5), 717-727.

Valentine, R.W. and Carpenter, J.L. 1990. Spleno-mesenteric-renal venous shunt in two dogs. Vet. Pathol. 27, 58-60.

Van den Ingh, T.S., Rothuizen, J. and Meyer, H.P. 1995a. Circulatory disorders of the liver in dogs and cats. Vet. Q. 17, 70-76.

Van den Ingh, T.S., Rothuizen, J. and Meyer, H.P. 1995b. Portal hypertension associated with primary hypoplasia of the hepatic portal vein in dogs. Vet. Rec. 137, 424-427.

Wilson, K., Scrivani, P. and Léveillé, R. 1997. What is your diagnosis? Portocaval and portoazygous shunts and microhepatia in a dog. J. Am. Vet. Med. Assoc. 211(4), 415-416.

11

Anaesthetic management of a unilateral adrenalectomy of an adrenocortical tumour in a dog

I.K. Wise[1,*] and S. Boveri[2]

[1]University of Cambridge, Department of Clinical Veterinary Medicine, Madingley Road, Cambridge, UK
[2]The University of Liverpool, School of Veterinary Science, Neston, UK

Abstract

Adrenalectomies in dogs are being more commonly performed, however anaesthetic management of such cases can be challenging due to the multiple aetiologies of adrenal tumours and the physiological role of adrenal glands. This case report describes the anaesthetic management of a dog with clinical signs of hyperadrenocorticism that underwent unilateral adrenalectomy via laparotomy and discusses anaesthetic preparedness, protocol selection and management of complications for dogs undergoing adrenalectomy.

Keywords: Adrenal neoplasia, Adrenalectomy, Canine.

Introduction

Adrenalectomy is the treatment of choice for canine adrenal tumours for a good long-term outcome (Lang et al., 2011). Surgical techniques for adrenalectomies in dogs are increasingly reported (Kyles et al., 2003; Jiménez Peláez et al., 2008; Lang et al., 2011; Massari et al., 2011; Gójska-zygner et al., 2012; Smith et al., 2012; Barrera et al., 2013; Naan et al., 2013). However, anaesthetic management of these cases has rarely been described (Kyles et al., 2003; Jiménez Peláez et al., 2008; Lang et al., 2011; Massari et al., 2011). Complications reported for adrenalectomies are hypotension, hypertension, tachycardia, ventricular arrhythmias and haemorrhage, with a reported incidence of 35 to 100% (Lang et al., 2011). Perioperative mortality rates for adrenalectomies have been reported as 6% for elective procedures increasing to 50% when performed in emergencies (Lang et al., 2011). These mortality rates are higher than that of 1.33% in dogs classified as American Society of Anesthesiologists (ASA) physical status 3-5 in the Confidential Enquiry into Perioperative Small Animal Fatalities (Brodbelt et al., 2008).

The most common primary adrenal tumours are adrenocortical adenomas or adenocarcinomas, and phaeochromocytomas (Massari et al., 2011). Less commonly, myelolipomas, aldosteronomas, deoxycorticosterone- or sex hormone- secreting adrenal tumours are found (Massari et al., 2011). Adrenal tumours may be endocrinologically active (Gójska-zygner et al., 2012); thus the presenting clinical signs and the physiological response to anaesthesia and surgery may reflect the type of tumour present.

Case Details

A 6-year-old female neutered 33 kg Airedale was referred to the Queens Veterinary Hospital, University of Cambridge, for investigation of an 18-month history of lethargy, weight gain with abdominomegaly, polyuria, polydipsia (PU/PD) and polyphagia. There had been concurrent thinning of the coat with hyperpigmentation of the skin. On examination, the dog was quiet, alert and responsive with a left-sided head tilt and left-sided facial muscle weakness suggestive of facial nerve paralysis. Cardiorespiratory examination was unremarkable. Complete haematology and a comprehensive biochemistry profile showed the following significant abnormalities: PCV 60% (reference range 37–55); total protein 84 g/dL (60–80); urea 9.5 mmol/L (2.5–7.5); ALT 283 iu/L (14–67); ALP 561 iu/L (26–107); cholesterol 14.1 mmol/L (3.3–6.5). Urinalysis of a free catch sample showed isosthenuria (urine specific gravity 1.008). A right adrenal mass was the only abnormality detected by abdominal ultrasonography. A total body computer tomography scan with iodinated contrast confirmed the presence of a well circumscribed hyperplastic right adrenal gland and a hypoplastic left adrenal gland with no evidence of vascular infiltration or metastatic disease. The owners declined further clinical pathology tests. A right-sided adrenocortical tumour causing clinical signs of hyperadrenocorticism was presumptively diagnosed. The patient was scheduled for right adrenalectomy via laparotomy and was assigned an ASA physical status of 3.

The patient was premedicated with medetomidine (1 µg kg-1, Sedator; Dechra Veterinary Products, Skipton, UK) and methadone (0.3 mg kg-1, Comfortan; Dechra Veterinary Products, Skipton, UK) intramuscularly (IM) followed by the placement of a 20G catheter in the cephalic vein. After preoxygenation, general anaesthesia was induced with propofol (PropoFlo Plus; Zoetis, Tadworth, UK) 2.7 mg kg-1 and diazepam

(Diazemuls; Actavis UK Ltd, Barnstable, UK) 0.2 mg kg⁻¹ intravenously (IV). After oro-tracheal intubation with a 10 mm diameter cuffed tube, anaesthesia was maintained with isoflurane (IsoFlo; Zoetis, Tadowrth, UK) in oxygen. Monitoring included electrocardiography (ECG), pulse oximetry (SpO_2), invasive blood pressure, oesophageal temperature, end-tidal (ET) gas analysis and capnography. Active warming was provided using a semi-conductive heating device (Hot Dog; Augustine Temperature Management, Eden Prairie, USA) to maintain normothermia.

In anticipation of intraoperative haemorrhage, an 18G catheter was placed in the contralateral cephalic vein to enable rapid fluid administration. Blood products, hetastarch and crystalloids were placed in theatre. Intravenous fluid therapy (IVFT) consisted of Hartmann's solution (Compound Sodium Lactate for Infusion BP; Baxter, Staines-upon-Thames, UK) administered at 5 ml kg⁻¹ hr⁻¹ during surgical preparation, doubled during the surgical procedure. Intraoperative blood loss was monitored using a combination of haemoglobin concentration measurement in the suction system and the swab gravimetric method.

Atracurium (Tracrium; GlaxoSmithKline, Uxbridge, UK) 0.2 mg kg⁻¹ was administered IV to facilitate the surgical approach. The neuromuscular blockade was monitored with accelerometry (TOF watch™; Wardray Premise, Thames Ditton, UK) placed across the ulnar nerve. Additional atracurium 0.1 mg kg⁻¹ IV was administered as needed during the procedure to maintain a train of four (TOF) reading of one. The dog was mechanically ventilated to maintain normocapnia.

Analgesia was provided using lidocaine (Lidocaine 2% BP; Hameln Pharmaceuticals Ltd, Gloucester, UK) and fentanyl (Sublimaze; Janssen-Cilag Ltd, High Wycombe, UK) IV infusions, respectively at 40 µg kg⁻¹ min⁻¹ and 2-15 µg kg⁻¹ hr⁻¹, both preceded by loading boluses of 1 mg kg⁻¹ and 2 µg kg⁻¹ IV respectively. Paracetamol (Perfalgan; Bristol-Myers Squibb Pharmaceutical Ltd, Uxbridge, UK) 10 mg kg⁻¹ was administered IV towards conclusion of surgery and bupivicaine (Marcain 0.5% Polyamp Steripack; AstraZeneca, Luton, UK) 10 ml was splashed on the rectus abdominus muscles once sutured. Cefuroxime (Zinacef; GlaxoSmithKline, Uxbridge, UK) 20 mg kg⁻¹ IV was administered every 90 minutes throughout surgery.

Approximately 30 minutes after commencement of surgery, when the mass was being manipulated via blunt dissection around the adrenal capsule, the dog became acutely hypertensive (systolic 200 mmHg and diastolic 110 mmHg) with an increased HR of 110 bpm and premature supraventricular complexes. Thus a fentanyl bolus of 2 µg kg⁻¹ IV was administered followed by an increased infusion rate of 15 µg kg⁻¹ hr⁻¹. Methadone 0.3 mg kg⁻¹ IV was also administered. These

interventions resolved the arrhythmia and reduced the systolic blood pressure to 100 mmHg. During further manipulation of the mass, a sudden increase in systolic pressure (200 mmHg) occurred with concurrent severe bradycardia (30 bpm) with third-degree atrioventricular blocks. Promotion of vasodilation by increasing the isoflurane percentage and administering acepromazine (ACP Injection; Novartis Animal Health, Basingstoke, UK) 5 µg kg⁻¹ IV increased the heart rate to 60 bpm and reduced the systolic blood pressure to between 80 and 90 mmHg. The patient remained stable for the remainder of anaesthesia as the right adrenal gland and associated tumour were excised en mass via further blunt dissection and vessel ligation.

Prior to recovery, a lumbosacral epidural injection of morphine (Morphine BP; Martindale Pharmaceuticals UK, Wockhart, UK) 0.15 mg kg⁻¹ diluted with sterile saline to a volume of 0.12 ml kg⁻¹ was administered and an 8 Fr Foley urinary catheter (Infusion Concept, Sowerby Bridge, UK) was placed. The neuromuscular blockade was not antagonized as two equal twitches in response to double burst stimulation were seen. Anaesthesia and surgery times were 290 minutes and 225 minutes, respectively.

The dog recovered from anaesthesia in the intensive care unit (ICU). Post-operative monitoring consisted of hourly assessments of pulse rate and quality, ECG, respiratory rate and pattern, Doppler blood pressure monitoring, mucous membrane colour and capillary refill time. Urinary output was monitored hourly and electrolytes levels were monitored every six hours for the first 24 hours. Pain was assessed every two hours using a modified Glasgow pain scale. If the pain score exceeded six, methadone 0.2 mg kg⁻¹ IM was prescribed as rescue analgesia. Paracetamol 10 mg kg⁻¹ was continued per os twice daily and lidocaine 40 µg kg⁻¹ h⁻¹ IV was infused for 24 hours. Prednisolone (Prednicare; Animalcare, Nether Poppleton, UK) 0.2 mg kg⁻¹ was administered once orally in the early postoperative period. Omeprazole, cefuroxime and vitamin A were prescribed by the attending clinicians. Two hours into the recovery period, the systolic blood pressure increased to 200 mmHg without concurrent arrhythmias. Therefore, acepromazine (ACP tablets; Elanco Animal Health, Basingstoke, UK) 1 mg kg⁻¹ was administered orally, which reduced the systolic pressure to 140 mmHg within 30 minutes. The patient had no further complications and was discharged from intensive care the following day. Histopathological analysis defined the resected mass as an adrenocortical carcinoma.

Discussion

Although adrenalectomy is the preferred treatment for adrenal tumours in dogs (Lang *et al.*, 2011), complications during anaesthesia and surgery are common and sometimes fatal. This case provides an opportunity to reflect on anaesthetic preparedness, protocol selection and management of possible complications that may occur in dogs undergoing anaesthesia for adrenalectomy.

A functional adrenocortical tumour may cause clinical signs of hyperadrenocorticism, such as PU/PD, abdominal enlargement, hypertension, prolonged healing, skin changes, lethargy, polyphagia and facial paralysis (Johnson and Norman, 2007). Uncommonly, adrenocortical tumours may also produce excess mineralocorticoids, causing clinical signs of Addison's disease. Phaeochromocytomas produce excess catecholamines which may cause hypertensive episodes. Phaeochromocytomas often invade adjacent blood vessels or organs, which may cause haemorrhage into the retroperitoneal space. Therefore, clinical signs of phaeochromocytoma are often nonspecific and include weakness, tachypnoea, collapse, tachyarrhythmias and seizures (Herrera et al., 2008). In our patient, the presence of many clinical signs of hyperadrenocorticism without evidence of hypertensive episodes or local tumour invasion lead to a preoperative presumptive diagnosis of an adrenocortical tumour producing excess cortisol. Further preoperative diagnostic testing such as adrenocorticotropic hormone stimulation testing and urine protein-to-creatinine ratio may have provided additional supporting evidence. As commonly occurs with adrenal tumours, a definitive diagnosis of adrenocortical adenocarcinoma was not made until postoperative histopathology was performed on the resected mass.

In patients suspected to have a phaeochromoytoma due to documented hypertensive episodes, preoperative stabilisation with phenoxybenzamine has been advocated to decrease perioperative mortality (Kyles et al., 2003; Herrera et al., 2008; Massari et al., 2011). Phenoxybenzamine, an α-adrenergic antagonist, irreversibly binds to α1 and α2 adrenergic receptors to block the response to circulating catecholamines (Herrera et al., 2008). Preoperative treatment of human patients is for at least two weeks (Kyles et al., 2003), while the literature for dogs reports time frames between 7 and 120 days (Herrera et al., 2008). As our patient had no preoperative clinical signs of hypertension, phenoxybenzamine was not prescribed.

The most common intraoperative complication reported is haemorrhage, more likely when a cavotomy is required. Preoperative blood typing would have been required if our patient had received previous blood transfusions (Tocci and Ewing, 2009). Preoperative coagulation parameters may allow for preoperative management of any abnormalities detected. Hypercoagulability has classically been described as a consequence of hyperadrenocorticism. However, this has recently been disputed in dogs (Klose et al., 2011). This patient had no preoperative clinical signs of

hyper- or hypo-coagulopathies, therefore coagulation parameters were not measured. Having pre-emptively placed large bore peripheral IV catheters in the patient and also the placement of resuscitative fluids in theatre meant that rapid treatment of major haemorrhage could occur. The swab gravimetric method has been reported to accurately quantify intraoperative haemorrhage in dogs (Lee et al., 2006). Therefore, the additional measurement of haemoglobin concentration of the suction fluid to approximate the volume of haemorrhage was likely unnecessary, as this technique is reportedly of similar accuracy to the gravimetric technique (Clark et al., 2010).

The ideal anaesthetic protocol for adrenalectomies should maintain homeostasis despite potential sudden physiological changes. Surgical manipulation of the adrenal gland can lead to a catecholamine surge and subsequent cardiovascular manifestations, regardless of the adrenal tumour type present (Lang et al., 2011). The anaesthetic protocol should also provide analgesia and muscle relaxation.

Premedication with a pure mu agonist such as methadone (Kyles et al., 2003; Massari et al., 2011) provides pre-emptive analgesia, sedation and a reduction in the required inhalant minimum alveolar concentration (MAC) with minimal cardiovascular effects. Previous studies report the use of an opioid-benzodiazepine combination in dogs undergoing adrenalectomy (Jiménez Peláez et al., 2008; Lang et al., 2011). Benzodiazepines cause minimal cardiovascular depression; however, in adult dogs the sedation can be unreliable and dysphoria may occur (Sanchez et al., 2013). Sedation with acepromazine may provide benefit to hypertensive patients due to the α-1 adrenergic blockade it produces (Monteiro et al., 2007). However, the prolonged and irreversible duration of action of acepromazine may impede the treatment of hypotension during anaesthesia. In this case, medetomidine was selected to provide sedation and MAC reduction of isoflurane beyond that of an opioid alone (Lerche and Muir III, 2006). An additional benefit of medetomidine is the profound sympatholytic effect attributable to central α2-adrenoreceptor activation, which may partially counteract the effect of a catecholamine surge (Väisänen et al., 2002). The marked cardiovascular effects caused by α-2 agonists such as decreased cardiac output and transient hypertension are dose-dependent and short acting, and an antagonist drug is available (Pypendop and Verstegen, 1998).

Previous studies describe the use of propofol (Jiménez Peláez et al., 2008), etomidate or propofol co-administered with midazolam (Lang et al., 2011) as induction agents prior to adrenalectomy. In a paper describing anaesthesia protocols for humans undergoing adrenalectomies, etomidate was avoided due to its ability to suppress the adrenocortical axis and thus production of mineralo- and gluco-corticosteroids (Domi and Sula, 2011). In contrast, Dabbagh *et al.* (2009) reported infusing etomidate to control the clinical signs of hyperadrenocorticism preoperatively. Our choice of co-induction with propofol and diazepam has been described in the veterinary literature (Robinson and Borer-Weir, 2013; Sanchez *et al.*, 2013), although the only benzodiazepine achieving a significant reduction in propofol dose has been midazolam. However, most patients in the study from Robinson and Borer-Weir (2013) were healthy dogs of ASA status 1 or 2, with an insufficient number of ASA 3 dogs in the treatment group to speculate association with ASA category. In our clinical experience, benzodiazepenes as co-induction agents at lower doses than those published often reduce the induction agent dose required in debilitated patients. All published reports utilise inhalant techniques for the maintenance of anaesthesia (Jiménez Peláez *et al.*, 2008; Lang *et al.*, 2011). Isoflurane was used in this case as the maintenance agent because sevoflurane was unavailable. The acute episode of severe vasoconstriction, hypertension and reflex bradycardia that occurred during adrenal gland manipulation was likely due to a catecholamine surge. The vasodilatory effect of isoflurane was utilised to manage this event. Ideally, anti-hypertensive drugs should be short-acting and titratable to effect. The use of sevoflurane may have allowed for more rapid changes in ET agent concentrations due to its lower blood-gas coefficient (Lopez *et al.*, 2009). Other reportedly used vasoactive drugs such as phentolamine (Kyles *et al.*, 2003), a short acting competitive α-1 adrenergic blocking drug, or sodium nitroprusside (SNP) (Kyles *et al.*, 2003; Lang *et al.*, 2011) were unavailable. One study reported that the vasodilation induced by isoflurane was advocated to maintain better overall tissue perfusion than SNP (Humm *et al.*, 2007). On this occasion, the short action of phentolamine would have been more suitable than acepromazine to provide additional vasodilation. Acepromazine likely contributed to the subsequent mild hypotension. Furthermore, the long and irreversibly action of acepromazine may have impeded management of blood pressure were it to worsen (Monteiro *et al.*, 2007). If the reflex bradycardia had not responded to the induction of vasodilation, treatment with an anticholinergic such as atropine would have been indicated.

Tachyarrhythmias commonly occur due to adrenal gland manipulation, nociceptive input or in response to hypotension. Supraventricular tachycardias (SVT) and ventricular arrhythmias (Kyles *et al.*, 2003; Lang *et al.*, 2011) have been reported during adrenalectomy. In this instance, opioids successfully treated the supraventricular tachycardia by reducing both sympathetic tone and nociception as reported in older studies. A more recent paper (Garofalo

et al., 2008) failed to demonstrate a protective effect of remifentanil against ventricular arrhythmias induced by adrenaline in halothane-anaesthetised dogs. Myocardial sensitization to catecholamine-induced arrhythmias by halothane as used in Garofalo's study may have made tachyarrythmias more difficult to treat compared to isoflurane. The second-line treatment for SVT would have been ultra short-acting beta-blockers such as esmolol (Kyles *et al.*, 2003; Lang *et al.*, 2011). If ventricular arrhythmias had occurred, treatment with higher doses of lidocaine or with procainamide would have been indicated (Lang *et al.*, 2011).

Multimodal analgesia was provided with the co-administration of fentanyl and lidocaine; the latter also for its MAC sparing (Valverde *et al.*, 2004) and antiarrhythmic properties (Bruchim *et al.*, 2012). Opioids have been used in all published studies, with hydromorphone, methadone, morphine and fentanyl infusions reported (Jiménez Peláez *et al.*, 2008; Lang *et al.*, 2011). Nonsteroidal anti-inflammatory drugs (NSAIDs) were avoided as they may precipitate gastrointestinal ulceration in patients with excess glucocorticoids (Kukanich *et al.*, 2012). To avoid this, paracetamol was preferred as an adjunctive analgesic in this case (Benitez *et al.*, 2015).

Neuromuscular blockade may facilitate surgical approaches to deep structures during laparotomies (Clarke *et al.*, 2014) but has only been described in one veterinary paper describing adrenalectomies (Lang *et al.*, 2011). In a case report of two human adrenalectomies (Domi and Sula, 2011), cis-atracurium was selected for its short duration of action and plasma degradation; for similar reasons, atracurium was administered to our patient.

Post-operative complications occur with high incidence following adrenalectomies (30% according to Lang *et al.* (2011)), necessitating close monitoring in ICU settings. Reported complications include hypo- or hyper-tension, arrhythmias, vomiting, oesophagitis, seizures, pancreatitis, acute renal failure, haemoperitoneum, hyperthermia, hypokalaemia, tachypnoea and cardiopulmonary arrest (Kyles *et al.*, 2003; Lang *et al.*, 2011 Gójska-zygner *et al.*, 2012). Many complications relate to inadequate function of the remaining adrenal gland, leading to acute adrenal insufficiency and crisis. Corticoid administration using various protocols in the perioperative period features in all published studies. Most commonly reported is glucocorticoid supplementation with dexamethasone once the adrenal tumour is removed, followed by administration of prednisolone in the recovery period (Kyles *et al.*, 2003; Lang *et al.*, 2011). In this case, as commonly occurs, it was unknown whether the remaining hypoplastic adrenal gland was capable of producing sufficient corticoids postoperatively. Therefore, a single postoperative dose of prednisolone was administered to provide additional glucocorticoid support for recovery from the physiological stress of anaesthesia and surgery. Close monitoring of vital signs was undertaken to detect signs of an adrenal crisis, such as cardiovascular shock or vomiting. Serum electrolytes were measured every six hours in the early postoperative period to identify any acute mineralocorticoid deficiency and prompt treatment if required. The only identified postoperative complication in our case was mild hypertension, which responded to the administration of acepromazine.

In conclusion, the anaesthetic management for adrenalectomies is challenging because of the high incidence of severe complications. A good understanding of the physiological derangements that may be induced by both the tumour itself and the surgical procedure is required. Adequate preparations for anticipated problems, including availability of resuscitative fluids and short-acting drugs, will minimize patient morbidity and mortality.

References

Barrera, J.S., Bernard, F., Ehrhart, E.J., Withrow, S.J. and Monnet, E. 2013. Evaluation of risk factors for outcome associated with adrenal gland tumors with or without invasion of the caudal vena cava and treated via adrenalectomy in dogs: 86 cases (1993-2009). J. Am. Vet. Med. Assoc. 242(12), 1715-1721.

Benitez, M.E., Roush, J.K., McMurphy, R., KuKanich, B. and Legallet, C. 2015. Clinical efficacy of hydrocodone-acetaminophen and tramadol for control of postoperative pain in dogs following tibial plateau leveling osteotomy. Am. J. Vet. Res. 76(9), 755-762.

Brodbelt, D.C., Blissitt, K.J., Hammond, R.A., Neath, P.J., Young, L.E., Pfeiffer, D.U. and Wood, J.L. 2008. The risk of death: Confidential Enquiry into Perioperative Small Animal Fatalities. Vet. Anaesth. Analg. 35(5), 365-373.

Bruchim, Y., Itay, S., Shira, B.H., Kelmer, E., Sigal, Y., Itamar, A. and Gilad, S. 2012. Evaluation of lidocaine treatment on frequency of cardiac arrhythmias, acute kidney injury, and hospitalization time in dogs with gastric dilatation volvulus. J. Vet. Emerg. Crit. Care 22(4), 419-27.

Clark, L., Corletto, F. and Garosi, L.S. 2010. Comparison of a method using the Hemocue near patient testing device with a standard method of haemorrhage estimation in dogs. Vet. Anaesth. Analg. 37(1), 44-47.

Clarke, K.W., Trim, C.M. and Hall, L.W. (eds). 2014. Veterinary Anaesthesia, 11th ed. London: Saunders Elsevier, pp: 169-194.

Dabbagh, A., Sa'adat, N. and Heidari, Z. 2009. Etomidate infusion in the critical care setting for suppressing the acute phase of Cushing's syndrome.

Anesth. Analg. 108(1), 238-239.

Domi, R. and Sula, H. 2011. Cushing syndrome and the anesthesiologist, two case reports. Indian J. Endocrinol. Metab. 15(3), 209-213.

Garofalo, N.A., Teixeira-Neto, F.J., Schwartz, D.S., do Carmo, F., Vailati, M. and Steagall, P.V.M. 2008. Effects of the opioid remifentanil on the arrhythmogenicity of epinephrine in halothane-anesthetized dogs. Can. J. Vet. Res. 72(4), 362-366.

Gójska-zygner, O., Lechowski, R. and Zygner, W. 2012. Functioning unilateral adrenocortical carcinoma in a dog. Can. Vet. J. 53(6), 623-625.

Herrera, M.A., Mehl, M.L., Kass, P.H., Pascoe, P.J., Feldman, E.C. and Nelson, R.W. 2008. Predictive factors and the effect of phenoxybenzamine on outcome in dogs undergoing adrenalectomy for pheochromocytoma. J. Vet. Intern. Med. 22(6), 1333-1339.

Humm, K.R., Senior, J.M., Dugdale, A.H. and Summerfield, N.J. 2007. Use of sodium nitroprusside in the anaesthetic protocol of a patent ductus arteriosus ligation in a dog. Vet. J. 173(1), 194-196.

Jiménez Peláez, M., Bouvy, B.M. and Dupré, G.P. 2008. Laparoscopic adrenalectomy for treatment of unilateral adrenocortical carcinomas: technique, complications, and results in seven dogs. Vet. Surg. 37(5), 444-453.

Johnson, C. and Norman, E.J. 2007. 'Endocrine disease', in Seymour, C. and Duke-Novakovski, T. (eds), BSAVA Manual of Canine and Feline Anaesthesia and Analgesia, 2nd edn. Gloucester, UK: British Small Animal Veterinary Association.

Klose, T.C., Creevy, K.E. and Brainard, B.M. 2011. Evaluation of coagulation status in dogs with naturally occurring canine hyperadrenocorticism. J. Vet. Emerg. Crit. Care 21(6), 625-632.

KuKanich, B., Bidgood, T. and Knesl, O. 2012. Clinical pharmacology of nonsteroidal anti-inflammatory drugs in dogs. Vet. Anaesth. Analg. 39(1), 69-90.

Kyles, A.E., Feldman, E.C., De Cock, H.E., Kass, P.H., Mathews, K.G., Hardie, E.M., Nelson, R.W., Ilkiw, J.E. and Gregory, C.R. 2003. Surgical management of adrenal gland tumors with and without associated tumor thrombi in dogs: 40 cases (1994-2001). J. Am. Vet. Med. Assoc. 223(5), 654-662.

Lang, J.M., Schertel, E., Kennedy, S., Wilson, D., Barnhart, M. and Danielson, B. 2011. Elective and emergency surgical management of adrenal gland tumors: 60 cases (1999-2006). J. Am. Anim. Hosp. Assoc. 47(6), 428-435.

Lee, M.H., Ingversten, B.T., Kirpensteijn, J., Jensen, A.L. and Kristensen, A.T. 2006. Quantification of surgical blood loss. Vet. Surg. 35(4), 388-393.

Lerche, P. and Muir III, W.W. 2006. Effect of medetomidine on respiration and minimum alveolar concentration in halothane- and isoflurane-anesthetized dogs. Am. J. Vet. Res. 67(5), 782-789.

Lopez, L.A., Hofmeister, E.H., Pavez, J.C. and Brainard, B.M. 2009. Comparison of recovery from anesthesia with isoflurane, sevoflurane, or desflurane in healthy dogs. Am. J. Vet. Res. 70(11), 1339-1344.

Massari, F., Nicoli, S., Romanelli, G., Buracco, P. and Zini, E. 2011. Adrenalectomy in dogs with adrenal gland tumors: 52 cases (2002-2008). J. Am. Vet. Med. Assoc. 239(2), 216-221.

Monteiro, E.R., Teixeira Neto, F.J., Castro, V.B. and Campagnol, D. 2007. Effects of acepromazine on the cardiovascular actions of dopamine in anesthetized dogs. Vet. Anaesth. Analg. 34(5), 312-321.

Naan, E.C., Kirpensteijn, J., Dupré, G.P., Galac, S. and Radlinsky, M.G. 2013. Innovative approach to laparoscopic adrenalectomy for treatment of unilateral adrenal gland tumors in dogs. Vet. Surg. 42(6), 710-715.

Pypendop, B.H. and Verstegen, J.P. 1998. Hemodynamic effects of medetomidine in the dog: a dose titration study. Vet. Surg. 27(6), 612-622.

Robinson, R. and Borer-Weir, K. 2013. A dose titration study into the effects of diazepam or midazolam on the propofol dose requirements for induction of general anaesthesia in client owned dogs, premedicated with methadone and acepromazine. Vet. Anaesth. Analg. 40(5), 455-463.

Sanchez, A., Belda, E., Escobar, M., Agut, A., Soler, M. and Laredo, F.G. 2013. Effects of altering the sequence of midazolam and propofol during co-induction of anaesthesia. Vet. Anaesth. Analg. 40(4), 359-366.

Smith, R.R., Mayhew, P.D. and Berent, A.C. 2012. Laparoscopic adrenalectomy for management of a functional adrenal tumor in a cat. J. Am. Vet. Med. Assoc. 241(3), 368-372.

Tocci, L.J. and Ewing, P.J. 2009. Increasing patient safety in veterinary transfusion medicine: an overview of pretransfusion testing. J. Vet. Emerg. Crit. Care 19(1), 66-73.

Väisänen, M., Raekallio, M., Kuusela, E., Huttunen, P., Leppäluoto, J., Kirves, P. and Vainio, O. 2002. Evaluation of the perioperative stress response in dogs administered medetomidine or acepromazine as part of the preanesthetic medication. Am. J. Vet. Res. 63(7), 969-975.

Valverde, A., Doherty, T.J., Hernández, J. and Davies, W. 2004. Effect of lidocaine on the minimum alveolar concentration of isoflurane in dogs. Vet. Anaesth. Analg. 31(4), 264-271.

12

Contagious equine metritis in Portugal: A retrospective report of the first outbreak in the country and recent contagious equine metritis test results

T. Rocha*

Bacteriology Laboratory, National Reference Laboratory for CEM, Instituto Nacional de Investigação Agrária e Veterinária- INIAV (National Institute of Agrarian and Veterinary Research), Avenida da República, Quinta do Marquês, 2784-157 Oeiras, Portugal

Abstract

Contagious equine metritis (CEM), a highly contagious bacterial venereal infection of equids, caused by *Taylorella equigenitalis*, is of major international concern, causing short-term infertility in mares. Portugal has a long tradition of horse breeding and exportation and until recently was considered CEM-free. However, in 2008, *T. equigenitalis* was isolated at our laboratory from a recently imported stallion and 2 mares from the same stud. Following this first reported outbreak, the Portuguese Veterinary Authority (DGAV) performed mandatory testing on all remaining equines at the stud (n=30), resulting in a further 4 positive animals. All positive animals were treated and subsequently tested negative for *T. equigenitalis*. Since this outbreak, over 2000 genital swabs from Portuguese horses have been tested at our laboratory, with no further positive animals identified. The available data suggests that this CEM outbreak was an isolated event and we have no further evidence of CEM cases in Portugal, however, an extended and wider epidemiological study would be needed to better evaluate the incidence of the disease in Portuguese horses.

Keywords: Contagious disease, Contagious equine metritis, Equine, Reproduction, *Taylorella equigenitalis*.

Introduction

Contagious equine metritis (CEM), a highly contagious venereal disease of horses, is of major international concern, with important repercussions for the horse industry. It was first reported as a previously undescribed disease of horses in the United Kingdom and Ireland (Crowhurst, 1977; Platt *et al.*, 1977), where it ravaged the Thoroughbreds racing industry in the late 70's and early 80's. Since then, the disease has been recorded in various horse breeds world-wide (Timoney, 1996; Ozgur *et al.*, 2001). The causative agent of CEM was first described as *Haemophilus equigenitalis* (Taylor *et al.*, 1978) and later classified into a new genus as *Taylorella equigenitalis* (Sugimoto *et al.*, 1983). Two biotypes have been identified, either sensitive or resistant to streptomycin (Platt and Taylor, 1982). The acute infection in mares can cause endometritis, cervicitis or vaginitis of variable severity (with a mucopurulent vaginal discharge ranging from minimal to copious), that usually result in temporary infertility and, rarely, in abortion; clinical recovery occurs in the majority of cases, but some mares may become carriers and foals infected at foaling can become long-term, sub-clinical carriers (Eaglesome and Garcia, 1979; Timoney and Powell, 1982; Timoney, 1996). Many primary cases of infection with *T. equigenitalis* in the mare are subclinical and a frequent indicator of infection is a mare returning to oestrus prematurely after being bred to a putative carrier stallion (OIE, 2012). Infected stallions are not clinically affected and act as asymptomatic carriers for months or years if not treated, transmitting the disease to mares by sexual contact or artificial insemination. Transmission can also occur through inadvertent contamination of fomites during handling of the equines at time of breeding (Timoney, 1996; Schulman *et al.*, 2013). The isolation and identification of *Taylorella equigenitalis* is the OIE (World Organization for Animal Health) approved method for diagnosis and the prescribed method for the international trade (OIE, 2012).

Portugal has a long tradition of horse breeding and exportation to many countries, and there is an increasing interest in the Lusitano horse, both within the country and internationally. Until recently, Portugal was considered CEM-free, however, in May 2008, *T. equigenitalis* was isolated for the first time (Rocha, 2014). This communication reports on the laboratory findings of this outbreak and subsequent follow up, as well as routine CEM testing data at the Instituto Nacional de Investigação Agrária e Veterinária (INIAV) for the following years, up to the present date.

Materials and Methods

Animals tested

Following the detection of the first positive case of *T. equigenitalis* in Portugal, from an imported stallion, in May 2008 (Rocha, 2014) and from 2 mares at the same stud in June, mandatory testing of all remaining equines

*Corresponding Author: Teresa Rocha. Instituto Nacional de Investigação Agrária e Veterinária- INIAV, Avenida da República, Quinta do Marquês, 2784-157 Oeiras, Portugal. Email: *teresa.rocha@iniav.pt*

on the premises was performed by the Portuguese veterinary authority in Portugal (Direcção Geral de Alimentação e Veterinária - DGAV), consisting of 30 animals, 8 stallions and 22 mares. In addition to the animals involved in the outbreak, a total of 2070 swabs from apparently healthy Portuguese equines, 437 (21.1%) from mares and 1633 (78.9%) from stallions, were tested in our laboratory between May 2008 and the end of 2015. These swabs were taken from horses due for export or prior to breeding or semen collection and exportation. The 2070 samples corresponded to a total of unique 736 animals (413 stallions and 323 mares). The geographical distribution of those 736 horses can be seen in Figure 1. Most of the horses originated from the main horse breeding regions in continental Portugal: Lisboa e Setúbal (43.3%), Estremadura e Ribatejo (26.8%) and Alentejo (17.4%).

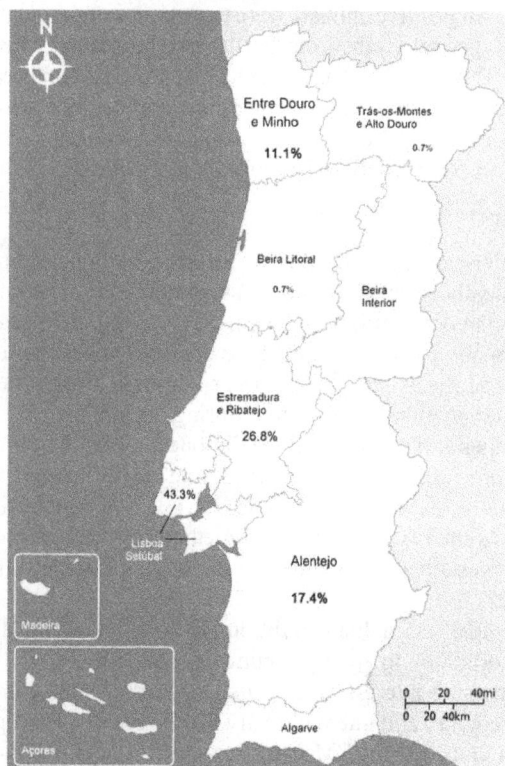

Fig. 1. Geographical distribution of the 736 horses (2070 samples) submitted for routine CEM testing at the INIAV between 2008 and 2015.

In what concerns the breeds of the tested animals, all outbreak animals were from the Lusitano breed; From the 736 horses further tested for CEM screening, only 326 of them had mention to the race on the files submitted to our laboratory and 71% of those were the Lusitano breed, while the remaining belonged to several breeds, like Arabian, Selle Francais, Holsteiner, Hanoverian, Portuguese Cruzado, Portuguese-sport-horse, Pure Spanish Race and Dutch KWPN.

Quality control at our laboratory

T. equigenitalis is very difficult to isolate owing to its fastidious nature and the concomitant presence of commensal or other bacteria and possibly fungi in the genital tract of the horse. INIAV is the national reference laboratory for CEM in Portugal and since 2006 has participated in a Quality Assessment Scheme organized by the OIE reference laboratory for CEM (VLA, Bury St. Edmunds, UK),

Sampling and transport of samples to the laboratory

During the outbreak investigation, swabs were taken from the clitoral fossa and uterus in mares (2 swabs/anatomical site/mare) and in stallions 2 swabs were taken, one from the urethra and urethral fossa (fossa glandis) and another from the penis and penile sheath (prepuce). The swabbing protocols in screening for CEM diagnosis and recommended anatomical sites have been described previously and these procedures are a part of the veterinary practice in handling equines (Watson, 1997; HBLB, 2004). The 2070 samples for routine testing were, in mares, from the clitoris/clitoral fossa and, in stallions from the above mentioned anatomical sites as well as semen. However, occasionally only preputial/penis samples were submitted from the stallions.

All swabs were submerged in Amies charcoal transport medium and transported under cool conditions to the laboratory to be cultured within 48 hours of collection (HBLB, 2004; OIE, 2012). Only swabs under those conditions are accepted for CEM testing at the INIAV. The sterile swabs in Amies charcoal transport medium for sampling are available commercially, so they can be purchased by the veterinaries, but most of them were collected from our laboratory, since they are always granted by the INIAV when requested by the veterinaries as part of each of the analysis to be done at the INIAV.

Bacteriological isolation methods and identification of positives

Culture media were prepared at the INIAV and both the culturing and the identification of *T. equigenitalis* isolates were performed according to recommended procedures (OIE, 2012), including latex agglutination (Monotayl, Bionor Laboratories, Skien, Norway). Three different "chocolate" blood agar media were used, one with no inhibitors (inhibitors may prevent the isolation of some strains of *T. equigenitalis*), one containing streptomycin sulphate (200 µg/ml) to allow for the differentiation of Streptomycin-sensitive or resistant biotypes, and the third medium according to Timoney *et al.* (1982), a medium with inhibitors, containing 1 µg/ml trimethoprim, 5µg/ml clindamycin and 5 µg/ml amphotericin B, which allows the growth of both streptomycin resistant and sensitive biotypes and is particularly useful to suppress growth of commensal bacteria and inhibit fungal growth (OIE, 2012).

Plates were incubated at 37° C in a 5% (v/v) CO_2 incubator and an incubation period of 10 days with no growth of suspect colonies was allowed before considering specimens negative for *T. equigenitalis.*

The first T. equigenitalis strain isolated in Portugal (strain 18456) (Rocha, 2014) was sent for confirmation to the OIE reference laboratory for CEM (VLA, Bury St. Edmunds, UK), which was done both by observation of the phenotypic characteristics and by real-time PCR (Wakeley *et al.*, 2006). All other 6 isolates obtained during the outbreak investigation, from the first 2 positive mares (M1 and M2) and the next 3 positive mares and 1 stallion (M3, M4, M5 and St2), besides the phenotypic and monoclonal antibodies identification as *T. equigenitallis*, were further tested at the INIAV according to the method described by Anzai *et al.* (1999), a single step PCR test in a 2% agarose gel, using the primer set P1-N2, which amplifies a 445-bp DNA fragment of *T. equigenitallis*, allowing for its specific detection (Fig. 2).

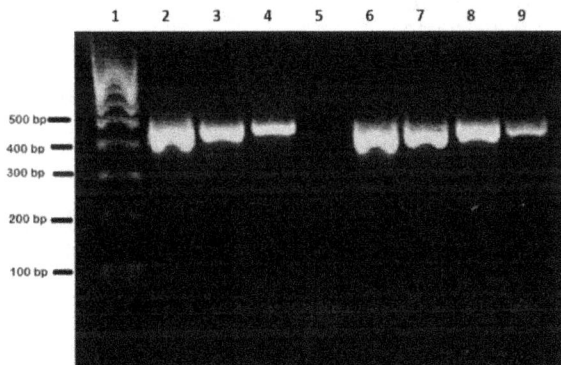

Fig. 2. PCR amplification of total DNAs of *T. equigenitalis* field isolates obtained from the CEM outbreak by single-step PCR with primer set P1-N2 in 2% agarose gel. Lane 1: Molecular weight marker *HyperLadder IV*-100bp; Lane 2: M1; Lane 3: M2; Lane 4: St 2; Lane 5: Negative control (water); Lane 6: M3; Lane 7: M4; Lane 8: M5; Lane 9: Positive control (*T. equigenitalis* strain from Veterinary Laboratories Agency-VLA, Bury St. Edmunds, UK).

Treatment of positive animals and collection of samples after treatment

Stallions and mares were treated by thoroughly cleaning the extended penis (stallions) or the clitoral area (mares) with chlorhexidine surgical scrub and then applying nitrofurazone ointment. The treatment is done daily for 5 days, and the animals retested 8-10 days after treatment. Following treatment, 3 sets of genital swabs from all positive horses, taken approximately 10 days apart, were submitted for the bacteriological testing for *T. equigenitalis.*

All treatment and swab collection was undertaken by a competent veterinary surgeon designated by the DGAV.

Results

The identity of the first *T. equigenitalis* isolation in Portugal (strain 18456, from a recently imported stallion) was confirmed by the OIE reference laboratory for CEM (VLA, Bury St. Edmunds, UK). In addition to 2 positive mares identified in June 2008, mandatory testing of all remaining equines at the stud (n=30) resulted in the isolation of *T. equigenitalis* from a further 4 animals, 3 mares and 1 stallion. All strains were sensitive to streptomycin.

Following treatment, all *T. equigenitalis*-positive equines tested negative on 3 serial cultures of genital swabs taken 10 days apart.

Since May 2008 to date, all bacteriological cultures performed at our laboratory of 2070 genital swabs from stallions and mares from various Portuguese stud farms, have yielded negative results for *T. equigenitalis.*

Discussion

Since CEM was first recognized as an emergent disease of equids in 1977, the causal agent, *T. equigenitalis*, has attained worldwide distribution owing to the shipment of carrier stallions and mares both within and between countries and sporadic epizootics have been confirmed in equine populations in over 29 countries in Europe and North and South America, as well as in Japan and Australia (Timoney, 2011; Schulman *et al.*, 2013). Horse importing countries outside Europe, like the USA, have considered all countries of the European Union, and a small number of other European countries outside the EU, to be affected with this disease (USDA-APHIS, 2014), despite that information on its occurrence in Europe is scarce.

International transparency regarding the presence of CEM in a country, as well as on the actions undertaken to prevent and control its spread would be very beneficial to individual horse breeders and to the international equine trade as a whole and will ultimately assist in preventing the spread of the disease and improving the general health status of equines worldwide.

Portugal has a long tradition of horse breeding and exportation to many countries, (including the UK, Brazil, Colombia and the U.S.A.). There is increasing interest in the Lusitano horse, both within the country and internationally, and there is also an increased demand for assisted reproductive techniques such as artificial insemination in the horse industry. The control of venereally-transmitted diseases is crucial to any breeding program or for successful export, and genital swabs are regularly collected from Portuguese horses and submitted to our laboratory for *T. equigenitalis* screening.

The isolation of *T. equigenitalis* in Portugal for the first time in 2008 produced major concern in the equine industry. *T. equigenitalis* was first isolated from a recently imported stallion from Germany, which entered Portugal with a negative certificate for *T. equigenitalis*. The exact origin of this infection could not be confirmed with the information available to the INIAV. Although 2 positive mares were detected on the same premises shortly after the stallion, it could not be confirmed whether the stallion was used for breeding prior to testing at our laboratory, thereby acquiring *T. equigenitalis* from those mares, or if the stallion was a carrier of *T. equigenitalis* despite his negative CEM certificate and had in fact transmitted the infection to the mares.

Outbreak investigation confirmed a further 4 *T. equigenitalis*-positive animals and following treatment and repeat serial negative post-treatment testing, the outbreak was considered controlled by the DGAV.

The isolation of *T. equigenitalis* from a stallion believed to be negative for *T. equigenitalis* reinforces the insidious nature of this disease and reiterates the fact that effective prevention and control of CEM must include a comprehensive testing program to allow for early detection and treatment of carriers animals, particularly stallions.

This paper reports the first occurrence of *T. equigenitalis* in Portugal, a country previously considered free of CEM. This outbreak was limited to one stud, where all positive animals were subsequently treated and tested negative on following up testing. These facts and the subsequent negative testing of over 2000 equine samples from 2008 to present at our laboratory, suggest that this was an isolated outbreak. However, a more extensive monitoring would be useful and required to monitor the incidence of CEM and identify possible further incursions of the disease into Portugal, given the insidious nature of the disease, the international trade in horses across borders and the constant presence of *T. equigenitalis* in neighboring European countries (Fig. 3) creating ideal conditions for spread of the disease.

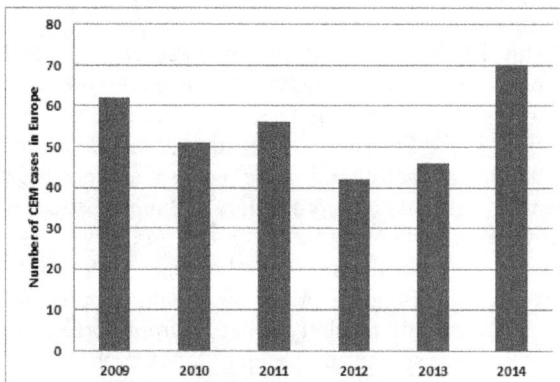

Fig. 3. Number of CEM cases in Europe, 2009-2014. (Source: EU Reference Laboratory for equine diseases, Anses, France).

Conflict of interest:
The author declares that there is no conflict of interest.

Acknowledgments
The author wishes to thank Conceição Baptista and Ana Vaz for the preparation of media for *T. equigenitalis* isolation; Mr. Paul Todd, Work Group Leader and OIE Test consultant for CEMO (VLA, Bury St. Edmunds) for technical advice and both Mr. Paul Todd and the VLA team for the confirmation of the identification of strain 18456, the first *T. equigenitalis* isolate in Portugal; Lurdes Clemente for technical help in further testing the *T. equigenitalis* isolates by PCR; Sandrine Petry, from the EU Reference Laboratory for Equine Diseases for the granting of data on number of cases of CEM in European countries.

References

Anzai, T., Eguchi, M., Sekizaki, T., Kamada, M., Yamamoto, K. and Okuda, T. 1999. Development of a PCR test for rapid diagnosis of contagious equine metritis. J. Vet. Med. Sci. 61, 1287-1292.

Crowhurst, R.C. 1977. Genital infection in mares. Vet. Rec. 100(22), 476.

Eaglesome, M.D. and Garcia, M.M. 1979. Contagious Equine Metritis: A Review. Can. Vet. J. 20, 201-206.

HBLB. 2004. HORSERACE BETTING LEVY BOARD Codes of Practice on Contagious equine metritis (CEM), Equine viral arteritis (EVA), Equine herpesvirus (EHV), Guidelines on strangles. Edited by: L. Archer and J.F. Wade.

OIE. 2012. Chapter 2.5.2 : Contagious Equine Metritis. OIE Terrestrial Manual. http://www.oie.int/fileadmin/Home/fr/Health_stan dards/tahm/2.05.02_CEM.pdf.

Ozgur, N.Y., Ikiz, S., Carioglu, B., Kilicarslan, R., Yilmaz, H., Akay, O. and Ligaz, A. 2001. Contagious equine metritis in Turkey: first isolation of *Taylorella equigenitalis* from mares. Vet. Rec. 149, 120-122.

Platt, H. and Taylor, C.E.D. 1982. Contagious Equine Metritis. In: Med. Microbiol., Vol. I. Eds: Easmon, C.S.F. and Jeljaszewicz, J., Academic Press, London, pp: 49-96.

Platt, H., Atherton, J.G., Simpson, D.J., Taylor, C.E.D., Rosenthal, R.O., Brown, D.F.J. and Wreghitt, T.G. 1977. Genital infection in mares. Vet. Rec. 101, 20.

Rocha, T. 2014. Metrite Contagiosa Equina em Portugal: Diagnóstico Laboratorial, primeiros casos positivos e dados subsequentes. In the Proceedings of the VIth Congress of the Portuguese Society of Veterinary Medicine, INIAV Oeiras, Portugal, 3-5 April 2014, pp: 233.

Schulman, M.L., May, C.E., Keys, B. and Guthrie, A.J. 2013. Contagious equine metritis: Artificial reproduction changes the epidemiologic paradigm. Vet. Microbiol. 167(1-2), 2-8.

Sugimoto, C., Isayama, Y., Sakazaki, R. and Kuramochi, S. 1983. Transfer of *Haemophilus equigenitalis* Taylor et al., 1978 to the genus *Taylorella* gen. nov. as *Taylorella equigenitalis* comb.-nov. Curr. Microbiol. 9, 155-162.

Taylor, C.E., Rosenthal, R.O., Brown, D.F.J., Lapage, S.P., Hill, L.R. and Legros, R.M. 1978. The causative organism of contagious equine metritis 1977: proposal for a new species to be known as *Haemophilus equigenitalis*. Equine Vet. J. 10(3), 136-144.

Timoney, P.J. 1996. Contagious equine metritis. Comp. Immunol. Microbiol. Infec. Dis. 19(3), 199-204.

Timoney, P.J. 2011. Horse Species Symposium: Contagious Equine Metritis: An insidious threat to the horse breeding industry in the United States. J. Anim. Sci. 89(5), 1552-1560.

Timoney, P.J. and Powell, D.G. 1982. Isolation of the contagious equine metritis organism from colts and fillies in the United Kingdom and Ireland. Vet. Rec. 111, 478-482.

Timoney, P.J., Shin, S.J. and Jacobson, R.H. 1982. Improved selective medium for isolation of the contagious equine metritis organism. Vet. Rec. 111, 107-108.

USDA-APHIS. 2014. United States Department of Agriculture - Animal and Plant Health Inspection Service (USDA-APHIS) Factsheet, May 2014.

Wakeley, P.R., Errington, J., Hannon, S., Roest, H.I.J., Carson, T., Hunt, B., Sawyer, J. and Heath, P. 2006. Development of a real-time PCR for the detection of *Taylorella equigenitalis* directly from genital swabs and discrimination from *Taylorella asinigenitalis*. Vet. Microbiol. 118, 247-254.

Watson, E. 1997. Swabbing protocols in screening for contagious equine metritis. Vet. Rec. 140, 268-271.

13

Cryptosporidium varanii infection in leopard geckos (*Eublepharis macularius*) in Argentina

A. Dellarupe[1,2], J.M. Unzaga[1,]*, G. Moré[1,2], M. Kienast[3], A. Larsen[4], C. Stiebel[5], M. Rambeaud[1,2] and M.C. Venturini[1]

[1]*Laboratorio de Inmunoparasitología, Facultad de Ciencias Veterinarias, Universidad Nacional de La Plata, 60 y 118, 1900 La Plata, Argentina*
[2]*Consejo Nacional de Investigaciones Científicas y Técnicas (CONICET), Buenos Aires, Argentina*
[3]*Instituto de Genética Veterinaria (IGEVET), CCT La Plata, CONICET, Facultad de Ciencias Veterinarias, Universidad Nacional de La Plata, La Plata, Argentina*
[4]*Cátedra de Inmunología Veterinaria, Facultad de Ciencias Veterinarias, Universidad Nacional de La Plata, La Plata, Argentina*
[5]*Dpto. Zoonosis, Municipalidad Gral. San Martín, Prov. de Buenos Aires, Argentina*

Abstract

Cryptosporidiosis is observed in reptiles with high morbidity and considerable mortality. The objective of this study was to achieve the molecular identification of *Cryptosporidium* spp. in pet leopard geckos (*Eublepharis macularius*) from a breeder colony in Buenos Aires, Argentina. Oocysts comparable to those of *Cryptosporidium* spp. were detected in three geckos with a history of diarrhea, anorexia and cachexia. Molecular identification methods confirmed the presence of *Cryptosporidium varanii* (syn. *C. saurophilum*). This agent was considered to be the primary cause of the observed clinical disease. This is the first description of *C. varanii* infection in pet reptiles in Argentina.

Keywords: Argentina, *Cryptosporidium* spp., Leopard gecko (*Eublepharis macularius*), PCR, Sequencing.

Introduction

Cryptosporidium infection (referred as cryptosporidiosis) is a zoonosis of worldwide distribution that affects the gastrointestinal tract of a range of vertebrate hosts, including mammals, reptiles, birds and fish (Fayer, 2010). Cryptosporidiosis in humans is a cause of diarrhea, mainly in children, and could cause a severe disease in immunocompromised patients (Xiao *et al.*, 2004a). Cryptosporidiosis has been described in many different reptile species, and is especially important in snakes and lizards. Two main *Cryptosporidium* species have been identified in reptiles: *C. serpentis* and *C. varanii* (syn. *C. saurophilum*). *C. serpentis* is a gastric parasite found mainly in snakes, and frequently associated with prominent clinical signs like anorexia, postprandial regurgitation, lethargy, mid-body swelling, and weight loss, while infections in lizards are usually asymptomatic (Fayer *et al.*, 1997). *C. varanii* is an intestinal parasite found primarily in lizards (Pavlasek and Ryan, 2008; Xiao *et al.*, 2004b) and can cause anorexia, progressive weight loss, abdominal swelling and high mortality, particularly in juvenile lizards (Koudela and Modry, 1998). Other *Cryptosporidium* spp. have been described in reptiles like *C. muris, C. parvum, C. parvum* mouse genotype (syn. *C. tyzzeri*). However, these *Cryptosporidium* spp. oocyst could represent a passage of parasites from ingested prey or feeder mice (Xiao *et al.*, 2004b).

Reptiles are becoming popular pets worldwide; however, little is known about the presence and control of cryptosporidiosis in this animal population. In the last several years, cryptosporidiosis has caused important economic losses for commercial reptile breeders. Therefore, the objective of this study was to perform molecular characterization of *Cryptosporidium* spp. from naturally infected leopard geckos (*Eublepharis macularius)* in Argentina.

Materials and Methods

Animals and samples

A pooled stool sample from 3 leopard geckos (*E. macularius)* was collected and submitted to La Plata University for molecular studies. Three geckos (two females and 1 male) (Fig. 1) were received by veterinary practitioners from a breeder colony in Buenos Aires, Argentina with a history of diarrhea, anorexia and cachexia. Faecal samples were first placed in a 15-ml tube. The tube was partially filled with sucrose solution and mixed in a vortex for approximately 5 sec each tube was centrifuged at 252 g for 10 min. An aliquot was taken from the surface and spread on a slide and examined for the presence of *Cryptosporidium* spp. oocysts by light microscopy (Deming *et al.*, 2008). The modified Ziehl-Neelsen stain for fecal smears was performed essentially as described previously (Henriksen and Pohlenz, 1981); were evidenced several round oocysts of 4-5 µm in diameter compatible with *Cryptosporidium* spp. (Fig. 2). The pooled sample was subjected to a sugar flotation technique (sucrose solution

*Corresponding Author: Juan Manuel Unzaga. Laboratorio de Inmunoparasitología, Facultad de Ciencias Veterinarias, Universidad Nacional de La Plata, 60 y 118, 1900, La Plata, Argentina. Email: junzaga@fcv.unlp.edu.ar

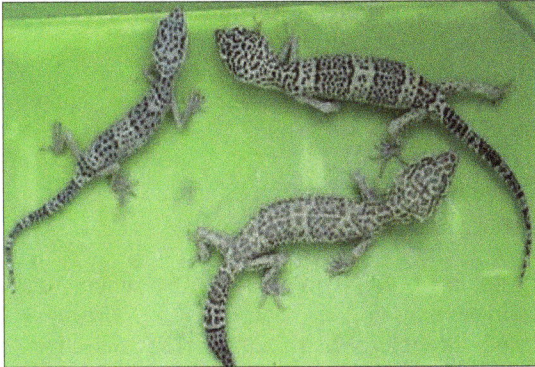

Fig. 1. Three leopard geckos (two females and 1 male) received by veterinary practitioners from a breeder colony in Buenos Aires, Argentina with a history of diarrhea, anorexia and cachexia.

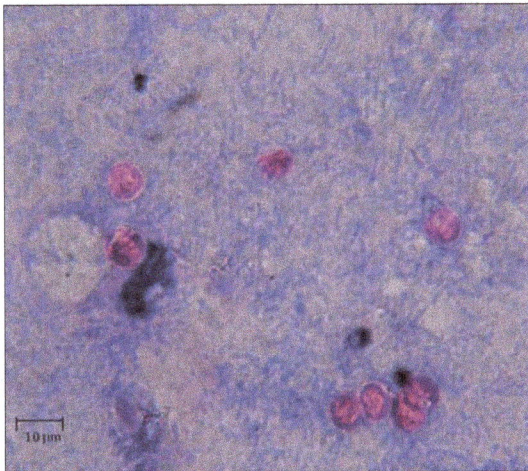

Fig. 2. Fecal smear of leopard geckos (Modified Ziehl-Neelsen technique): round oocysts of 4-5 μm diameter compatible with *Cryptosporidium* spp.

without formaldehyde) and water sedimentation as described previously for concentration of coccidian oocysts (Ortega-Mora *et al.*, 2007). Concentrated oocysts were re-suspended in 450 μl of nuclease free water.

DNA extraction

Oocyst disruption and DNA purification from the faecal sample (processed in triplicate) was performed with a DNA stool commercial kit (QIAamp DNA Stool Mini Kit, Qiagen, Hilden, Germany) according to the manufacturer's recommendations. A process control sample (extraction kit solutions and 150 μl of nuclease free water) was evaluated together with the stool samples.

Molecular identification

A nested PCR technique was performed for amplification of a polymorphic fragment of the 18S rDNA gene (Xiao *et al.*, 1999). Five μl aliquot of the internal PCR products was examined by electrophoresis

in 1% agarose gels and stained with ethidium bromide. Two of the amplicons obtained (which reach a gel estimated concentration of about 40 ng/μl), were purified using polyethylene glycol and sequenced in both directions using the Megabace 1000 Sequencing (GE Health care) at IGEVET, FCV, UNLP. Sequences were aligned and analyzed using GENEIOUS software (free available version 7.1, http://www.geneious.com). Consensus sequences obtained were compared with others published in GenBank by BLASTn megablast analysis.

Results and Discussion

Reptiles have become popular pets worldwide in recent years. The leopard gecko is a crepuscular ground-dwelling lizard naturally found in the deserts of Asia and throughout Pakistan, to the northwestern parts of India (Henkel *et al.*, 1995).

Upon ingestion of *Cryptosporidium* spp. oocysts by the host, sporozoites are released and invade epithelial cells. The protozoans multiply asexually and sexually causing death of the host cells. *Cryptosporidium* spp. infection is associated with hyperplastic and inflammatory lesions of the gastrointestinal tract in different animal species including geckos (Terrell *et al.*, 2003). Thus, Cryptosporidiosis has been associated with a wasting syndrome or "going light" in leopard geckos, characterized by chronic weight loss, diarrhea, lethargy, followed by anorexia and death (Deming *et al.*, 2008). In the present study, three leopard geckos from a breeder colony in Argentina showed a wasting syndrome and oocysts compatible with *Cryptosporidium* spp. were detected by Ziehl-Neelsen staining. Previous studies highlight the importance of molecular diagnostic methods to identify species level within the genus *Cryptosporidium* (Richter *et al.*, 2011). In Spain, Pedraza-Diaz *et al.* (2009) performed PCR and sequencing from seven leopard geckos stool samples with *Cryptosporidium* spp. oocysts, identifying *C. varanii* (n = 3), *C. serpentis* (n = 2) and *C. parvum* (n = 2). A similar study performed in Austria, detected *C. varanii* and *C. serpentis* (32/74 and 8/74 leopard geckos, respectively) (Richter *et al.*, 2011).

In the present study, molecular identification of *Cryptosporidium* spp. was performed by sequencing of a polymorphic fragment of the 18s rRNA gene. The nested PCR was positive (all 3 replicates), evidencing a product of around 830 bp. A consensus sequence of 748 bp was obtained and registered on GenBank under accession number KM610237. This sequence was compared with others published in GenBank by BLASTn megablast analysis and revealed a 99% sequence identity with *C. saurophilum* (GenBank EU553551, EU553552 and EF502042) from asymptomatic leopard geckos (*E. macularius)* and one snake *(Boa constrictor)* in Spain (Pedraza-Diaz *et al.*, 2009), and from symptomatic a adult snake

(*Elaphe guttata guttata*) from a private snake breeding colony from Japan (Plutzer and Karanis, 2007), respectively. The sequence evidenced similar identity (99%) with *C. varanii* (GenBank KJ000485) from an asymptomatic adult snake (*Pantherophis guttatus)* from the serpentarium of the Butantan Institute in São Paulo, Brazil (da Silva *et al.*, 2014), and *Cryptosporidium* spp. from a desert monitor (GenBank AF112573) from Missouri, USA (Xiao *et al.*, 1999).

C. varanii was initially named in 1995 by Pavlásek *et al.* (1995) to describe oocysts obtained from an Emerald monitor (*Varanus prasinus*) in the Prague Zoo. The description was based on oocyst morphology, histology of endogenous stages in the intestine, and failure to infect mice. The same species was subsequently identified in other lizards and in snakes (Pavlasek and Ryan, 2008). The nomenclature *C. saurophilum* was used in 1998 by Koudela and Modry (1998) for oocysts obtained from a Schneider's skink *(Eumeces schneideri).* Molecular comparison between *C. saurophilum* and *C. varanii* at the 18S rRNA and actin loci showed that they are genetically identical, but as *C. varanii* was described previously, it takes precedence over *C. saurophilum* which should be considered a junior synonym of *C. varanii* (Pavlasek and Ryan, 2008; Xiao *et al.*, 2004b). Considering the previous studies, the detected protozoan from leopard geckos in Argentina was identified as *C. varanii* (syn. *C. saurophilum*).

Cryptosporidium spp. obtained from a desert monitor was originally reported by Xiao *et al.* (1999). Morphologically, oocysts of the *Cryptosporidium* spp. desert monitor genotype were very similar to those of *C. varanii* in shape and size and significantly smaller than oocysts of *C. serpentis*. Molecular and biologic characterizations conducted in later studies identified the parasite as *C. saurophilum* (Xiao *et al.*, 2004b). This could explain why the sequence obtained in the present study evidenced 99% homology with the sequence GenBank AF112573 (Xiao *et al.*, 1999). The sequence names reported in GenBank should be revised in order to avoid further misinterpretations.

This is the first case report and molecular identification of *C. varanii* in leopard geckos in Argentina. Even though it was not possible to determine whether all three animals were infected with *C. varanii* since a pooled sample was received in the laboratory, it is possible to assume that all animals were infected by *C. varanii* as they all evidenced similar clinical signs compatible with cryptosporidiosis. Further studies should be conducted to identify the prevalence and implications of cryptosporidiosis in pet lizards from Argentina in order to generate awareness among commercial breeders, pet owners and clinical practitioners in Argentina. The present study evidenced the existence of clinical cryptosporidiosis in captive leopard geckos in Argentina and highlights the importance of molecular identification to species level of *Cryptosporidium* spp.-like oocysts found in fecal samples.

Acknowledgements

We gratefully acknowledge the technical support of Isidoro Ercoli.

Conflict of interest

The authors declare that there is no conflict of interest.

References

da Silva, D.C., Paiva, P.R., Nakamura, A.A., Homem, C.G., de Souza, M.S., Grego, K.F. and Meireles, M.V. 2014. The detection of *Cryptosporidium serpentis* in snake fecal samples by real-time PCR. Vet. Parasitol. 204, 134-138.

Deming, C., Greiner, E. and Uhl, E.W. 2008. Prevalence of cryptosporidium infection and characteristics of oocyst shedding in a breeding colony of leopard geckos *(Eublepharis macularius).* J. Zoo Wildl. Med. 39, 600-607.

Fayer, R. 2010. Taxonomy and species delimitation in *Cryptosporidium*. Exp. Parasitol. 124, 90-97.

Fayer, R., Speer, C.A. and Dubey, J.P. 1997. The general biology of Cryptosporidium. In: Fayer, R. (Ed.), Cryptosporidium and Cryptosporidiosis. Press, Boca Raton.

Henkel, F.W., Schmidt, J. and Hackworth, J. 1995. Geckoes: biology, husbandry, and reproduction. (Malabar, Florida, Krieger Publishing Co.).

Henriksen, S.A. and Pohlenz, J.F., 1981. Staining of cryptosporidia by a modified Ziehl-Neelsen technique. Acta Vet. Scand. 22, 594-596.

Koudela, B. and Modry, D. 1998. New species of *Cryptosporidium (Apicomplexa, Cryptosporidiidae)* from lizards. Folia Parasitologia 45, 93-100.
Levine, N.D. 1980. Some corrections of coccidian *(Apicomplexa: Protozoa)* nomenclature. J. Parasitol. 66, 830-834.

Ortega-Mora, L.M., Gottstein, B., Conraths, F.J. and Buxton, D., 2007. Protozoal Abortion in Farm Ruminants: Guidelines for Diagnosis and Control. CABI International, Wallingford (United Kingdom).

Pavlásek, I., Lávicková, M., Horák, P., Král, J. and Král, B. 1995. *Cryptosporidium varanii* n.sp. *(Apicomplexa: Cryptosporidiidae)* in Emerald monitor *(Varanus prasinus* Schlegal, 1893) in captivity in Prague zoo. Gazella, Zoo Praha. 22, 99-108.

Pavlasek, I. and Ryan, U. 2008. *Cryptosporidium varanii* takes precedence over *C. saurophilum*. Exp. Parasitol. 118, 434-437.

Pedraza-Diaz, S., Ortega-Mora, L.M., Carrion, B.A., Navarro, V. and Gomez-Bautista, M. 2009. Molecular characterisation of *Cryptosporidium* isolates from pet reptiles. Vet. Parasitol. 160, 204-210.

Plutzer, J. and Karanis, P. 2007. Molecular identification of a *Cryptosporidium saurophilum* from corn snake

(Elaphe guttata guttata). Parasitol. Res. 101, 1141-1145.

Richter, B., Nedorost, N., Maderner, A. and Weissenbock, H. 2011. Detection of *Cryptosporidium* species in feces or gastric contents from snakes and lizards as determined by polymerase chain reaction analysis and partial sequencing of the 18S ribosomal RNA gene. J. Vet. Diagn. Invest. 23, 430-435.

Terrell, S.P., Uhl, E.W. and Funk, R.S. 2003. Proliferative enteritis in leopard geckos *(Eublepharis macularius)* associated with *Cryptosporidium* sp. infection. J. Zoo Wildl. Med. 34, 69-75.

Xiao, L., Fayer, R., Ryan, U. and Upton, S.J. 2004a. *Cryptosporidium* taxonomy: recent advances and implications for public health. Clin. Microbiol. Rev. 17, 72-97.

Xiao, L., Morgan, U.M., Limor, J., Escalante, A., Arrowood, M., Shulaw, W., Thompson, R.C., Fayer, R. and Lal, A.A. 1999. Genetic diversity within *Cryptosporidium parvum* and related *Cryptosporidium* species. Appl. Environ. Microbiol. 65, 3386-3391.

Xiao, L., Ryan, U.M., Graczyk, T.K., Limor, J., Li, L., Kombert, M., Junge, R., Sulaiman, I.M., Zhou, L., Arrowood, M.J., Koudela, B., Modry, D. and Lal, A.A. 2004b. Genetic diversity of *Cryptosporidium spp.* in captive reptiles. Appl. Environ. Microbiol. 70, 891-899.

14

Exploiting serological data to understand the epidemiology of foot-and-mouth disease virus serotypes circulating in Libya

Ibrahim Eldaghayes[1,*], Abdunaser Dayhum[1], Abdulwahab Kammon[1], Monier Sharif[2], Giancarlo Ferrari[3], Christianus Bartels[4], Keith Sumption[4], Donald P. King[5], Santina Grazioli[6] and Emiliana Brocchi[6]

[1]Faculty of Veterinary Medicine, University of Tripoli, P. O. Box 13662, Tripoli, Libya
[2]Faculty of Veterinary Medicine, University of Omar Al-Mukhtar, Albeida, Libya
[3]Food and Agriculture Organization of the United Nations (FAO), Rome, Italy
[4]European Commission for the Control of Foot-and-Mouth Disease (EuFMD), Food and Agriculture Organization of the United Nations (FAO), Rome, Italy
[5]The Pirbright Institute, Ash Road, Surrey, UK
[6]Istituto Zooprofilattico Sperimentale della Lombardia e dell'Emilia Romagna (IZSLER), Brescia, Italy

Abstract

Sporadic outbreaks of foot-and-mouth disease (FMD) have occurred in Libya for almost fifty years. During the spring of 2013, a countrywide serosurvey was undertaken to assess the level of FMD virus circulation and identify FMD virus serotypes in the country. A total of 4221 sera were collected, comprising samples from large ruminants (LR; n=1428 samples from 357 farms) and small ruminants (SR; n=2793 samples from 141 farms). FMD sero-prevalence of NSP antibodies determined by ELISA were 19.0% (271/1428) with 95% CI (16.9 – 21.0) and 13.5% (378/2793) with 95% CI (12.3 – 14.8) for LR and SR samples, respectively. The sero-prevalence of NSP antibodies in LR was 12.3% and 19.8% for age group < 1 year and ≥ 1 year, respectively (X^2= 4.95, P= 0.026), while in SR was 3.7%, 13.6% and 21.3% for age group < 1 year, 1-2 year and > 2 year, respectively (X^2= 118.1, P= 0.000). These observed NSP serologic profiles support the hypothesis of an endemic level of FMD circulation in Libya. All positive sera were tested for SP antibodies for O, A and SAT-2 FMD virus serotypes. Serotype O was the dominant circulating serotype followed by serotype A, while evidence of SAT-2 was not found. These data provide an insight into the wider epidemiology of FMD in Libya, and contribute to field and laboratory investigations that during 2013 serotype O (O/ME-SA/Ind-2001 lineage) was isolated from clinical samples collected from the country.
Keywords: Foot-and-mouth disease, Large ruminants, Libya, Sero-prevalence, Small ruminants.

Introduction

Foot-and-mouth disease (FMD) is a highly contagious disease caused by FMD virus (FMDV), which belongs to the Picornaviridae family, genus *Aphthovirus*. FMDV has seven serotypes: O, A, C, Asia 1, SAT-1, SAT-2 and SAT-3 (OIE, 2012). FMD is known to be present in Libya, and periodic outbreaks have occurred since 1959 (Samuel *et al.*, 1999). As reported in the molecular epidemiology/genotyping reports of the World Reference Laboratory (WRLFMD; The Pirbright Institute, UK) only three serotypes have been confirmed in Libya: O (since 1959 and many following years until 2013), A (1979 and 2009) and SAT-2 (2003 and 2012) (Samuel *et al.*, 1999; Knowles *et al.*, 2016; WRLFMD, 2016). Libya currently is qualified in stage 1 of the Progressive Control Pathway (PCP-FMD) (FAO-OIE, 2012).

Following a huge number of FMD outbreaks in 2012 all over the country, mass vaccination was introduced in Libya by the end of 2012 using inactivated purified vaccine (Merial®) against serotypes O (strains: O Manisa + O 3039), A (strain: A Iran 05) and SAT-2 (strains: ERI + ZIM). Large ruminants (LR) were vaccinated against O, A and SAT-2, whereas small ruminants (SR) were vaccinated only against O and A. In order to gain a better understanding of the epidemiological situation in the country, a cooperation agreement was signed (in 2012) between the Libyan Ministry of Agriculture represented by the Libyan National Center of Animal Health (NCAH), and the Italian Government represented by Ministry of Health. Specific activities were designed and conducted in collaboration with the Istituto Zooprofilattico Sperimentale della Lombardia e dell'Emilia Romagna (IZSLER) in Brescia, Italy, an OIE/FAO FMD reference laboratory. A surveillance system was designed by Libyan, FAO, EuFMD and IZSLER experts, and was then implemented during the year 2013.

This project had a structure of three main components: (I) Collection of samples from clinically affected animals in FMD suspected outbreaks: samples

---

*Corresponding Author: Ibrahim Eldaghayes. Department of Microbiology and Parasitology, Faculty of Veterinary Medicine, University of Tripoli, P. O. Box 13662, Tripoli, Libya. Email: *ibrahim.eldaghayes@vetmed.edu.ly*

(vesicular epithelium, swabs, blood) for virus isolation and identification have been collected from suspected cases during the second half of 2013 from different areas in the country; (II) Evaluation of the immune response of vaccinated animals by collecting blood samples at the point of initial vaccination (day 1) and 30 days post vaccination, and (III) Investigation of the level of FMD virus circulation by detection of non-structural proteins (NSP) antibodies, and the serotypes present by detecting of structural proteins (SP) serotype-specific antibodies by the collection of sera samples from all over the country.

This study was focused mainly on the third of these components to measure the level of NSP antibodies as indicator of past or current FMDV infection, irrespective of the vaccination status. Subsequently SP antibodies were also tested to gather information on the circulating FMDV serotypes, furthermore, and for vaccinated animals, this will show the level of antibodies following vaccination. The wider aim of this work was to support surveillance activities that are required in order for the country to progress from PCP-FMD stage 1 to stage 2. These studies complemented phylogenetic analysis of sequences recovered from FMD virus positive samples collected from Libya that indicated a strain belonging to O/ME-SA/Ind-2001 lineage, which is derived from the Indian subcontinent, was circulating in the country (Valdazo-González et al., 2014; Knowles et al., 2016).

Materials and Methods

Study area
Libyan NCAH is responsible for seven regional animal health branches (Green Mountain, Benghazi, Middle Area, Zawiyah, Tripoli, West Mountain and Sabha). These animal health branches provide public veterinary services to cover the whole country. This study exploited samples from many Libyan cities that were collected by the National Veterinary Services.

Sampling strategy and study design
FMD susceptible animals in Libya are mainly cattle, sheep and goats. The LR (cattle) population in the country is around 150,000 and 6,500,000 for SR (sheep and goats). The sampling scheme varied according to the species. For each randomly selected owner, a questionnaire was completed by the veterinarian in order to get some basic information about the owner, the farm, collected samples and some risk factors.

For LR, a random selection of owners from different regions of the country was carried out. From each of the randomly selected farms, a maximum of 10 individual blood samples (the preferred age was 6-18 months) from the herd (all cows were sampled if the total number of animals was less than 10) were collected from two age categories: (I) 6-12 months of age and (II) over than 12 months of age. For SR, a two stage sampling design was carried out in order to randomly

select owners from all over the country who have at least 100 heads per herd. From each herd a total number of 48 samples were collected from three age categories: (I) 16 samples from the 6 months to less than 12 months age; (II) 16 from animals between 12 and 24 months of age and (III) 16 from animals that were more than 24 months of age.

Study animals and sample size
A total number of 4,221 serum samples were collected during the year 2013 from LR and SR in Libya. For LR, a total number of 1428 serum samples were collected from 357 farms from 29 cities. Whereas for SR, a total number of 2,793 serum samples were collected from 141 farms from 39 cities.

Serological testing
The samples were analysed in Brescia, Italy, at IZSLER, an OIE/FAO FMD reference laboratory. Different tests, developed at IZSLER, were used: (i) a NSP-ELISA (3ABC-ELISA) for the detection of antibodies against NSP; these are elicited after an infection and are common to all FMDV serotypes; (ii) a series of three competitive ELISAs for the detection and serotyping of antibodies to the SP of FMDV serotypes O, A and SAT-2, in order to indirectly identify the viral serotypes circulating in Libya.

NSP-ELISA
The serological assay used to detect anti-NSP antibodies was the previously validated 3ABC-trapping ELISA, (Brocchi et al., 2006), in the format of ready-to-use kit, with pre-sensitized ELISA immuno-plates, peroxidase-conjugated anti-ruminant IgG, control sera and TMB chromogen, produced at IZSLER, Brescia, Italy.

According to a previous validation study, the diagnostic performance of the IZSLER-Brescia kit are comparable to those of the OIE index test (Panaftosa-screening ELISA) described in the Diagnostic Manual of the World Organization for Animal Health. In particular, the specificity exceeds 99% and the sensitivity varies depending on the time elapsed after infection and on the previous vaccination status, achieving 100% for non-vaccinated cattle exposed to infection and 86.4% for the detection of carriers in vaccinated cattle (Brocchi et al., 2006).

Monoclonal antibody (MAb)-based Solid Phase Competitive ELISA (SPCE)
Ready-to-use kits developed and produced by IZSLER have been used for detection and titration of antibodies against FMDV serotypes O, A and SAT-2 (Brocchi et al., 2012; Dho et al., 2014).

The common principle of each assay corresponds to a solid phase competitive ELISA (SPCE) based on a peroxidase-conjugated, neutralizing monoclonal antibody (MAb), specific for a FMDV serotype. In the ready-to-use kit, ELISA microplates are supplied pre-coated with inactivated FMDV antigens captured by homologous serotype-specific MAbs. Appropriately diluted sera are incubated with the trapped antigen, enabling the specific antibodies present in the sample to bind to the antigen. Then, the anti-FMDV serotype-specific MAb, conjugated with peroxidase, is dispensed: its reaction with the homologous antigen will be inhibited by antibodies of positive sera previously bound to the virus, while in case of negative sera the conjugated MAb can bind to the FMDV antigen. After incubation, the unbound conjugate is removed by washing and the TMB substrate/chromogen solution is delivered into wells. A colorimetric reaction develops if the conjugated MAb has bound to the virus, i.e. if test serum is negative, while colour development is inhibited by positive sera. Antigen and conjugate concentrations are pre-calibrated in order to give a suitable reaction value (OD). After addition of a stop solution, the optical density of the developed color is read by a microplate photometer. Serum samples can be screened at a single dilution 1/10, to obtain a simple qualitative (positive/negative) result; in the present study all sera were titrated by analyzing serial dilutions and the end-point titre was calculated as the highest dilution inhibiting 50% reaction. The test can be applied to measure antibodies in serum or plasma samples of FMDV infected or vaccinated animals of any susceptible species. Since antibodies cross-reactive among different serotypes may be elicited and are detectable by ELISA assays, type-specificity cannot be perfect. However, significant differences in titres against different serotypes may help in interpretation.

Data analysis:

The data collected was entered into Microsoft Excel spreadsheet and coded for analysis. The sero-prevalence for FMD NSP antibodies was standardized by using the following formula:

Direct adjusted sero-prevalence= $\sum$ Sero-prevalence % (SP) X Reference population distribution (RPD) over all age group strata (Fleiss, 1973).

The NSP sero-prevalence in each age-group was estimated as $p = \dfrac{NSP +}{n}$

Where n is the total number of animals counted in the specific age-group considered. Whereas if at least one positive NSP animal was found in a one farm or a city, then this farm or city was considered as FMD positive. For each age-group; the age related risks of infection were estimated through the following equation (Vynnycky and White, 2010):

$$R_t = 1 - \frac{S_t}{S_{t-1}}$$

Where: S_t is the proportion of susceptible in the generic t age-group and S_{t-1} is the proportion of susceptible in

the preceding age-group. The age-specific monthly incidence rate m_t (monthly force of infection) was calculated according to the following:

$$m_t = \frac{-\ln(1 - R_t)}{a_t - a_{t-1}}$$

Where: The average age a_t of the SR in each age-group as well as the difference $(a_t - a_{t-1})$ between two adjacent age-groups were estimated. Pearson's chi-square tests were used to detect significant differences in seropositivity among and between age groups. Epidemiologic data (location and serotypes) were mapped. In all the analysis, the confidence level was set at 95% and p<0.05 set for significance. The Correlation between number of animals and the sero-prevalence of FMD at city level was calculated using Pearson Correlation.

Results

Using the NSP ELISA test, the sero-prevalence estimated in LR and SR was 19.0% (271/1428) with 95% CI (16.9-21.0) and 13.5% (378/2793) with 95% CI (12.3-14.8) respectively (Table 1). The age standardized sero-prevalence of FMD in the two species was 18.3 with 95% CI (2.4-34.3) and 15.5 with 95% CI (4.1-26.9) for LR and SR respectively (Table 2).

The distribution FMD sero-prevalence in NCAH branches:

The standardized sero-prevalence was calculated for the seven NCAH branches. For SR: the highest sero-prevalence was in Benghazi (25.8%) and Tripoli (22.1%) branches followed by West Mountain (13.2%), Middle Area (12.3%), Green Mountain (9.3%) and Sabha (7.7%) and the last Zawiyah (0.9%) (Fig. 1 and Table 3).

For LR: the highest sero-prevalence was in Green Mountain (28.4%) and Benghazi (23.2%) branches followed by Zawiyah (15.4%), Sabha (15.1%), Tripoli (14.8%) and West Mountain (6.8%) and last was in Middle Area (5.7 %) (Fig. 2 and Table 3).

The age distribution of sero-prevalence of FMD:

There were significant differences in the sero-prevalence estimated among the age groups in SR (X^2= 118.1, P= 0.000).

The sero-prevalence of FMD in SR was 3.7, 13.6 and 21.3 for age groups < 1 year, 1 - 2 year and > 2 year respectively. The prevalence risk ratio was 3.3 with 95% CI (2.3 - 4.9) and 5.7 with 95% CI (4.0 - 8.3) for age group 1 - 2 year and > 2 year respectively comparing to < 1 year (Table 4).

Also in LR, there were significant differences in the sero-prevalence estimated among the age groups (X^2= 4.95, P= 0.026). The sero-prevalence of FMD was 12.3 and 19.8 for age groups < 1 year and ≥ 1 year respectively with risk ratio 1.6 with 95% CI (1.04 - 2.5) as shown in Table 4.

Table 1. The sero-prevalence of FMD in Libya determined using NSP ELISA.

Species	No. of samples	No. of positive samples (%)	No. of farms	No. of positive farms (%)	No. of cities	No. of positive cities (%)
LR	1,428	271 (19%)	357	134 (37.5%)	29	20 (68.9%)
SR	2,793	378 (13.5%)	141	76 (53.9%)	39	30 (76.9%)
Total	4,221	649 (15.4%)	498	210 (42.9%)	44	43 (97.7%)

Table 2. The standardized sero-prevalence of FMD in Libya.

Species	Age group (months)	Sero-prevalence % (SP)	Reference population distribution (RPD)	Product (SP*RPD)	Standardized SP ∑ SP*RPD
LR	6 - < 12	12.3	0.2	2.46	18.3 (95% CI 2.4 – 34.3)
	≥ 12	19.8	0.8	15.84	
SR	6 - < 12	3.7	0.2	0.74	15.5 (95% CI 4.1 – 26.9)
	12-24	13.6	0.3	4.08	
	>24	21.3	0.5	10.65	

Table 3. The standardized sero-prevalence of FMD in LR and SR by branch.

Branch	No. of Farms		No. of infected farms (%)		No. of Samples		Sero-prevalence (%)	
	LR	SR	LR	SR	LR	SR	LR	SR
Green Mountain	133	25	57 (42.9)	12 (48.0)	368	572	28.4	9.3
Benghazi	18	35	7 (38.9)	22 (62.9)	106	834	23.2	25.8
Middle Area	7	19	2 (28.6)	5 (26.3)	42	87	5.7	12.3
Zawiyaha	72	8	20 (27.8)	1 (12.5)	227	182	15.4	0.9
Tripoli	88	15	38 (43.2)	12 (80.0)	516	282	14.8	22.1
West Mountain	33	20	6 (18.2)	16 (80.0)	132	610	6.8	13.2
Sabha	6	19	4 (66.7)	8 (42.1)	37	226	15.1	7.7
Total	357	141	134(37.5)	76 (53.9)	1428	2793	18.3	15.5

Table 4. Estimated prevalence risk of FMD in SR and LR by age group.

Age group	No. of Samples	No. of positive samples (%)	95% CI Lower-Upper	X^2	P-Value	RR (95% CI)
SR				118.1	0.000	
< 1 year*	804	30 (3.7)	2.5 – 5.3			
1 – 2 years	980	133 (13.6)	11.5 – 15.9			3.3 (2.3 – 4.9)
> 2 years	1009	215 (21.3)	18.8 – 24.0			5.7 (4.0 - 8.3)
LR				4.95	0.026	
< 1 year*	154	19 (12.3)	7.6 – 18.6			
≥ 1 year	1274	252 (19.8)	17.6 – 22.1			1.6 (1.04 -2.5)

*Reference group.

Table 5. Estimated monthly incidence rate per 1000 animals for FMD in SR for each age group.

Age-group (in months)	Prevalence (p)	Average age a_t (in months)	Proportion of susceptible $S_t = (1-p)$	Age related risks* $[1-(S_t/S_{t-1})]$	Age-specific monthly incidence rate/1000 animals $m_t = -ln(1-R_t)/(a_t - a_{t-1})$
6 - <12	0.037	8.86	0.963	0.037	4.2
12 - 24	0.136	19.84	0.864	0.103	9.9
>24	0.213	47.9	0.787	0.089	3.3

*Age related risks are estimated over different lengths of times within the different age-groups.

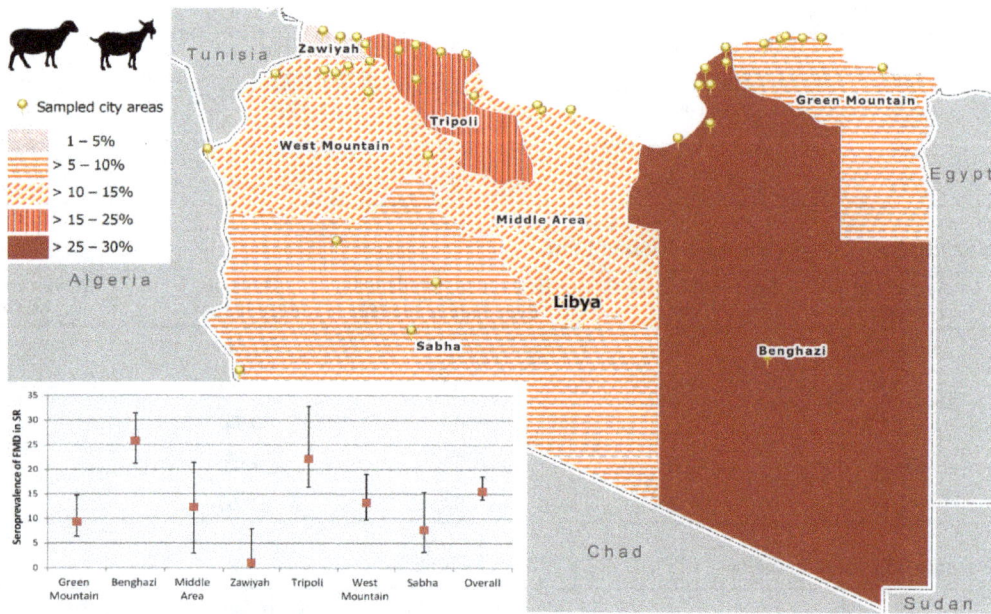

Fig. 1. Estimated sero-prevalence of FMD in SR by branch.

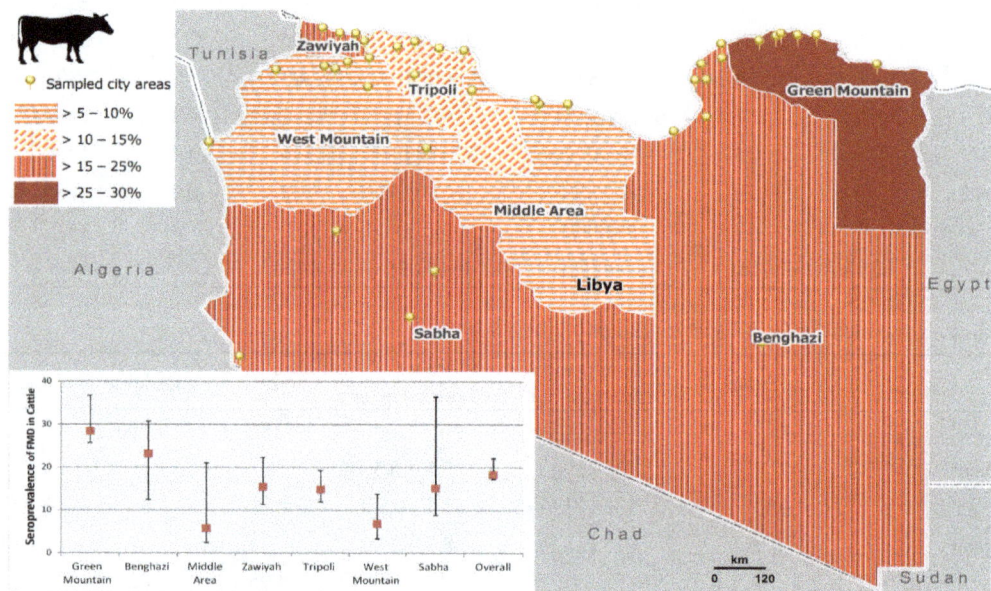

Fig. 2. Estimated Sero-prevalence of FMD in LR by branch.

The estimated monthly incidence rate was 4.2 per 1,000 animals between 0 and 8.9 months of age that increased up to 9.9 per 1,000 animals between 8.9 and 19.8 months and then dropped to 3.3 per 1,000 animals once the animals reached an average age of 47.9 months (Table 5).

Circulating FMD serotypes:

All NSP positive samples were subjected to SP ELISA for O, A and SAT-2 serotypes. The majority of the SR positive samples were serotype O (65.9%), then A (25.7%) and only 0.3% for SAT-2. The serotype O varied within the branches from 0 - 81.6% whereas

serotype A ranged from 12.3 to 100. In LR: the mean level of serotype O among NSP positive samples was 45.9% which ranged within the branches from 14.3 – 100%, whereas the mean level of serotype A was 41.7% ranging from 0 - 67.8%, while serotype SAT-2 was lower at 0.8%.

The overall percentage of O serotype in less than one-year age group for both SR and LR was almost two times higher than A serotype. The percentage of O serotype was higher in Green Mountain, Benghazi, Zawiyah and West Mountain whereas the percentage A serotype was higher in Middle Area, and Sabha Branch for SR (Table 6; Fig. 3 and 4). There was moderate correlation between the sero-prevalence of FMD in LR and the number of SR (Pearson Correlation value, 0.632 with p-value 0.000), low correlation between the sero-prevalence of FMD in cattle and the number of LR (Pearson Correlation value, 0.386 with p-value 0.042) and low correlation between the number of SR and cattle (Pearson Correlation value, 0.479 with p-value 0.002) as shown in Table 7.

Discussion

A surveillance study for FMD is an essential requirement before practical attempts are made to control the disease. For instance, in a vast country like Libya, with an area approaching 1,760,000 km^2, and six neighbouring countries where four FMDV serotypes (O, A, SAT-1, and SAT-2) are known to prevail (records), besides illegal animal movement along most of the borders, the task of FMD control is challenging.

Table 6. The distribution and the percentage of FMD serotypes of positive samples collected from SR and LR for age group less than one year.

Branches	Species	No. of Positive Samples	O	A	O,A	No serotype
Green Mountain	SR	2	2 (100)			
	LR	6	3 (50.0)	3 (50.0)		
Benghazi	SR	15	12 (80.0)	2 (13.3)	1 (6.7)	
	LR	0				
Middle Area	SR	1		1 (100)		
	LR	0				
Zawiyah	SR	0				
	LR	2	2 (100.0)			
Tripoli	SR	3	1 (33.3)	2 (66.7)		
	LR	10	5 (50.0)	2 (20.0)	3 (30.0)	
West Mountain	SR	6	3 (50.0)	2 (33.3)		1 (16.7)
	LR	1		1 (100.0)		
Sabha	SR	3	1 (33.3)	2 (66.7)		
	LR	0				
Over All	SR	30	19 (63.3)	9 (30.0)	1 (3.3)	1 (3.3)
	LR	19	10 (52.6)	6 (31.6)	3 (15.8)	

SAT-2 results were not included in the table due to that the two SAT2-positive results can be explained as cross-reactivity of type O-antibody with SAT-2 antigens.

Table 7: The correlation between the sero-prevalence of FMD and the number of SR and LR in 40 cities.

		% of FMD in SR	# of the LR	# of the SR
% of FMD in LR	Pearson Correlation	.171	.386*	.632**
	P-Value	.437	.042	.000
	N	23	28	28
% of FMD in SR	Pearson Correlation	1	-.020	-.043
	P-Value		.911	.803
	N		35	36
# of the LR	Pearson Correlation		1	.479**
	P-Value			.002
	N			40

* Correlation is significant at the 0.05 level (2-tailed)
** Correlation is significant at the 0.01 level (2-tailed).

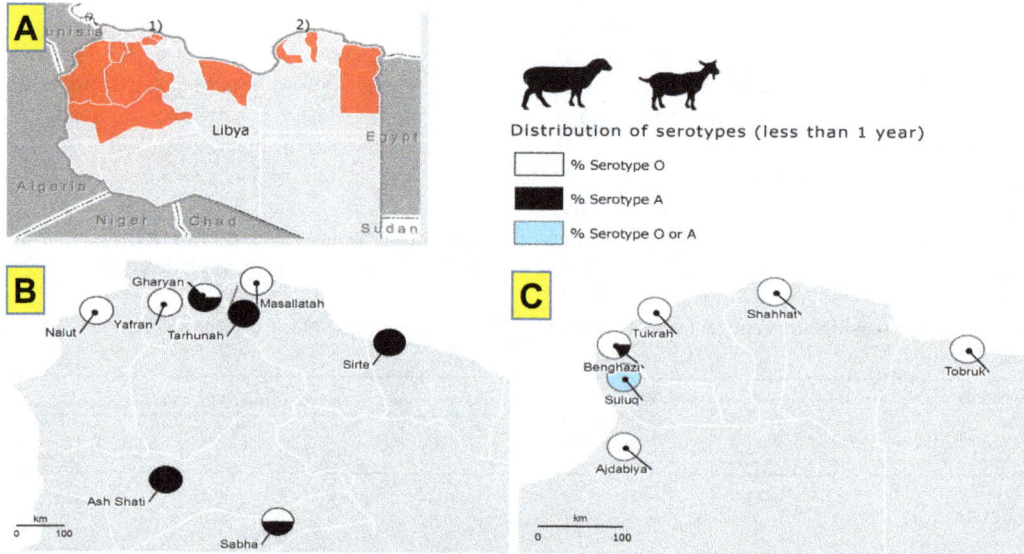

Fig. 3. Distribution of FMD serotypes in age group less than 1 year in SR as indication of recent FMD infections. (A): In the whole country. (B): In cities of the western part of the country. (C): In cities of the eastern part of the country.

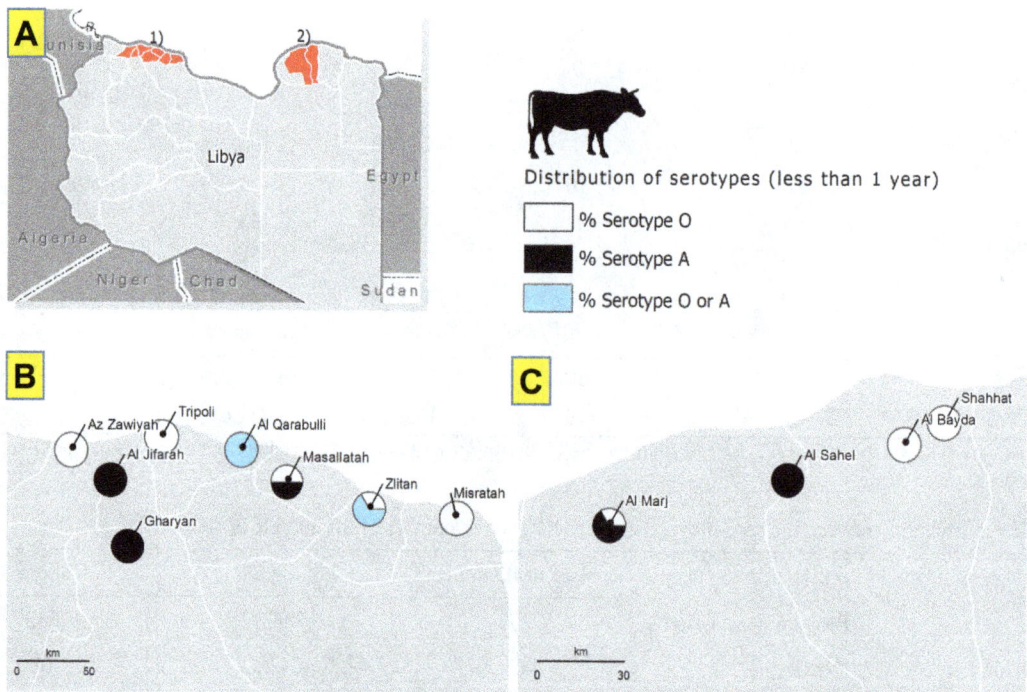

Fig. 4. Distribution of FMD serotypes in age group less than 1 year in LR as indication of recent FMD infections. (A): In the whole country. (B): In cities of the western part of the country. (C): In cities of the eastern part of the country.

The precise routes by which the new FMDV strain O/ME-SA/Ind-2001 was introduced into Libya in 2013 are not yet fully understood. This same virus strain has spread beyond Libya to Tunisia in April 2014 (WRLFMD, 2014a), then to Algeria in July 2014 (WRLFMD, 2014b) and more recently to Morocco in October 2015 (Bachanek-Bankowska *et al.*, 2016). Our results suggest that FMD is endemic in Libya and the working hypothesis is that the virus is maintained

mainly through the SR population. This hypothesis was supported by the profile of NSP antibodies in SR that showed a progressive increase in the sero-positivity concordant with the increasing average age of the animals tested with OR vary from 3.3 to 5.7 for age group 1-2 year and >2 years compared to <1 year age group, in contrast to LR where OR only 1.6 for ≥ 1 year age group compared to <1 year of age group. An additional reason that may lead to consider SR as candidate reservoirs of FMD virus in Libya is their relatively high number (6,500,000 approximately) in comparison with the estimated total population of LR (approximately 150,000 heads) with a ratio SR/LR ~44/1. Furthermore, the livestock movement and transhumance or nomadism practices of SR are common practice in Libya. Another relevant element identified through our study is that the correlation between number of animals and the sero-prevalence of FMD at city level was moderate between the sero-prevalence of FMD in LR and the number of SR (Pearson Correlation value, 0.632 with p-value 0.000) and low correlation between the sero-prevalence of FMD in cattle and the number of LR (Pearson Correlation value, 0.386 with p-value 0.042).

Such a combination of factors could determine that the clinical disease in SR (already difficult to be recognized) may go undetected, also because of the relatively low number of cases occurring in the overall population, the disease may then be clearly seen only once it spillovers in LR where the clinical signs are more apparent. For the above-mentioned reasons, sheep might act as a source of infection for cattle. Therefore, sheep vaccination would be an effective way to limit the spread of FMD outbreaks.

In general, vaccination against FMD in LR, and sometimes also in SR is the common strategy used in North Africa and Middle East in order to control the disease. Vaccines used in these countries were from a wide variety of sources, including producers based within the region, or from international vaccine producers.

FMD control in this region is not an easy task to be done due to the lack of relevant and harmonised surveillance programmes and the lack of transparency and collaboration between these countries. The long borders between countries in the region and the illegal animal movement between neighbouring countries make disease control even more difficult. Furthermore, some countries are not able to secure constant and continuous financial funding and budgets for FMD surveillance and control programmes.

Bravo de Rueda et al. (2015) developed a method to determine the (partial) reproduction ratios (R) for mixed populations of cattle and sheep by using published experimental transmission data and evaluated different vaccination strategies, and concluded that "vaccination of cattle only in mixed population consisting of sheep and cattle will in most cases be sufficient for controlling FMDV epidemics". In Libya, one possible approach for the vaccination programme could be: (i) to protect LR against clinical disease with an extensive vaccination programme; (ii) to better characterise risk hotspots and transmission pathways among the SR population which should possibly lead to formulate a preventive program

targeting the sub-populations where the risk of infection will be estimated to be higher. It will be extremely important, if such approach is adopted, to thoroughly review the definition of a suspected case among SR as the overall sensitivity for detecting FMD would significantly decrease if LR were vaccinated.

During the first quarter of 2012, Libya had an epidemic of FMD all over the country (in average of 18 FMD infected herds per day; unpublished data). A mass vaccination was introduced in Libya by the end of 2012 to reduce the negative economic impact of FMD.

In our results, both for SR and LR, serotype O was the highest followed by serotype A. In Sudan, the main FMDV circulation in seven states in 2010 in cattle was A (78.1%), O (69.4%), SAT-2 (44.0%) and SAT-1 (20.2%) whereas in sheep was O (27.5%), SAT-2 (9.1%), A (8.7%) and SAT-1 (5.1%) (Habiela et al., 2010). Another study in Khartoum state Sudan by Noureldin and Elfadil (2014) found that serotype O (82.6%) and SAT-2 (40%) were the main circulating FMDVs in cattle. Raouf et al. (2012) in a study conducted in western Sudan showed positive results for SAT-2 (40%) and O (25%). In Egypt, serotype O (19.5%) and A (14.9%) were detected in sheep (Hassan et al., 2011).

In this study, a sero-positive rate of 18.3% with 95% CI (2.4 – 34.3) was detected in cattle, which was similar to other studies conducted in Malaysia, Bangladesh and Somaliland (Hasaballa and Abbo, 2010; Sarker et al., 2011; Elnaker et al., 2012). These values are in contrast to the FMD sero-prevalence study conducted in the neighbouring country of Sudan where higher values of 79.2% (Habiela et al., 2010) and 25-56% in south of Sudan (Ochi et al., 2014) were detected.

It is not easy to compare the results for this study (Libya) with other studies due to the variety of different involving factors. Some examples of these factors would be: the differences in husbandry management, size of herd, total number of LR, presence of reservoirs (no buffaloes in Libya), the immunity status of cattle, the breed, the sampling design, the sensitivity and specificity of the diagnostic test, etc.

For LR, higher FMD sero-prevalence in the eastern part of the country might be associated with the transhumance and nomadism practices compared to other branches. Whereas, the lower sero-prevalence of FMD was in the Middle Area and West Mountain branches, that might be due to the small number of LR population in these areas.

The sero-prevalence in cattle revealed increasing of positive cases as the age increases (higher in older animals). This finding was similar to results obtained in other studies (Kahn et al., 2002; Gelaye et al., 2009; Sarker et al., 2011; Ochi et al., 2014). One explanation for that is that young cattle are always kept in pen and closed areas with less exposure and contact with other animals. Another study by Kahn *et al.* (2002), noticed that adult cattle that kept for long time with history of previous infection act as chronic carriers. The high prevalence in old age group is likely due to constant re-exposure to FMD and indicates the cumulative experience of the population with the agent (Murphy *et al.*, 1999). However, few other studies showed higher FMD sero-prevalence in calves than adult cattle (Perry *et al.*, 2003; Rufael *et al.*, 2008).

The standardized FMD sero-prevalence of 15.5% with 95% CI (4.1-26.9) was obtained for SR livestock. These results were almost similar to those reported in Egypt (18.4%) by Hassan *et al.* (2011) where higher prevalence was reported in males (29%) than females (13%). In India, 20.4% sheep and 13.6% goats were found to be FMD NSP positive (Rout *et al.*, 2014). Higher sero-prevalence was reported in Sudan (24.3%) (Habiela *et al.*, 2010). In another study conducted in India showed that the overall sero-prevalence was 38% in goats (Ranabijuli *et al.*, 2010).

For SR, the sero-prevalence varied between different Libyan NCAH branches. The highest FMD sero-prevalence reported in Benghazi and Tripoli branches (Tripoli and Benghazi are the two main cities of Libya with about 2/3 of the total Libyan inhabitants), might be associated with the herd management and movement of animals towards the two big cities as well as these two cities have large number of livestock markets.

The present study revealed that there was statistical association between age of SR animals and sero-positive rate for FMD (P<0001). In another study in South Sudan, Ochi *et al.* (2014) found that the FMD-sero-prevalence in sheep < one-year-old was 12.5% and 31% in age group > 3 year.

The age-related risks of infection for FMD in SR were estimated for the three age groups to evaluate the effect of the FMD vaccination that was applied during last quarter of the year 2012. Animals at age < one-year-old were not exposed to 2012 FMD outbreaks, therefore, these animals were expected to provide information about recent infections, whereas the older animals may have experienced the extensive 2012 FMD outbreaks. Before FMD outbreaks (the effect of years before 2012), the estimated monthly incidence rate per 1000 animals for FMD was 3.3 cases. During the year of the FMD outbreak (2012) the monthly incidence rate increased dramatically to 9.9 per 1000 animals. Following the vaccination, the monthly incidence rate decreased to 4.2 per 1000 animals. The results of the monthly incidence rate can be counted as an indicator and an indirect measurement for the efficacy and the success of the mass vaccination campaign.

In conclusion, the present study indicates that FMD has been circulating in large areas of Libya and the majority of the outbreaks were undetected because of inadequate national disease surveillance systems. The NSP serologic profile observed in both small and large ruminants supports the hypothesis of an endemic level of FMDV. While in 2013, serotype O (O/ME-SA/Ind-2001 lineage) was the only serotype isolated from clinical samples, a deeper evaluation of SP antibodies titers cannot rule out the concurrent presence of serotype A.

Further research should be conducted to get better understanding of the livestock production, data collection on the management system and risk factors analysis. Therefore, findings provide insight information on the epidemiology of FMD, scientifically sound strategies could be developed for disease control to limit the effect of FMD on Libyan animal livestock.

Acknowledgments
Authors are grateful to the staff of the Libyan National Center for Animal Health (NCAH) especially to those who contributed in collecting samples and filling questionnaires. Special thanks to Zohra Bensouliman, Khalid Aswaise, Saad Altayef and Ali Milad from NCAH who helped in organizing samples in Tripoli and helping by testing samples in IZSLER lab in Brescia. Authors are grateful to Giulia Conchedda and Giuseppina Cinardi from AGAL, FAO, Rome, for helping in preparing the maps. The authors would like to express their gratitude to the staff of the National Reference Centre for Vesicular Diseases, Biotechnology Department, OIE/FAO reference laboratories for FMD and for SVD, IZSLER, in Brescia, Italy, and also to the Italian Ministry of Health for providing the financial support for testing all samples in IZSLER lab.

Conflict of interest:
The author declares that there is no conflict of interest.

References
Bachanek-Bankowska, K., Wadsworth, J., Gray, A., Abouchoaib, N., King, D.P. and Knowles, N.J. 2016. Genome sequence of foot-and-mouth disease virus serotype O isolated from Morocco in 2015. Genome Announc. 4(2), e01746-15. doi:10.1128/genomeA.01746-15.

Bravo de Rueda, C., Dekker, A., Eble, P.L. and De Jong, M.C. 2015. Vaccination of Cattle Only is Sufficient to Stop FMDV Transmission in Mixed Populations of Sheep and Cattle. Epidemiol. Infect. 143(11), 2279-2286.

Brocchi, E., Bergman, I., Dekker, A., Paton, D., Sammin, D., Greiner, M., Grazioli, S., De Simone, F., Yadin, H., Haas, B., Bulut, N., Malirat, V., Neitzert, E., Goris, N., Parida, S., Sørensen, K. and De Clercq, K., 2006. Comparative evaluation of six ELISAs for the detection of antibodies to the non-structural proteins of foot-and-mouth disease. Vaccine 24(47-48), 6966-6979.

Brocchi, E., Spagnoli, E., Li, Y., Haas, B., De Clercq, K., Dho, G., Grazioli, S. and De Simone, F. 2012. Ready-to-use kits for detection of antibodies to FMDV serotypes O, A, Asia 1. Open Session of the standing technical and research committees of the EuFMD commission – Jerez de la Frontera, Spain, 29-31 October 2012.

Dho, G., Grazioli, S., Bugnetti, M., Pezzoni, G., Maree, F.F., Esterhuysen, J., Chitray, M., Scott, K. and Brocchi, E. 2014. "Ready-to-use kits for the detection of antibody to FMDV serotypes SAT1 and SAT2". Open Session of the Standing Technical and research Committees of EuFMD, Cavtat (Croatia), 29-31 October 2014, pp: 140-141.

Elnaker, Y.F., Sayed-Ahmed, M., El-Beskawy, M., El-Sawalhy, A.A. and Wabacha, J.K. 2012. Seroprevalence of FMD in cattle, sheep and goats in Somaliland. Bull. Anim. Health Prod. Africa 60(4), 383-392.

FAO-OIE. 2012. The Progressive Control Pathway for FMD control (PCP-FMD): Principles, Stage Descriptions and Standards. 2012. http://www.fao.org/fileadmin/user_upload/eufmd/docs/PCP/PCP_Guidelines_Eng_2012web.pdf.

Fleiss, J.L. 1973. Statistical method for rates and proportions. Torinto, Canada: John Wiley & Sons, pp: 155-164.

Gelaye, E., Ayelet, G., Abere, T. and Asmare, K. 2009. Seroprevalence of foot and mouth disease in Bench Maji zone, Southwestern Ethiopia. J. Vet. Med. Anim. Health 1(1), 5-10.

Habiela, M.M., Alamin, A.G., Raouf, Y.A. and Ali, Y.H. 2010. Epizootiological study of foot and mouth disease in the Sudan: the situation after two decades. Vet. Archiv. 80(1), 11-26.

Hasaballa, H. and Abbo, A. 2010. Prevalence of Foot and Mouth Disease and Evaluation of Effectiveness of Vaccination in Malaysian Cattle. Master thesis, Universiti Putra Malaysia.

Hassan, A.I., Ebeid, M.H., Hamoda, F.K. and Azab, A.M.H. 2011. Studies on Foot and Mouth Disease Virus type O1, A in Sheep. PhD thesis, Benha University, Egypt.

Kahn, S., Geale, D.W., Kitching, P.R., Bouffard, A., Allard, D.G. and Duncan, J.R. 2002. Vaccination against foot-and-mouth disease: the implications for Canada. Can. Vet. J. 43(5), 349-354.

Knowles, N.J., Bachanek-Bankowska, K., Wadsworth, J., Mioulet, V., Valdazo-González, B., Eldaghayes, I.M., Dayhum, A.S., Kammon, A.M., Sharif, M.A., Waight, S., Shamia, A.M., Tenzin, S., Wernery, U., Grazioli, S., Brocchi, E., Subramaniam, S., Pattnaik, B. and King, D.P. 2016. Outbreaks of Foot-and-Mouth Disease in Libya and Saudi Arabia During 2013 Due to an Exotic O/ME-SA/Ind-2001 Lineage Virus. Transbound. Emerg. Dis. 63(5), e431-435.

Murphy, A.F., Gibbs, J.E., Horzinec, C.M. and Studdert, J.M. 1999. Foot and Mouth Disease. In: Veterinary Virology. 3rd edition California, Acadamic press USA, pp: 512-537.

Noureldin, A.M.M.A. and Elfadil, A.A.M. 2014. Prevalence and Risk Factors of Foot and Mouth Disease of Cattle in Khartoum State - Sudan. Master thesis, Sudan University of Science and Technology.

Ochi, E.B., Suliman, M.A. and Ismail, A.O. 2014. A Review on Epidemiology of Foot and Mouth Disease (FMD) in South Sudan. Report Opinion 6(11), 13-16.

OIE. 2012. "OIE Manual of Diagnostics for Foot and Mouth Disease: chapter 2.1.5," http://www.oie.int/fileadmin/Home/eng/Health_standards/tahm/2.01.05_FMD.pdf.

Perry, B.D., Randolph, T.F., Ashley, S., Chimedza, R., Forman, T., Morrison, J., Poulton, C., Sibanda, L., Stevens, C., Tebele, N. and Yngstrom, I. 2003. The Impact and Poverty Reduction Implications of Foot and Mouth Disease Control in South Africa with Special Reference to Zimbabwe. Proceedings of the 10th International Symposium on Veterinary Epidemiology and Economics, Available at: www.sciquest.org.nz.

Ranabijuli, S., Mohapatra, J.K., Pandey, L.K., Rout, M., Sanyal, A., Dash, B.B., Sarangi, L.N., Panda, H.K. and Pattnaik, B. 2010. Serological Evidence of Foot-and-Mouth Disease Virus Infection in Randomly Surveyed Goat Population of Orissa, India. Transbound. Emerg. Dis. 57(6), 448-454.

Raouf, Y.A., Tamador, M.A.A., Nahid, A.I. and Shaza, M. 2012. A survey for antibodies against current infection of foot-and-mouth disease virus in Sudanese cattle, sheep and goats using neutralization test. Bull. Anim. Health Prod. Africa 60(3), 351-358.

Rout, M., Senapati, M.R., Mohapatra, J.K., Dash, B.B., Sanyal, A. and Pattnaik, B. 2014. Serosurveillance of foot-and-mouth disease in sheep and goat population of India. Prev. Vet. Med. 113, 273-277.

Rufael, T., Catley, A., Bogale, A., Sahle, M. and Shiferaw, Y. 2008. Foot and mouth disease in the Borana pastoral system, southern Ethiopia and implications for livelihoods and international trade. Trop. Anim. Health Prod. 40(1), 29-38.

Samuel, A.R., Knowles, N.J. and MacKay, D.K. 1999. Genetic analysis of type O viruses responsible for epidemics of foot-and-mouth disease in North Africa. Epidemiol. Infect. 122(3), 529-538.

Sarker, S., Talukder, S., Haque, M.H., Islam, M.H. and Gupta, S.D. 2011. Epidemiological Study on Foot-and-Mouth Disease in Cattle: Prevalence and Risk

Factor Assessment in Rajasthan, Bangladesh. Wayamba J. Anim. Sci. 71-73.

Valdazo-González, B., Knowles, N.J. and King, D.P. 2014. Genome Sequences of Foot-and-Mouth Disease Virus O/ME-SA/Ind-2001 Lineage from Outbreaks in Libya, Saudi Arabia, and Bhutan during 2013. Genome Announc. 2(2), e00242-14.

Vynnycky, E. and White, R.G. 2010. An introduction to Infectious Disease Modelling. Oxford University Press, Oxford, UK.

WRLFMD. 2014a. Genotyping report: FMDV type O. Country: Tunisia. FAO World Reference Library for Foot-and-Mouth Disease (WRLFMD), the Pirbright Institute, Surrey, United Kingdom: http://www.wrlfmd.org/fmd_genotyping/2014/WRLFMD-2014-00029%20O%20Tunisia%202014.pdf.

WRLFMD. 2014b. Genotyping report: FMDV type O. Country: Algeria. FAO World Reference Library for Foot-and-Mouth Disease (WRLFMD), the Pirbright Institute, Surrey, United Kingdom: http://www.wrlfmd.org/fmd_genotyping/2014/WRLFMD-2014-00028%20O%20Algeria%202014.pdf.

WRLFMD. 2016. The FAO World Reference Laboratory for Foot-and-Mouth Disease. http://www.wrlfmd.org/fmd_genotyping/africa/lib.htm. Accessed: 02/02/2016.

15

Cataracts and strabismus associated with hand rearing using artificial milk formulas in Bengal tiger (*Panthera tigris* spp *tigris*) cubs

Rogério Ribas Lange[1], Leandro Lima[1], Erika Frühvald[1], Vera Sônia Nunes da Silva[2], Aparecida Sônia de Souza[2] and Fabiano Montiani-Ferreira[1,*]

[1]*Universidade Federal do Paraná (UFPR), Departamento de Medicina Veterinária, Rua dos Funcionários, 1540, Bairro Juvevê, 80035-050, Curitiba – PR, Brazil*
[2]*Universidade Estadual de Campina (UNICAMP), Centro de Ciência e Qualidade de Alimentos ITAL, Avenida Brasil, 2880, Campinas – SP, Brazil*

Abstract
The aim of this investigation is to describe the potential contributing nutritional factors involved in the development of ophthalmic and dermatologic changes in four Bengal tiger (*Panthera tigris* spp *tigris*) cubs fed an artificial milk formula. The affected animals were compared with two other tiger cubs that had been nursed by their dam naturally. After the first clinical signs appeared, the tiger cubs underwent ophthalmic evaluation. Severe symmetric generalized alopecia over the trunk, sparing the head and distal portion of the front and rear limbs, bilateral cataracts and strabismus were noticed. Milk and blood from the mother, as well as blood from the healthy and affected cubs were collected in order to evaluate complete blood counts, serum chemistry values, and amino acid levels. The amino acid concentrations in the artificial formula were also evaluated for comparison to the milk from the dam. The concentration of taurine, arginine, phenylalanine, tryptophan and histidine were very low in the artificial formulas as compared to the dam´s milk. The tiger cubs that received the artificial formula had lower levels of the amino acids listed previously as compared to those that nursed from the dam naturally. Taurine, as well as arginine, phenylalanine, tryptophan and histidine deficiency appeared to be possible causes of the development of skin problems, cataracts and strabismus in the tiger cubs fed with these particular artificial milk replacers. In the future, special attention should be given in order to make sure that adequate levels of these amino acids are present in artificial milk for tiger cubs.
Keywords: Alopecia, Amino acids, Lens opacity, Wild felid, Zoo animal.

Introduction

Wild felids are commonly kept in zoos and large felids such as lions, tigers and cheetahs are popular among visitors and attract the population's interest worldwide. Large felids breed commonly in captivity and occasionally neonates of these species are not able to be raised by their dams. Optimum nutrition for suckling neonates is provided by the natural milk from the dam (Baines, 1981; Remillard et al., 1993).
When species-specific milk is not available, nutritional formulation are extrapolated from the milk of related species (Baines, 1981; McManamon, 1993; Remillard et al., 1993). The milk composition of the following felids has been investigated: domestic cat (*Felis catus*) (Adkins et al., 1997; Jacobsen et al. 2004), lion (*Panthera leo*) (BenShaul, 1962; De Waal et al., 2004), cheetah (*Acinonyx jubatus*) (Osthoff et al., 2006), serval (*Felis serval*) (Osthoff et al., 2007) and clouded leopard (Senda et al., 2010).
However, no information is available regarding the composition of tiger (*Panthera tigris*) milk. These previous publications show that protein and fat content vary considerably among different species of wild felids.
In zoos, an option frequently used is to provide cow´s milk or even other non-related species' milk-replacer formulas (Tilson and Seal, 1988; Osthoff et al., 2006, 2007). There are numerous protocols for hand rearing tigers using natural milk from another species (Tilson and Seal, 1988), artificial formulas and even mixtures of both (Baines, 1981; Remillard et al., 1993; Adkins et al., 1997).
Cataracts, dietary intolerance and reduced weight gain have been anecdotally attributed to differences in protein, fatty acid and carbohydrate composition between natural tigress milk and milk replacers' formulas (Tilson and Seal, 1988; Remillard et al., 1993; Osthoff et al., 2007). Specific nutritional requirements or optimal surrogate milk composition for tiger neonates have not yet been characterized.
The aim of this article is to describe the potential contributing nutritional factors involved in the development of the dermatologic and ophthalmic changes in tiger cubs fed artificial milk formulas.

*Corresponding Author: Fabiano Montiani-Ferreira. Universidade Federal do Paraná (UFPR), Departamento de Medicina Veterinária, Rua dos Funcionários, 1540, Bairro Juvevê, 80035-050, Curitiba – PR, Brazil. Email: montiani@ufpr.br

Case details

Clinical history

Six Bengal tigers (*Panthera tigris* ssp. *tigris*) cubs and two adult tigresses living at Pomerode's Zoo (Pomerode City, Santa Catarina State, Brazil) were investigated. The cubs were conceived naturally and born in three different litters, two successive litters from Tigress 1 (Fig. 1a) and a litter from Tigress 2. Two out of three litters were separated from the dam by the Zoo employees due to the dam's history of killing its cubs.

The first litter (litter 1) from Tigress 1 yielded cub 1A (male) and cub 1B (female) that were separated from the dam at 3 days of age and hand-raised with a homemade artificial milk replacer (MR1) and subsequently developed clinical abnormalities. The second litter (litter 2) from Tigress 2 yielded cub 2A (male) and cub 2B (male), which also were separated from the dam at 3 days of age and hand-raised with a different artificial milk replacer (MR2) that was formulated in an attempt to avoid the clinical abnormalities noted in cubs 1A and 1B. A third litter (litter 3) from Tigress 1 yielded cub 3A (male) and 3B (male). This time, a successful attempt to leave the cubs to be raised by the dam was made and the cubs received natural tiger milk.

Litter 1

The tiger cubs 1A and 1B were fed MR1 for the first 60 days after birth. During the first days of life, the cubs received a volume of MR1 via bottle-feeding (Fig. 1b), which was calculated based on body weight as recommended in the literature (Binczik *et al.*, 1988; Tilson and Seal, 1988). The cubs' eyelids opened by 7 days of age (cub 1B) and 10 days of age (cub 1A). During the first 30 days of age, cubs 1A and 1B developed dermatological abnormalities; generalized erythema, dry skin, and alopecia. Both of these cubs developed all these signs but the alopecia was more severe in the cub 1A.

The alopecia was severe (about 60% of the body surface), symmetrical, generalized over the trunk but sparing the head and distal portions of the front and rear limbs (Fig. 1c), which began to resolve around 60 days of age (Fig. 1d). At the end of the second month, cub 1B weighed 7.0 kg and cub 1A 6.0 k. A set of sharp and fine teeth started to appear after the first seven days of age. At about 60 days of age, the teeth were notably thicker and larger and the cubs started to receive a supplement of raw meat (without bones).

When cubs 1A and 1B were 70 days of age, the Comparative Ophthalmology Laboratory of the Veterinary Teaching Hospital of Federal University of Paraná (LABOCO-HV-UFPR), Curitiba, Paraná State, Brazil, performed an ophthalmic evaluation in the cubs to assess suspected visual impairment, noticed when they were about 30 days of age.

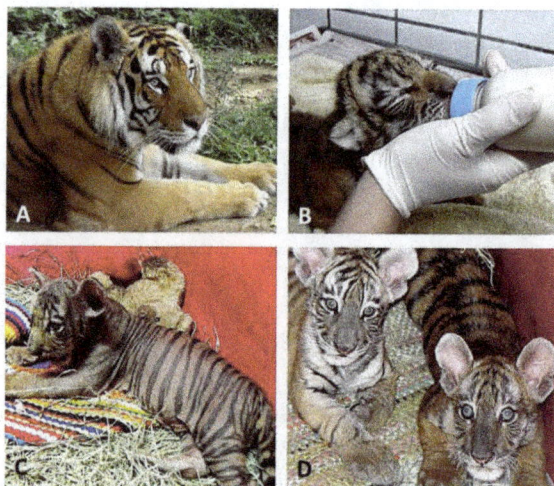

Fig. 1. Sequential photographs of some of the *Panthera tigris* spp. *tigris* involved. (A): Tigress 1 in the external zoo enclosure after giving birth. (B): Male cub (1A) at 14 days of age receiving milk replacer from a bottle. (C): Cub 1A at 30 days of age demonstrating severe symmetric generalized alopecia over the trunk, sparing the head and distal portion of the front and rear limbs. (D): Cub 1A (right) and Cub 1B (left) with cataracts and strabismus at 70 days of age. Note that the fur was already starting to grow at this time point.

During ophthalmic evaluation, bilateral mature (cub 1A) and immature (cub 1B) cataracts were diagnosed in addition to unilateral exotropia (also known as divergent strabismus) in the right eye of cub 1A (Fig. 2a) and bilateral exotropia for cub 1B. The eyes were examined with a slit lamp biomicroscope (Hawk Eye; Dioptrix, L'Union, France) to evaluate the anterior segment. Neither cub had a menace response. Pupillary and consensual light reflexes were normal in both eyes. The cornea, anterior chamber, aqueous humor and iris were normal in both cubs. The cataracts in both cubs showed no anterior capsular opacities and there were no signs of lens subluxation. The cataracts precluded posterior segment evaluation. With the exception of cataracts and strabismus, no other ocular abnormalities were noted.

Litter 2

Cubs 2A and 2B also were separated from the dam at 3 days of age and fed with a different artificial milk formula (MR2). At this point a nutritional problem was already a suspicion. MR2 was developed empirically by the staff of another zoo who claimed to have successfully used it to hand-rear tiger cubs in the past. So the information for the MR2 formula was communicated and this formula was tried in cubs 2A and 2B, in an empiric attempt to prevent the clinical signs seen in Litter 1.

MR2 formula, nevertheless, was similar to MR1. Basically it is MR1 formula with a multivitamin supplement and a commercially available milk powder for small animals added. Further details of MR2 are discussed below. However, cubs 2A and 2B developed similar clinical signs to the cubs from the first litter (cubs 1A and 1B).

Both cubs developed alopecia at 25 days of age, however, alopecia was milder than the first litter. At the end of the second month, cub 2A weighed 5.8 kg and cub 2B weighed 7 kg. When these animals were about 50-days-old their teeth also were evident and they started receiving raw meat in order to empirically supplement the MR2 possible diet deficiencies, since a nutritional cause was suspected. The alopecia began resolving on its own at approximately 60 days of age, like cubs 1A and 1B. Ophthalmic findings of cubs 2A and 2B included bilateral immature cataracts and mild bilateral esotropia (convergent strabismus) (Fig. 2b).

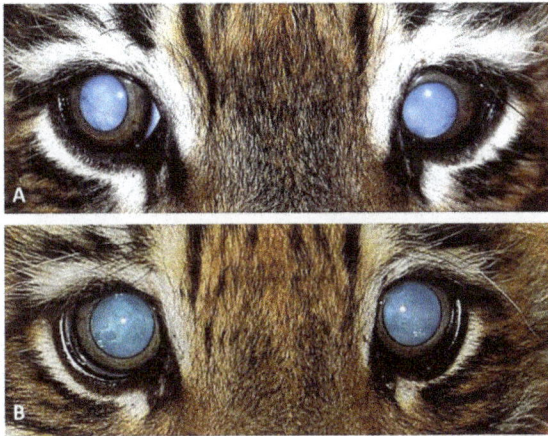

Fig. 2. Bengal tiger (*Panthera tigris* spp. *tigris*) cubs affected with cataracts. (A): Cub 1A, fed with artificial milk replacer 1 (MR1) demonstrating unilateral divergent strabismus (OD) and bilateral mature cataracts. (B): Cub 2A, fed with MR2 showing bilateral immature cataracts and mild bilateral convergent strabismus. Note the faint blue tapetal reflex and nuclear and cortical lens opacity.

Litter 3

The cubs from the third litter (cubs 3A and 3B) were parent raised and received natural tigress milk for eight weeks. These cubs did not develop dermatological or ophthalmic signs. At the end of the second month of life, the weight of cub 3A was 5.3 kg and 3B was 4.75 kg.

Milk replacer formulas

Two milk replacer formulas (MR1 and MR2) were prepared based on previous supposedly effective experiences by other Brazilian zoos. There were small differences between the components of MR1 and MR2. Tables 1 and 2 list the ingredients used in the MR1 and MR2 recipes. The cubs were fed these diets from the third day of life and the composition of MR1 and MR2 did not vary over time.

Table 1. Ingredients used in MR1 recipe.

- 500 ml of 4% fat whole milk - ultra-high-temperature-pasteurized (UHT) cow's milk (Leite Líquido NINHO Forti+ Integral, Nestlé Ltda, PR, Brazil).
- 500 ml of 90% reduced lactose cow's milk (Leite Líquido NINHO Forti+ Zero Lactose, Nestlé Ltda, PR, Brazil).
- 10 ml of cod-liver oil (Emulsão de Scott Regular, Laboratório GlaxoSmithKline, RJ, Brazil). Each 10 ml also contains vitamin A (2,530 IU) and vitamin D (253 IU)
- 75 mg – equivalent of 1 ml of dimethicone oral emulsion (Luftal, Bristol-Myers Squibb, SP, Brazil).
- 1 ml of a probiotic supplement for dogs and cats containing *Saccharomyces cerevisiae*, *Lactobacillus acidophillus*, *Bifidobacterium bifidum*, *Enterococcus faecium*, *Lactobacillus plantarum* (Probiótico Vetnil, Vetnil Indústria e Comércio, PR, Brazil).
- 15 g of canned cat food (Hill's a/d Science Diet, Hills Pet Nutrition INC, SP, Brazil).
- 10 ml of a multivitamin oral suspension (Clusivol, Wyeth Indústria Farmacêutica Ltda, SP, Brazil). Each 10 ml contained: Retinyl Palmitate (vitamin A) 2,500 IU; Cholecalciferol (vitamin D3) 200 IU; Ascorbic Acid (vitamina C) 32.50 mg; Cyanocobalamin (vitamin B12) 3.00 mcg; Thiamine Chloride (vitamin B1) 0,75 mg; Riboflavin (as riboflavin 5'-phosphate) (vitamin B2) 0.85 mg; Pyridoxine Hydrochloride (vitamin B6) 1.00 mg; Nicotinamide 10.00 mg; Dexpanthenol (d-panthenol) 6.00 mg; Inositol 5.00 mg. Amino acids: L-lysine Hydrochloride 25.00 mg; Choline Tartrate 5,00 mg. Mineral salts: Iron (as ferrous gluconate) 3.00 mg; Calcium (as calcium lactate and calcium hypophosphite) 40.00 mg; Phosphorus (as calcium hypophosphite) 30.00 mg; Iodine (as potassium iodide) 75.00 mcg; Potassium (as potassium gluconate) 2.50 mg; Manganese (as manganese gluconate) 0.52 mg; Zinc (as zinc lactate) 0.50 mg; Magnesium (as magnesium gluconate) 3.00 mg.

Table 2. Ingredients used in MR2 recipe.

- 500 ml of 4% fat whole milk - ultra-high-temperature-pasteurized (UHT) cow's milk (Leite Líquido NINHO Forti+ Integral, Nestlé Ltda, PR, Brazil).
- 500 ml of 90% reduced lactose cow's milk (Leite Líquido NINHO Forti+ Zero Lactose, Nestlé Ltda, PR, Brazil).
- 10 ml of cod-liver oil (Emulsão de Scott Regular, Laboratório GlaxoSmithKline, RJ, Brazil). Each 10 ml also contains vitamin A (2,530 IU) and vitamin D (253 IU).
- 75 mg – equivalent of 1 ml of dimethicone oral emulsion (Luftal, Bristol-Myers Squibb, SP, Brazil).
- 1 ml of a probiotic supplement for dogs and cats containing *Saccharomyces cerevisiae*, *Lactobacillus acidophillus*, *Bifidobacterium bifidum*, *Enterococcus faecium*, *Lactobacillus plantarum* (Probiótico Vetnil, Vetnil Indústria e Comércio, PR, Brazil).
- 4 g of a commercially available milk powder for dogs and cats (PetMilk, Vetnil Indústria e Comércio, PR, Brazil).
- 5 ml a multivitamin suspension (Supre Gatos, Syntec, SP, Brazil) Each 5 ml contained: Folic Acid 0.045 mg; Choline Tartrate 35 mg; Copper 0.114 mg; Pantothenic Acid 4 mg; Zinc 0.35 mg; Vitamin A 1479 IU/g; Iron 0.75 mg; Magnesium 0.004 mg; Vitamin B1 1.5 mg; Phosphorus 0.04 g; Manganese 0.24 mg; Vitamin B6 1.51 mg; Biotin 0.012 mg; Vitamin B2 1.50 mg; Vitamin B12 5.886 mcg; Calcium 0.061 g; Niacin 7.4 mg; Vitamin K 0.77 mg; Iodine 0.28 mg; Potassium 0.09 mg; Vitamin D3 148 IU/g; Sodium 0.001 g; Taurine 1 mg; Vitamin E 6.7 mg; Inositol 1.5 mg.

Sampling

Blood samples from two of the affected cubs (2A and 2B) were collected in order to evaluate the amino acid levels. Additionally, milk and blood from Tigress 1 and blood from the two healthy cubs (3A and 3B) were collected to serve as controls. Furthermore, complete blood counts (CBC), serum biochemical analyses of these animals and amino acid analysis of MR1 and MR2 were evaluated. Milk was obtained from Tigress 1 during the eighth week of lactation. The tigress was five years old and fed 5 kg per day of a beef and chicken meat mixture which was supplemented with a commercial mineral and vitamin C veterinary supplement (Aminomix pet performance; Vetnil Indústria e Comércio de Produtos Veterinários LTDA, SP, Brazil). To collect milk samples, Tigress 1 was anesthetized by darting with an intramuscular combination of ketamine (10 mg/kg) (Ketamin S(+), Laboratório Cristália – Produtos Químicos e Farmacêuticos, SP, Brazil) and midazolam (0.5 mg/kg) (Midazolam; Eurofarma Laboratórios LTDA, SP, Brazil). Once anesthetised, blood samples were collected from the cephalic vein, and a bolus of oxytocin (0.25 IU/kg [ocitocina; Vetnil Indústria e Comércio de Produtos Veterinários LTDA, SP, Brazil]), was injected intravenously. The milk sample (150 mL) was collected immediately after oxytocin injection by manual compression and then divided into three 50-ml plain tubes (Falcon, Becton Dickinson, Lincoln Park, NJ). The milk was then frozen for one week at -20 C until the amino acid analysis was performed.

Blood samples of all cubs were collected from the femoral veins into plain 3 ml tubes using manual restraint when the cubs were 60 (cubs 3A and 3B) and 58 (cubs 2A and 2B) days old. Whole blood was allowed to clot and then immediately centrifuged. The serum was then collected and frozen until analyzed. Blood samples were processed by the Clinical Pathology Laboratory of the Federal University of Paraná (Curitiba City, Paraná State, Brazil), and milk and blood serum amino acid analyses were performed by the State University of Campinas, Center of Science and Food Quality (Centro de Ciência e Qualidade de Alimentos ITAL, Campinas, SP, Brazil).

Milk and serum analyses results

Concerning the CBC and serum biochemistry, no significant findings or pertinent differences between the cubs were observed on the blood work.

Lactose was measured in milk and MR samples and the results are expressed in mg/100 mL. The natural tigress milk had 2.77 lactose, compared to the 2.46 of MR2 and 1.55 of MR1. All amino acids evaluated in tigress milk and MRs are presented in Table 3, and the content of free amino acids in serum of Tigress 1 and cubs (cubs 2A, 2B, 3A and 3B) can be seen in Table 4.

Table 3. Qualitative and quantitative amino acid analysis of tigress milk and milk replacers (MR1* and MR2**).

Amino acids	Total amino acids (mg/100 mL of sample)		
	MR1*	MR2**	Tigress milk
Alanine	146.96	121.87	413.92
Arginine	144.62	137.53	732.14
Aspartic acid	301.02	287.83	1092.02
Cystine	91.00	89.29	306.29
Glutamic acid	737.85	763.39	2638.78
Glycine	112.97	74.73	151.35
Histidine	98.46	94.40	426.54
Isoleucine	188.96	186.82	631.67
Leucine	360.94	354.67	1558.20
Lysine	333.09	316.60	944.97
Methionine	72.83	67.09	219.10
Phenylalanine	185.98	177.81	503.05
Proline	308.75	321.14	1085.74
Serine	197.52	193.11	542.71
Taurine	3.58	0.06	90.00
Threonine	169.97	165.09	808.36
Tryptophan	121.38	124.96	276.94
Tyrosine	179.70	177.71	670.49
Valine	225.47	219.72	741.86
Total	3981.07	3873.83	13834.15

*MR1 – Milk Replacer 1.
**MR2 –Milk Replacer 2.

All of the amino acids measured in MR1 and MR2 were present in lower quantities as compared to tigress milk. Compared to tigress milk, taurine levels were particularly low in both MRs but levels of arginine, phenylalanine, tryptophan and histidine were also low. Inferential statistical analyses were not performed due to the small sample numbers.

In Table 4, the comparison between free amino acids in serum of the cubs fed with MR2 (2A and 2B) and cubs fed with tigress milk (3A and 3B) revealed that the levels of some amino acids were higher in the cubs fed MR2 as compared to those fed tigress milk, but a lower level of taurine. Nevertheless, the level of serum taurine in affected cubs was similar to that in the tigress.

Discussion

Cataracts, strabismus and alopecia were diagnosed in four tiger cubs that had been fed with different artificial formulas during the initial weeks of development.

Table 4 – Content of free amino acids in serum of Tigress 1 and cubs.

Amino Acids	Free amino acids (mg/100 mL of sample)				
	Tigress 1	Cub 3A*	Cub 3B*	Cub 2A**	Cub 2B**
Alanine	5.51	3.33	2.44	5.19	6.63
Arginine	2.70	2.98	2.77	3.43	3.49
Aspartic acid	0.01	0.39	0.21	0.43	0.43
Cystine	3.59	4.67	3.39	3.67	3.78
Glutamic acid	0.92	1.92	1.51	3.49	3.57
Glycine	3.12	2.19	2.03	3.84	4.05
Histidine	1.93	2.73	2.13	2.86	3.60
Isoleucine	0.82	1.49	0.88	1.18	1.03
Leucine	1.19	2.92	1.69	2.00	1.66
Lysine	1.83	1.68	1.22	1.87	1.67
Methionine	0.91	1.14	0.97	1.89	2.31
Phenylalanine	0.63	1.02	1.06	1.28	1.14
Proline	1.10	3.31	1.80	3.17	3.09
Serine	5.9	6.69	5.65	7.91	11.47
Taurine	3.87	6.31	5.92	3.75	2.81
Threonine	0.93	2.68	1.59	1.42	1.36
Tryptophan	1.49	1.96	1.86	2.10	1.97
Tyrosine	0.72	1.67	1.04	1.31	1.02
Valine	1.44	2.66	1.72	2.13	1.89
Total	38.61	51.74	39.88	52.92	56.97

*Cubs 3A and 3B were raised by their dam and received only natural tiger milk.
**Cubs 2A and 2B were raised by hand and received milk replacer 2 (MR2).

Amino acid analyses of the milk formulas and natural milk from the dam were performed. The concentration of taurine, arginine, phenylalanine, tryptophan and histidine were very low in the artificial formulas as compared to the dam´s milk.

Intrinsic limitations in this investigation are absence of a controlled environment and availability of these animals to be examined at matched ages in a controlled environment. Nevertheless, taurine, as well as arginine, phenylalanine, tryptophan and histidine deficiency appeared to be possible causes of the development of skin problems, cataracts and strabismus in the tiger cubs fed with these particular artificial milk replacers.

Cataracts associated with nutritional deficiencies in immature animals have been reported in dogs (Vainisi et al., 1981; Martin and Chambreau, 1982; Glaze and Blanchard, 1983; Ranz et al., 2002), cats (Frankel, 2001), wolves (Vainisi et al., 1981), rabbits (Devi et al., 1965), guinea pigs (VonSallman et al., 1959), rats (Albanese, 1952; Bagghi, 1959; Bunce et al., 1978, 1984; Koch et al. 1982), and fish (Poston et al., 1977; Poston and Rumsey, 1983; Richardson et al., 1985). In

these species, there are different nutritionally related causes involved in cataract development. Amino acid imbalances can alter the physiological milieu of the body's tissues and cells leading to severe pathophysiologic states (Raju et al., 2007). Deficiencies of valine, histidine, arginine and phenylalanine amino acids may cause cataracts in dogs, cats and wolves hand-reared on commercial or empirically produced milk replacers (Vainisi et al., 1981; Martin and Chambreau, 1982; Glaze and Blanchard, 1983; Frankel, 2001). Tryptophan, phenylalanine and histidine deficiency also were associated with cataract formation in immature rats (Pike, 1951; Albanese, 1952).

Nutritional cataracts resulting from a deficiency of essential amino acids and certain vitamins or an excess of particular carbohydrates, have been observed in different species in the last several decades (Malone et al., 1993).

The mechanism of cataract development for most amino acid deficiencies observed in rats was apoptosis of lens epithelial cells due to lowered intracellular pH or to disruption of lysosomes (Wegener et al., 2002; Raju et al., 2007). Nutritional cataracts caused by artificial milk replacers in large felids are not a rare occurrence in zoos and most experienced zoo workers are at least aware of this possible complication. Paradoxically, there are several anecdotal reports and non-scientific publications on the subject but not very many scientific publications about this apparently common phenomenon.

A report links the use of milk replacers and the occurrence of cataracts in an African lion (Sardari et al., 2007). Yet, the exact deficient amino acid involved in the development of cataracts in large felids has not been identified (Magrane and VanDeGrift, 1975; Benirschke et al., 1976). Heritable cataracts have not yet been demonstrated in tiger cubs, making amino acid deficiency a likely important cause for cataract development in these animals. Nevertheless, some authors have suggested the occurrence heritable cataracts in lions and clouded leopards (Cooley, 2001). Although these are not the same species, they are large wild felids facing similar breeding challenges in captivity such as low genetic diversity and consequently more chances to demonstrate genetic diseases.

In fact, interesting progresses have been made in the area of heritable cataracts in large felids bred in zoos. For instance the genomic sequences of 4 crystalline genes CRYAA, CRYAB, CRYBB2, and CRYBB1 was analyzed in inbred Angolan lions kept in German zoos. In addition, 10 candidate genes were analyzed using adjacent microsatellites (Philipp et al., 2010). As a result, these genes were excluded as responsible for the familial primary cataract in these Angolan lions.

Nutritional cataracts caused by inappropriate formulation of artificial milk formulas were studied in laboratory rats (Sonnenber et al., 1982). Twenty percent of rat pups fed an artificial milk substitute developed cataracts. These rat pups also had atypical amino acid levels and low concentrations of several amino acids in the blood. In particular, only traces of taurine were found, (Sonnenber et al., 1982) and it was speculated that taurine deficiency leads to the development of cataracts in these rats.

In our investigation, amino acid analysis of the blood showed higher concentration of arginine, glutamic acid, glycine and methionine and a lower level of taurine in the cubs fed MR as compared to those fed natural tigress milk. Higher concentrations of any of these amino acids has not been associated with cataract formation in other animal species; however, since taurine deficiency has been associated with cataract development in other species (Poston et al., 1977; Bunce et al., 1978, 1984; Sonnenber et al., 1982; Poston and Rumsey, 1983; Richardson et al., 1985; Raju et al., 2007), it is possible that the lower level of taurine is involved in the cataract development in the tiger cubs.

Quantitative analysis of rat eye tissues revealed that taurine was the most abundant amino acid in the retina, vitreous, lens, cornea, iris, and ciliary body (Ripps and Shen, 2012). However, physiological mechanisms mediating the actions of taurine in the eye are not fully known (Ripps and Shen, 2012). Results of an in vitro study using intact lenses of rabbits incubated in tissue culture media containing galactose and taurine, and galactose alone, showed that galactose without taurine significantly increased the rate of cataract development compared to galactose with taurine. In this study, taurine appeared to protect the lens against the development of sugar-induced cataracts and may have exerted this effect by decreasing oxidative damage (Malone et al., 1993; Rathore and Gupta, 2010). The role of taurine deficiency in cataract development has been studied by a number of other groups (Zhang and Chen, 1998; Son et al., 2007; Hsu et al., 2012). It is possible that the deficiency of taurine in the cubs receiving the two different artificial milk formulas may have exposed their lenses to an oxidative effect. However, levels of lipid peroxidation products, galactose and lactose in the blood were not measured.

A thorough investigation of retinal function was not performed in the cubs, though taurine deficiency is known to cause retinal degeneration in domestic cats. A single case report of a white Bengal tiger with a central retinal defect compared the affected animal's taurine levels with those of orange Bengal tigers and taurine-deficient domestic cats with resulting central retinal degeneration. Nonetheless, the authors concluded that though the affected white Bengal tiger's

taurine was lower, it was not as low as affected domestic cats and thus, the low taurine levels were unlikely to have caused that animal's lesion (Pickett et al., 1990).

Although the cubs fed with MR2 and cubs fed with tigress milk revealed lower levels of taurine, the level of serum taurine in affected cubs was similar to that in the tigress. However, the converted tigress' serum value (309.25μmol/L) was lower than the only previous report of a normal range for Bengal tigers of (320–620 μmol/L) (Hedberg et al., 2007). While the domestic cat appears to be an acceptable physiologic model for wild felids, it is often difficult to assess taurine status in zoo feeding programs owing to scattered data on feed taurine content as well as a lack of normal ranges for assessment of taurine in biological tissues (Hedberg et al., 2007). Additionally, it is known that individual domestic cats vary greatly in their capacity to regulate taurine metabolism and occasionally do well with diets containing less than ideal taurine levels (Hedberg et al., 2007). According to Hedberg et al. (2007) one blood sample might not be enough to confirm inadequate taurine levels unless the diet offered is severely deficient, which is the case in the present report.

The characteristics of nutritional cataracts in tiger cubs have not been previously described in the literature. We believe this is because these animals are not frequently examined in zoos until they develop severe ophthalmic changes (like vision loss and/or intense lens opacity). In our cubs fed with milk replacer, the ophthalmic evaluation revealed an initial nuclear opacity of the lens that appeared to progress quickly in a matter of few weeks to involve the cortex during the cataract development. This pattern is very different to that observed in domestic puppies fed with diets deficient in arginine and phenylalanine, which are both essential amino acids. The opacities in this case were described as a nuclear–cortical junction ring with some vacuolization of the equatorial fibers and Y-sutures (Ranz et al., 2002). This pattern was not observed in the tiger cubs presently described.

Some authors do not recommend surgery in tigers with nutritional cataracts because they considered these cataracts to be self-limiting (Tilson and Seal, 1988). However, cataract development certainly varies according to the type and intensity of the nutritional imbalance in question. The opacities observed in these cubs did not appear to be self-limiting, as in other descriptions, and instead were unquestionably progressive.

It is important to determine the possible origin of lens opacities when a veterinary ophthalmologist evaluates any animal, but it is especially important for zoo animals because the diagnosis of nutritional cataracts may have a different clinical course compared to those due to metabolic, inflammatory, traumatic, hereditary or congenital causes. In some zoos, the diagnosis of a hereditary or congenital cataract may result in castration, exclusion from reproduction and even euthanasia (Tilson and Seal, 1988). This is important for the protection of the species by eliminating affected animals from the gene pool (Seitz and Weisse, 1979; Tilson and Seal, 1988).

Cataract surgery might be considered an option to improve the quality of life of affected individuals as in the case reported in a Siberian tiger (Seitz and Weisse, 1979). The tiger cubs that developed cataracts had normal globe positions until they reached 30 days of life. Divergent strabismus was noted after 45 days of age.

In another case report of a white Bengal tiger cub born with convergent strabismus and poor vision, the possible causes considered for strabismus were an adaptation to genetically abnormal visual pathways linked to lack of pigment, abnormalities of the abducens nerve and mechanical restricting conditions of the medial rectus muscles (Bernays and Smith, 1999; Pachaly and Montiani-Ferreira, 2003). In this Bengal tiger, no nutritional causes were speculated as it was born with strabismus.

The occurrence of cataracts and strabismus in the cubs fed with MRs was the main focus of the present study. Nevertheless, transitory alopecia also was a conspicuous clinical sign observed in these animals. Protein and amino acid deficiency is well known to cause loss of body hair in wild animals in captivity (Novak and Meyer, 2009). Although vitamin and mineral imbalances have been postulated as a possible cause of body hair loss (Novak and Meyer, 2009), the nutritional parameters that might regulate hair production in animals and humans were not completely characterized. Moderate to severe zinc deficiency has been associated with alopecia in children (Alhaj et al., 2007). Zinc, vitamin D and vitamin A deficiencies are known to cause alopecia in animals and humans (Rushton, 2002; Ginn et al., 2007).

Interestingly, deficiency of tryptophan also has been reported to lead to a very rapid formation of cataracts and alopecia in rats (Wegener et al., 2002). The amino acid deficiency presented here as the main candidate for the development of cataracts and strabismus, possibly contributed to the occurrence of alopecia as well. Vitamin and mineral levels were not objectively assessed in the cubs reported here. Nevertheless, the authors believe that imbalances of vitamins and minerals also might have contributed to the transient alopecia observed in these animals.

The tiger cubs presently reported were born with normal globe position, and strabismus became evident after other dermatological and ophthalmological clinical signs were also evident. The influence of amino acids in the pathophysiology of the tiger strabismus is still unknown and it must be studied in the future.

Considering nutrition of captive tigers, some zoos formulate diets from basic ingredients so the components are relatively constant. However, nutritional analysis on the finished product is rarely conducted. Diets should be weighed and daily records kept as to how much is offered to each individual tiger and how much is consumed. It is possible that the tiger cubs consumed a different quantity of milk replacer than the quantity calculated for the size of the cub. Because of this, it is difficult to say if in the early stages of growth, the quantity of amino acids absorbed by the tiger cubs were the same as those measured in the amino acid analysis at 60 days of age.

In the literature, there is no amino acid requirement information for growing cubs or even adult tigers. Even though taurine deficiency was believed to be involved in the cataract formation in these cubs, it is possible that altered levels of other amino acids, vitamins and even fat, carbohydrates or protein, may have contributed to the pathophysiology as well. In fact, a previous evaluation of two milk replacers fed to hand-reared cheetah cubs indicated that both formulas were low in the majority of essential amino acids compared with domestic cat maternal milk (Bell et al., 2011).

The difficulty in evaluating wild animals, particularly in large felids, during lactation, the quantity of milk samples to collect and the high costs of a complete milk analysis are factors that understandably inhibit investigations such as this. Limitations of our study include a small number of animals investigated and the analysis of a milk sample from only one tigress. However, it can be used in the future as a general guideline, reference and as a catalyst for other nutritional investigations with tigress milk and artificial formulations, including other tests like fat, carbohydrate and protein analysis.

Taurine deficiency appeared to be a possible cause of the development of cataracts in the tiger cubs fed with these particular artificial milk replacers. In the future, special attention should be given in order to make sure that adequate levels of taurine, arginine, phenylalanine, tryptophan and histidine are present in artificial milk for tiger cubs.

We believe that the present report provides important information that could help zoo veterinarians prevent the development of nutritional cataracts in neonatal tiger cubs.

Acknowledgments

The authors would like to thank Dr. Marianna Bacellar Teodoro da Silva, Michigan State University for her help in the research and Dr. Gillian Shaw, University of Wisconsin, Madison, WI, USA, for her invaluable help in the preparation of this manuscript.

References

Adkins, Y., Zicker, S.C., Lepine, A. and Lönnerdal, B. 1997. Changes in nutrient and protein composition of cat milk during lactation. Am. J. Vet. Res. 58, 370-375.

Albanese, A.A. 1952. The effects of amino acid deficiencies in man. Am. J. Clin. Nutr. 1, 44-51.

Alhaj, E., Alhaj, N. and Alhaj, N.E. 2007. Diffuse alopecia in a child due to dietary zinc deficiency. Skinmed 6, 199-200.

Bagghi, K. 1959. The effects of methionine sulphoxamine induced methionine deficiency on the crystalline lens in albino rats. Indian J. Med. Res. 47, 437-447.

Baines, F.M. 1981. Milk substitutes and the hand rearing of orphan puppies and kittens. J. Small Anim. Pract. 22, 555-578.

Bell, K.M., Rutherfurd, S.M., Cottam, Y.H. and Hendriks, W.H. 2011. Evaluation of two milk replacers fed to hand-reared cheetah cubs (Acinonyx jubatus): nutrient composition, apparent total tract digestibility, and comparison to maternal cheetah milk. Zoo Biol. 30, 412-426.

Benirschke, K., Griner, L.A. and Staltzstein, S.L. 1976. Pathological findings in Siberian tigers. Internationalen Symposiums uber die Erkrankungen der Zootiere. 18, 263-274.

BenShaul, D.M. 1962. The composition of the milk of wild animals. Int. Zoo Yearb. 4, 333-342.

Bernays, M.E. and Smith, R. 1999. Convergent strabismus in a white Bengal tiger. Aust. Vet. J. 77, 152-155.

Binczik, G.A., Reindl, N.J., Taylor, R., Seal U.S. and Tilson, R.L. 1988. A neonatal growth model for captive Amur tigers. In: Tilson RL, Seal US. Tigers of the World: The biology, biopolitics, management, and conservation of an endangered species. Park Ridge, NJ: Noyes Publications.

Bunce, G.E., Hess, J.L. and Davis, D. 1984. Cataract formation following limited amino acid intake during gestation and lactation. Proc. Soc. Exp. Biol. Med. 176, 485-489.

Bunce, G.E., Hess, J.L. and Fillnow, G.M. 1978. Investigation of low tryptophan induced cataract in weanling rats. Exp. Eye Res. 26, 399-405.

Cooley, P.L. 2001. Phacoemulsification in a clouded leopard (Neofelis nebulosa). Vet. Ophthalmol. 4, 113-117.

Devi, A., Raina, P.L. and Singh, A. 1965. Abnormal protein and nucleic acid metabolism as a cause of cataract formation induced by nutritional deficiency in rabbits. Br. J. Ophthalmol. 49, 271-275.

De Waal, H.O., Osthoff, G., Hugo, A., Myburgh, J. and Botes, P. 2004. The composition of African lion (Panthera leo) milk collected a few days postpartum. Mamm. Biol. 69, 375-383.

Frankel, D.J. 2001. Malnutrition-induced cataracts in an orphaned kitten. Can. Vet. J. 42, 653-654.

Ginn, P.E., Mansell, J.E.K.L. and Rakich, P.M. 2007. Skin and appendages, p.553-781. In: Maxie M.G. (Ed.), Jubb, Kennedy, and Palmer's Pathology of Domestic Animals. Vol.1. 5th ed. Saunders Elsevier, Philadelphia.

Glaze, M.B.; Blanchard, G.L. 1983. Nutritional cataracts in a Samoyed litter. J. Am. Anim. Hosp. Assoc.19, 951-954.

Hedberg, G.E., Dierenfeld, E.S. and Rogers, Q.R. 2007. Taurine and zoo felids: considerations of dietary and biological tissue concentrations. Zoo Biol. 26, 517-531.

Hsu, Y.W., Yeh, S.M., Chen, Y.Y., Chen, Y.C., Lin, S.L. and Tseng, J.K. 2012. Protective effects of taurine against alloxan-induced diabetic cataracts and refraction changes in New Zealand White rabbits. Exp. Eye Res. 103, 71-77.

Jacobsen, K.L., DePeters, E.J., Rogers, Q.R. and Taylor, S.J. 2004. Influences of stage of lactation, teat position and sequential milk sampling on the composition of domestic cat milk (Felis catus). J. Anim. Physiol. Anim. Nutr. 88, 46-58.

Koch, H.R., Ohrloff, C., Bours, J., Riemann, G., Dragomireseu, V. and Hockwin, O. 1982. Separation of lens proteins in rats with tryptophan deficiency cataracts. Exp. Eye Res. 34, 479-486.

Magrane, W.G. and VanDeGrift, E.R. 1975. Extracapsular extraction in a Siberian tiger (Panthera tigris altaica). J. Zoo. Wildl. Med. 6, 11-12.

Malone, J.I., Benford, S.A. and Malone, J.Jr. 1993. Taurine prevents galactose-induced cataracts. J. Diabetes Complications 7, 44-48.

Martin, C.L. and Chambreau, T. 1982. Cataract production in experimentally orphaned puppies fed a commercial milk replacement for bitch's milk. J. Am. Anim. Hosp. Assoc.18, 115-119.

McManamon, R. 1993. Practical tips in nursery rearing of exotic cats. J. Small Exot. Anim. Med. 2, 137-140.

Novak, M.A., Meyer, J.S. 2009. Alopecia: Possible Causes and Treatments, Particularly in Captive Nonhuman Primates. Comp. Med. 59, 18-26.

Osthoff, G., Hugo, A. and de Wit, M. 2006. The composition of cheetah (Acinonyx jubatus) milk. Comp. Biochem. Physiol. B Biochem. Mol. Biol. 145, 265-269.

Osthoff, G., Hugo, A. and de Wit, M. 2007. The composition of serval (Felis serval) milk during mid-lactation. Comp. Biochem. Physiol. B Biochem. Mol. Biol. 147, 237-241.

Pachaly, J.R. and Montiani-Ferreira, F. 2003. Convergent strabismus in a white bengal tiger (Panthera tigris) - Case Report. Arq. Ciênc. Vet. Zool. UNIPAR. 6, 184-187.

Philipp, U., Steinmetz, A. and Distl, O. 2010. Development of feline microsatellites and SNPs for evaluating primary cataract candidate genes as cause for cataract in Angolan lions (Panthera leo bleyenberghi). J. Hered. 101, 633-638.

Pickett, J.P., Chesney, R.W., Beehler, B., Moore, C.P., Lippincott, S., Sturman J. and Ketring, K.L. 1990. Comparison of serum and plasma taurine values in Bengal tigers with values in taurine sufficient and deficient domestic cats. J. Am. Vet. Med. Assoc. 196, 342-346.

Pike, R.L. 1951. Congenital cataract in albino rats fed different amounts of tryptophan and niacin. J. Nutr. 44, 191-204.

Poston, G.A., Riis, R.C., Rumsey, G.I. and Ketola, H.G. 1977. The effect of supplemental dietary amino acids, minerals and vitamins on salmonids fed cataractogenic diet. Cornell Vet. 67, 472-509.

Poston, H.A. and Rumsey, G.L. 1983. Factors affecting dietary requirement and deficiency signs of L-tryptophan in rainbow trout. J. Nutr. 113, 2568-2577.

Raju, T.N., Kanth, V.R. and Reddy, U.M. 2007. Influence of kynurenines in pathogenesis of cataract formation in tryptophan-deficient regimen in Wistar rats. Indian J. Exp. Biol. 45, 543-548.

Ranz, D., Gutbrod, F., Eule, C. and Kienzle, E. 2002. Nutritional lens opacities in two litters of newfoundland dogs. J. Nutr. 132, 1688-1689.

Rathore, M.S. and Gupta, V.B. 2010. Protective effect of amino acids on eye lenses against oxidative stress induced by hydrogen peroxide. Asian J. Pharm. Clin. Res. 3, 166-169.

Remillard, R.L., Pickett, J.P., Thatcher, C.D. and Davenport, D.J. 1993. Comparison of kittens fed queen's milk with those fed milk replacer. Am. J. Vet. Res. 54, 901-907.

Richardson, N.L., Higgs, D.A., Beames, R.M. and McBride, J.R. 1985. Influence of dietary calcium, phosphorus, zinc and sodium phytate level on cataract incidence, growth and histopathology in juvenile Chinook salmon (Onconrhynchus tshawytscha). J. Nutr. 115, 553-567.

Ripps, H. and Shen, W. 2012. Review: taurine: a "very essential" amino acid. Mol. Vis. 18, 2673-2686.

Rushton, D.H. 2002. Nutritional factors and hair loss. Clin. Exp. Dermatol. 27, 396-404.

Sardari, K., Emami, M.R., Tabatabaee, A.A. and Ashkiani, A. 2007. Cataract surgery in an African lion (Panthera leo) with anterior lens luxation. Comp. Clin. Pathol. 16, 65-67.

Seitz, R. and Weisse, I. 1979. Operation on a congenital cataract in a Siberian tiger. Ophthalmologica 178, 56-65.

Senda, A., Hatakeyama, E., Kobayashi, R., Fukuda, K., Uemura, Y., Saito, T., Packer, C., Oftedal, O.T. and Urashima, T. 2010. Chemical characterization of milk oligosaccharides of an African lion (Panthera leo) and a clouded leopard (Neofelis nebulosa). Anim. Sci. J. 81, 687-693.

Son, H.Y., Kim, H.H. and Kwon, Y. 2007. Taurine prevents oxidative damage of high glucose-induced cataractogenesis in isolated rat lenses. J. Nutr. Sci. Vitaminol. (Tokyo). 53, 324-330.

Sonnenber, N., Bergstrom, J.D., Ha, Y.H. and Edmond, J. 1982. Metabolism in the artificially reared rat pup: effect of an atypical rat milk substitute. J. Nutr. 112, 1506-1514.

Tilson, R.L. and Seal, U.S. 1988. Tigers of the World: The biology, biopolitics, management, and conservation of an endangered species. Park Ridge, NJ: Noyes Publications.

Vainisi, S.J., Edelhauser, H.F., Wolf, E.D., Cotlier, E. and Reeser, F. 1981. Nutritional cataracts in timber wolves. J. Am. Anim. Hosp. Assoc.179, 1175-1180.

VonSallman, L., Reid, M.E., Grimes, P.A. and Collins, E.M. 1959. Tryptophan-deficiency cataracts in guinea pigs. Arch. Ophthalmol. 62, 662-672.

Wegener, A., Golubnitschaja, O., Breipohl, W., Schild, H.H. and Vresnsen, G.F.J.M. 2002. Effects of dietary deficiency of selective amino acids on the function of the cornea and lens in rats. Amino Acids 23, 337-342.

Zhang, W. and Chen, C. 1998. A study on the prevention of selenite cataract with taurine. Zhonghua Yan Ke Za Zhi. 34, 208-210.

16

Central vestibular syndrome in a red fox (*Vulpes vulpes*) with presumptive right caudal cerebral artery ischemic infarct and prevalent midbrain involvement

Mario Ricciardi[1,*], Floriana Gernone[1], Antonio De Simone[2] and Pasquale Giannuzzi[1]

[1] *"Pingry" Veterinary Hospital, via Medaglie d'Oro 5, 70126 Bari, Italy*
[2] *"Chisimaio" Veterinary Clinic, via Chisimaio 32, 00199 Roma, Italy*

Abstract

A wild young male red fox (*Vulpes vulpes*) was found in the mountainous hinterland of Rome (Italy) with a heavily depressed mental status and unresponsive to the surrounding environment. Neurological examination revealed depression, left circling, right head tilt, ventromedial positional strabismus and decreased postural reactions on the left side. Neurological abnormalities were suggestive of central vestibular syndrome. Two consecutive MRIs performed with 30 days interval were compatible with lacunar ischemic infarct in the territory of right caudal cerebral artery and its collateral branches. The lesion epicentre was in the right periaqueductal portion of the rostral mesencephalic tegmentum. Neuroanatomical and neurophysiological correlation between lesion localization and clinical presentation are discussed.

Keywords: Mesencephalon, Midbrain, MRI, Stroke, *Vulpes vulpes*.

Introduction

Cerebral ischemic stroke is a sudden interruption of arterial blood flow in a limited area of the brain caused by vascular obstruction, impaired vasodilation or increased blood viscosity leading to neuronal injury and parenchymal necrosis (Garosi *et al.*, 2006; Higgins *et al.*, 2006; Hillock *et al.*, 2006; Wessmann *et al.*, 2009; Giannuzzi *et al.*, 2014). Depending on the size of the involved vessel, cerebral infarcts are distinct in territorial infarcts, associated with disease of superficial, large diameter blood vessels and lacunar infarcts, deriving from disease of small, intraparenchymal, penetrating arteries (Garosi *et al.*, 2006). Clinical signs of focal ischemic encephalopathy are variable and ultimately related to the involved brain area (telencephalon; thalamus or midbrain; cerebellum; brainstem) (Hillock *et al.*, 2006). Although a large percentage, more or less 40%, of ischemic strokes have an unknown etiology, several underlying causes have been recognized in dogs and cats including, hypertension, endocrine, kidney, heart, metastatic diseases, parasitic thromboembolism (Garosi, 2010) and Evans' syndrome (Giannuzzi *et al.*, 2014). Focal ischemic encephalopathy is frequently diagnosed in companion animals and, in the last decade, it has been more commonly recognized likely because of both increased awareness of it as a potential neurologic disorder and increased availability of magnetic resonance imaging (MRI) and computed tomography (Dewey, 2003; Hillock *et al.*, 2006). However, despite the large amount of medical data regarding ischemic stroke in dogs, description of such condition in wild canids is lacking in veterinary literature.

In this paper, the authors describe the clinical signs, MRI findings and follow up of a presumptive focal ischemic encephalopathy in a wild red fox (*Vulpes vulpes*) in Southern Italy.

Case details

A wild young male red fox (*Vulpes vulpes*) weighting 10 kg was found in the mountainous hinterland of Rome (Italy) with a heavily depressed mental status and unresponsive to the surrounding environment. The animal was able to stand, with pronounced right head tilt, showing no aggressiveness nor fear towards humans. The fox received a single dose of dexamethasone and amoxicillin-clavulanic acid by the first examiner veterinarian and three days later the animal was referred to the Pingry Veterinary Hospital of Bari with an improved reactivity towards the surrounding environment. On physical examination, no abnormalities were observed. Neurological examination revealed depression, circling to the left, right sided head tilt and decreased postural reactions on the left side. Ventromedial positional strabismus was the most reliable abnormality detectable on cranial nerves examination (Fig. 1). The menace response was questionable on both eyes. Neurological abnormalities suggested a multifocal encephalic neuroanatomic localization with right forebrain and central vestibular system involvement. Because of the lack of a reliable clinical history, creating an appropriate differential diagnosis list was not possible.

*Corresponding Author: Dr. Mario Ricciardi. "Pingry" Veterinary Hospital, via Medaglie d'Oro 5, 70126 Bari, Italy.
Email: *ricciardi.mario@alice.it*

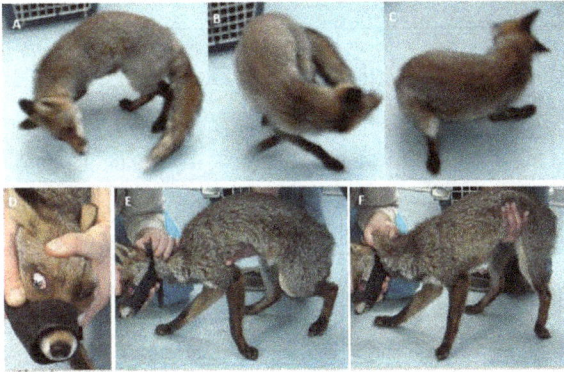

Fig. 1. Neurological examination. (A,B,C): Major neurological examination included depression, left circling with right head tilt. (D): Ventromedial positional strabismus on the right eye. (E,F): decreased postural reactions on the left side. Neurological abnormalities suggested a multifocal encephalic neuroanatomic localization with right forebrain and central vestibular system involvement.

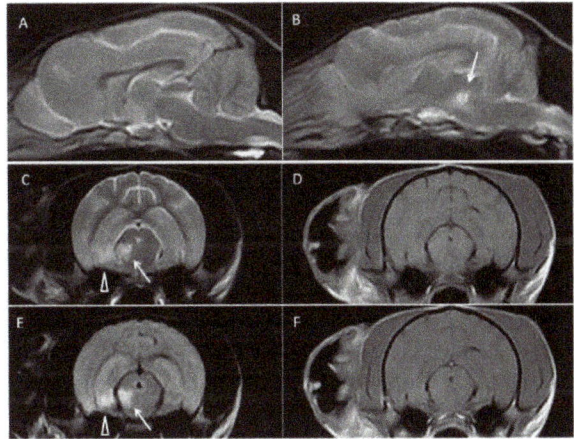

Fig. 2. First MRI of the brain. (A): midsagittal and (B): right parasagittal T2-weighted MRI images. (C): Transverse T2-weighted, (D): T1-weighted, (E): FLAIR and (F): contrast-enhanced T1-weighted MRI images obtained at the level of the rostral midbrain. T2W ad FLAIR images show a sharply hyperintense well demarcated lesion affecting the ventrolateral portion of mesencephalic tegmentum (arrows) and adjacent caudo-ventro-lateral portion of the right thalamus (not shown). The lesion extends to the medial surface of the right temporal lobe with involvement of cerebral cortex of the parahippocampal gyrus and ventral portion of right hippocampus (arrowheads).The lesion appears isointense on T1-W images with faint and irregular enhancement after contrast medium administration. No mass effect is evident.

Brain MRI was performed using a 0.25Tesla permanent magnet (ESAOTE VET-MR GRANDE, Esaote, Genoa, Italy) with the fox under general anesthesia. MRI sequences used included a Fast SE T2-W acquired in sagittal and transverse plane, a fluid attenuated inversion recovery (FLAIR) image, and a SE T1-W acquired in transverse plane before and after intravenous administration of paramagnetic contrast medium (Magnegita, gadopentetate dimeglumine 500mmol/mL, insight agents; 0.15mmol/kg BW).

T2W and FLAIR images showed a sharply hyperintense, well demarcated lesion at the ventro-medial surface of the right temporal lobe with focal involvement of the ventrolateral portion of mesencephalic tegmentum and adjacent caudo-ventro-lateral portion of the right thalamus (Figs. 2, 3).

In the temporal lobe signal changes involved both gray and white matter with major involvement of cerebral cortex of the parahippocampal gyrus and ventral portion of right hippocampus. The lesion appeared isointense on T1-W images with mild and irregular enhancement after contrast medium administration (Fig. 2). No mass effect was evident. The distribution of the lesion matched the territory of the right caudal cerebral artery and its paramedian branches with possible involvement of caudal perforating arteries arising from basilar bifurcation. These findings were primarily suggestive of vascular ischemic lesion while inflammatory conditions were considered less likely.

Protein levels (14 mg/dl; reference interval: < 30 mg/dl) and cell count (3 cell/μl; reference interval: 0-3 cell/μl) of a CSF sample collected from the cerebellomedullary cistern were apparently normal. Fecal flotation test was positive for ascarids eggs and two consecutive Baermann tests were negative for strongyles and Crenosoma vulpis larvae.

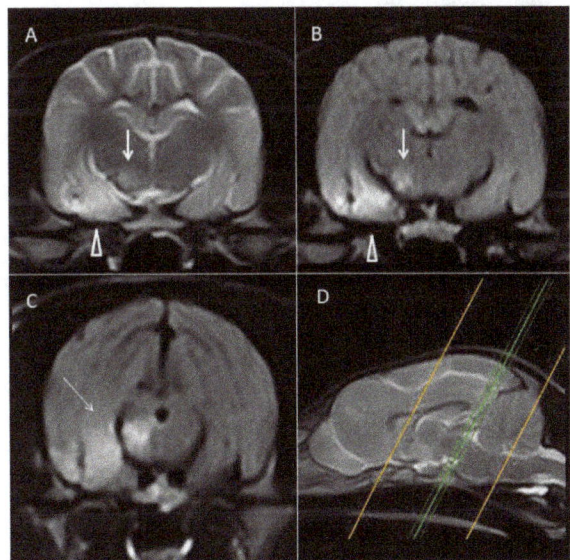

Fig. 3. First MRI of the brain. (A): Transverse T2-weighted and (B): FLAIR MRI images obtained at the level of the caudal thalamus. The mesencephalic lesion extended cranially with focal involvement of the caudo-ventro-lateral portion of the right thalamus (arrows). In the temporal lobe signal changes involved both gray and white matter of the parahippocampal gyrus. (C): Oblique-transverse FLAIR image at level of cross reference in image (D), showing in detail the mesencephalic and telencephalic lesion extension (thin arrow).

Table 1. Hemato-biochemical findings.

Analyte	Value	Reference intervals for juvenile Urocyon Littoralis (§)	Mean values for Vulpes velox (¶)	Reference intervals for adult dogs (*)
RBC (x10^6/ µl)	14.94	5.9-8.4	9.46 ± 0.92	5.7-8.56
Hb (g/dl)	17.6	11.4-16.2	17.95 ± 1.84	14.1-21.2
HCT (%)	61.9	37.4-54.2	51.15 ± 4.84	39.0-59.2
MCV (fl)	41.4	57-71	53.65 ± 2.33	63.1-72.6
MCH (pg)	11.8	17.6-20.7	18.57 ± 0.61	21.8-25.4
MCHC (g/dl)	28.4	27.7-34.5	34.47 ± 1.19	33.3-36.8
NRBC (/100 WBC)	0	0-6	n.a.	0-0
WBC (x10^3/ µl)	5.92	6.7-15.7	5.05 ± 1.354	5.45-12.98
Absolute segmented neutrophils (/µl)	2424	3567-10836	n.a.	3555-9314
Absolute band neutrophils (/µl)	0	0-110	n.a.	0-286
Absolute lymphocytes (/µl)	1858	666-5217	n.a.	1169-3810
Absolute monocytes (/µl)	550	66-1026	n.a.	186-798
Absolute eosinophils (/µl)	1047	87-2882	n.a.	104-1164
Absolute basophils (/µl)	41	0-429	n.a.	0-106
PLT (x10^3/ µl)	418	-	n.a.	176-479
ALP (U/l)	81	13-184	53.43 ± 76.25	24-40
ALT (U/I)	304	45-305	n.a.	30-60
AST (U/l)	52	27-154	n.a.	19-29
CK (U/l)	142	94-3045	n.a.	49-126
TP (g/dl)	6.5	4.9-7.6	6.28 ± 0.63	5.9-71
Albumin (g/dl)	2.6	2.6-3.8	2.83 ± 0.26	3.0-3.4
Globulin (g/dl)	3.9	2.2-4.4	3.45 ± 0.68	2.6-3,4
Total bilirubin (mg/dl)	0.2	0.0-0.2	0.17 ± 0.16	0.13-0.2
BUN (mg/dl)	35	10-36	23.35 ± 6.77	21-48
Creatinine (mg/dl)	0.82	0.4-1.0	0.79 ± 0.63	0.76-1.09
Cholesterol (mg/dl)	200	107-197	n.a.	175-248
Glucose (mg/dl)	120	91-199	100.87 ± 48.61	100-109
Calcium (mg/dl)	10.2	8.0-10.3	11.57 ± 1.78	9.5-10.7
Phosphorus (mg/dl)	6.2	3.3-8.8	5.69 ± 1.26	2.1-3.8
Bicarbonate (mEq/l)	22.9	10-21	n.a.	17.4-24.2
Chloride (mEq/l)	113	105-118	n.a.	110-115
Potassium (mEq/l)	5.0	3.7-5.5	5.0 ± 0.66	4.2-4.5
Sodium (mEq/l)	147	141-154	148.78 ± 4.64	145-148

(WBC): white blood cell; (RBC): red blood cell; (Hb): hemoglobin; (HCT): hematocrit; (MCV): mean corpuscular volume; (MCH): mean corpuscular hemoglobin; (MCHC): mean corpuscular hemoglobin concentration; (NRBC): nucleated red blood cell; (PLT): platelets; (ALP): alkaline phosphatase; (ALT): alanine transaminase; (AST): aspartate transaminase; (CK): creatine kinase; (TP): total protein; (BUN): blood urea nitrogen; (n.a.): not available.

(§) Biochemical and hematologic reference intervals for the island fox (*Urocyon littoralis*) (Inoue *et al.*, 2012).

(¶) Mean values for haematology and serum biochemistry from a population of swift foxes (*Vulpes velox*) (Mainka, 1988).

(*) Reference values provided by a certified veterinary laboratory (San Marco Veterinary Laboratory, Padova, Italy)

Complete blood (cell) count (CBC), and biochemical profile were also carried out. Hemato-biochemical analysis apparently revealed erythrocytosis, microcytosis, hypochromic red blood cells and mild neutropenia (Table 1 - hemato-biochemical results were compared with the reference values of the island fox and dogs, and with mean values available for Vulpes velox).

Within 30 days of hospitalization the fox showed progressive clinical improvement without medical therapy. A second neurological examination revealed normalization of vestibular signs and left side postural reactions with residual mild left circling.

A MRI of the brain was repeated using the same sequence protocol. The second imaging examination showed significant reduction in size of the primary lesions and fluid replacement of T2 and FLAIR hyperintense mesencephalic areas previously detected (Fig. 4).

Based on MRI pattern of distribution and evolution of the lesions, spontaneous improvement of neurological signs and CSF analysis, a presumptive diagnosis of ischemic infarct in the territory of right caudal cerebral artery and its collateral branches was made. Involvement of right caudal perforating arteries arising from basilar bifurcation was also considered.

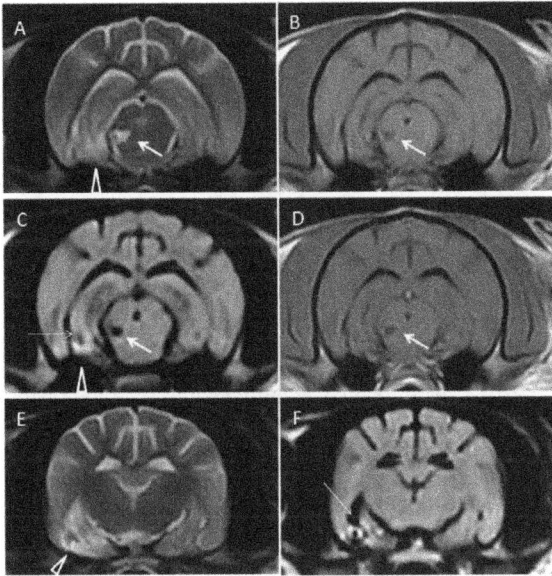

Fig. 4. Repeat MRI of the brain acquired 30 days after the first examination. **(A):** Transverse T2-weighted, **(B):** T1-weighted, **(C):** FLAIR and **(D):** contrast-enhanced T1-weighted MRI images obtained at the level of the rostral midbrain. There is significant reduction in size of the primary lesions and fluid replacement of T2 and FLAIR hyperintense mesencephalic areas previously detected (arrows). **(E):** Transverse T2-weighted and **(F):** FLAIR MRI images obtained at the level of the caudal thalamus showing normal parenchymal signal intensity of the thalamic area previously involved by the lesion. Slight residual hyperintensity is observed at the level of parahippocampal gyrus (arrowheads) with fluid signal at the level of the ventral portion of right hippocampus (thin arrows).

Discussion

Canidae is one of the most studied mammalian groups. From comparative studies on their neuroanatomy it has been clarified that the external cerebrum morphology of the modern Canidae is extremely uniform and, except for small differences in the shape and size of frontal gyri (sigmoid and proreal gyrus), characterized by lack of important differences between the genera (Radinsky, 1969, 1973, 1978; Lyras and Van Der Geer, 2003). Such uniformity can also be observed from the comparison of cross-sectional anatomy of the red fox and dog brain as revealed by previous MRI studies in both species (Kassab and Bahgat, 2007; Leigh *et al.*, 2008).

As reported in dogs (Garosi *et al.*, 2006), the imaging findings (shape and distribution of the lesions, absence of mass effect, signal intensity and evolution of the lesions) in the fox herein examined were suggestive of ischemic infarct in the territory of the right caudal cerebral artery (CCA).

In dogs, the CCAs arise from the caudal communicant arteries of the cerebral arterial circle (circle of Willis) and run caudo-laterally supplying blood to the caudal and medial surface of each telencephalic hemisphere.

Along their course the CCAs give rise to small branches to the ventro-medial portion of temporal lobes, to the caudo-lateral part of the thalamus and to the lateral mesencephalon (perforating arteries) (Barone, 2003; Garosi *et al.*, 2006; Hillock *et al.*, 2006).

The same territorial distribution of the CCAs have been proven in detailed anatomical studies on the vascular brain anatomy in the red fox and pampas fox (Pseudalopex gumnocercus).

In particular, specific collateral CCA branches to the piriform lobe, parahippocampal gyrus, thalamus and mesencephalon have been described in such species (Depedrini and Campos, 2003, 2007; Ozudogru *et al.*, 2012).

The distribution of the lesions observed on MRI in the ventrolateral mesencephalon, ventrolateral caudal thalamus, piriform lobe and para-hippocampal gyrus confirmed the course of the collateral CCA branches as also described in foxes (Depedrini and Campos, 2003, 2007; Ozudogru *et al.*, 2012) and matched the most commonly affected regions reported in dogs with CCA infarction (Garosi *et al.*, 2006).

However, for thalamic and midbrain lesions, concomitant involvement of caudal perforating arteries arising from basilar bifurcation could not be ruled out (Garosi *et al.*, 2006).

In this fox, the presence of vestibular signs resulted apparently unsolved and speculative.

In cats, unilateral experimentally-induced mesencephalic lesions, resulted in lateral tilt of the head toward the opposite side, while bilateral lesions induced dorsiflexion of the head (Fukushima *et al.*, 1987). Anatomical basis associated with these abnormal head posture involve dysfunction of the interstitial nucleus of Cajal (INC) (in the rostral midbrain adjacent to the periaqueductal gray matter), interstitiospinal fibres (that run in the medial longitudinal fasciculus) (Nyberg-Hansen, 1966) and their control on the rostral cervical muscles (Fukushima *et al.*, 1987).

In particular, unilateral induced lesion in INC or in its descending fibres up to the caudal region of mesencephalon, cause an increase in activity of the major ipsilateral dorsal neck muscles and in the contralateral obliquus capitis caudalis resulting in controlateral head tilt (Fukushima *et al.*, 1985, 1987; Kavaklis *et al.*, 1992).

Bilateral lesions induce activation of dorsal neck muscles producing dorsiflexion of the head (Fukushima *et al.*, 1987; Fukushima-Kudo *et al.*, 1987).

In dogs, mesencephalic dysfunction has been related with different abnormal neck and head posture (Garosi *et al.*, 2006; Goncalves *et al.*, 2011, Canal *et al.*, 2015). In dogs with ventrolateral thalamic infractions, the lesions were associated with mesencephalic involvement resulting in controlateral or ipsilateral head tilt as prevailing vestibular sing (Goncalves *et al.*, 2011).

Moreover, in two dogs with intracranial expansive lesions exerting bilateral compression of dorsal mesencephalon, permanent neck extension (retrocollis) has been observed and attributed to bilateral INC dysfunction (Canal *et al.*, 2015). Interestingly, neurological signs detected in this fox perfectly reflected those reported for ventrolateral thalamic infractions with mesencephalic involvement in dogs (Garosi *et al.*, 2006; Goncalves *et al.*, 2011).

In this fox, as well as in previously reported canine cases, while compulsive circling and controlateral proprioceptive deficit were well explained by prosencephalic lesions, the neuroanatomic explanation of the concomitant ipsilateral vestibular signs is consistent with unilateral involvement of nucleus of Cajal in the rostral mesencephalon.

Thalamic dysfunction is also suspected to cause vestibular signs in dogs, especially after acute lesions (de Lahunta and Glass, 2009). The pathways for conscious balance perception involving a relay from a thalamic nucleus seems implicated in the vestibular thalamic syndrome (Brandt and Dieterich, 1999).

In attempt to identify possible underling risk factors for brain infarction, hemato-biochemical analysis were performed. Unfortunately, normal reference values for red foxes (*Vulpes vulpes*) are not available in veterinary medical literature.

To the author's knowledge hemato-biochemical reference intervals for wild foxes are available only for the island fox (urocyon littoralis) (Inoue *et al.*, 2012). In addition hematologic and serum chemistry mean values are available for the species Vulpes velox (Mainka, 1988). From the analysis of hemato-biochemical abnormalities detected in our fox using the reference values of the island fox and dogs, and by the comparison with mean values available for Vulpes velox species, erythrocytosis associated with microcytosis and hypochromic red blood cells and mild neutropenia were apparently detectable (Table 1). However, taking into account the possible variability existing among these different species, such abnormal findings were considered of doubtful interpretation.

Thus, in this fox the possible cause of brain infarction remains unclear due to the lack of further diagnostic evaluations (blood pressure measurement, thoracic and abdominal imaging evaluation, urinalysis, endocrine tests) and the equivocal relevance of hematobiochemical abnormalities.

Finally, this case is the first report of a presumptive thalamic and midbrain infarction in a fox showing multifocal encephalic syndrome with predominant vestibular dysfunction. This case suggests not only an anatomic but also a neurophysiologic analogy between dogs, cats and foxes.

Acknowledgments

The authors wish to thank all the staff of the Pingry Veterinary Hospital of Bari, Italy for their assistance with data collection.

Conflict of interest

The authors declare that there is no conflict of interests.

References

Barone, R. 2003. Anatomia comparata dei mammiferi domestici: Neurologia, Vol. 6, 3rd ed. Edagricole, Bologna.

Brandt, T. and Dieterich, M. 1999. The vestibular cortex: its locations, functions, and disorders. Ann. N. Y. Acad. Sci. 871, 293-312.

Canal, S., Baroni, M., Falzone, C., De Benedictis, G.M. and Bernardini, M. 2015. Dorsal midbrain syndrome associated with persistent neck extension: clinical and diagnostic imaging findings in two dogs. Can. Vet. J. 56, 1261-1265.

de Lahunta, A. and Glass, E. 2009. Veterinary Neuroanatomy and Clinical Neurology. 3rd ed. Elsevier, St. Louis, Miss, USA, pp: 324.

Depedrini, J.S. and Campos, R. 2003. A systematic study of the brain base arteries in the pampas fox (Dusicyon gymnocercus). Braz. J. Morphol. Sci. 20, 181-188.

Depedrini, J.S. and Campos, R. 2007. Systematization, distribution and territory of the caudal cerebral artery on the surface of the brain in pampas foxes (Pseudalopex gymnocercus). Braz. J. Morphol. Sci. 24, 126-136.

Dewey, C.W. 2003. Vascular encephalopathies in the dog and cat. Proc. 21st ACVIM Forum, pp: 398-400.

Fukushima, K., Fukushima, J. and Terashima, T. 1987. The pathways responsible for the characteristic head posture produced by lesions of the interstitial nucleus of Cajal in the cat. Exp. Brain Res. 68, 88-102.

Fukushima, K., Takahashi, K., Kudo, J. and Kato, M. 1985. Interstitialvestibular interaction in the control of head posture. Exp. Brain Res. 57, 264-270.

Fukushima-Kudo, J., Fukushima, K. and Tashiro, K. 1987. Rigidity and dorsiflexion of the neck in progressive supranuclear palsy and the interstitial nucleus of Cajal. J. Neurol. Neurosurg. Psych. 50, 1197-1203.

Garosi, L., McConnell, J.F., Platt, S.R., Barone, G., Baron, J.C., de Lahunta, A. and Schatzberg, S.J. 2006. Clinical and topographic magnetic resonance characteristics of suspected brain infarction in 40 dogs. J. Vet. Intern. Med. 20, 311-321.

Garosi, L.S. 2010. Cerebrovascular disease in dogs and cats. Vet. Clin. North Am. Small Anim. Pract. 40, 65-79.

Giannuzzi, A.P., DeSimone, A., Ricciardi, M. and Gernone, F. 2014. Presumptive Ischemic Brain

Infarction in a Dog with Evans' Syndrome. Case Reports in Veterinary Medicine. Volume 2014, Article ID 456524.

Goncalves, R., Carrera, I., Garosi, L., Smith, P.M., Fraser McConnell, J. and Penderis, J. 2011. Clinical and topographic magnetic resonance imaging characteristics of suspected thalamic infarcts in 16 dogs. Vet. J. 188, 39-43.

Higgins, M.A., Rossmeisl, J.H. Jr. and Panciera, D.L. 2006. Hypothyroid-associated central vestibular disease in 10 dogs: 1999-2005. J. Vet. Intern. Med. 20, 1363-1369.

Hillock, S.M., Dewey, C.W., Stefanacci, J.D. and Fondacaro, J.V. 2006. Vascular encephalopathies in dogs: incidence, risk factors, pathophysiology, and clinical signs. Compend. Contin. Educ. Pract. Vet. 28, 196-207.

Inoue, H., Clifford, D.L., Vickers, T.W., Coonan, T.J., Garcelon, D.K. and Borjesson, D.L. 2012. Biochemical and hematologic reference intervals for the endangered island fox (Urocyon littoralis). J. Wildl. Dis. 48, 583-592.

Kassab, A. and Bahgat, H. 2007. Magnetic Resonance Imaging and cross-sectional anatomy of the brain of the red fox (Vulpes vulpes).Vet. Med. J. Giza. 55, 779-786.

Kavaklis, O., Shima, F., Kato, M. and Fukui, M. 1992. Ipsilateral pallidal control of the sternocleidomastoid muscle of cats: Relationship to the side of thalamotomy for torticollis. Neurosurgery 30, 724-730.

Leigh, E.J., Mackillop, E., Robertson, I.D. and Hudson, L.C. 2008. Clinical anatomy of the canine brain using magnetic resonance imaging. Vet. Radiol. Ultrasound. 49, 113-121.

Lyras, G.A. and Van Der Geer, A.A.E. 2003. External brain anatomy in relation to phylogeny of Caninae (Carnivora: Canidae). Zool. J. Linn. Soc. 138, 505-522.

Mainka, S.A. 1988. Hematology and serum biochemistry of captive swift foxes (Vulpes velox). J. Wildl. Dis. 24, 71-74.

Nyberg-Hansen, R. 1966. Sites of termination of interstitiospinal fibers in the cat. An experimental study with silver impregnation methods. Arch. Ital. Biol. 104, 98-111.

Ozudogru, Z., Can, M. and Balkaya, H. 2012. Macro-Anatomical Investigation of the Cerebral Arterial Circle (Circle of Willis) in Red Fox (Vulpes vulpes Leunnoleus, 1758). J. Anim. Vet. Adv. 11, 2861-2864.

Radinsky, L.B. 1969. Outlines of canid and felid brain evolution. Ann. N. Y. Acad. Sci. 167, 277-288.

Radinsky, L.B. 1973. Evolution of the canid brain. Brain Behav. Evol. 7, 169-202.

Radinsky, L.B. 1978. The evolutionary history of dog brains. Museologia 10, 25-29.

Wessmann, A., Chandler, K. and Garosi, L. 2009. Ischaemic and haemorrhagic stroke in the dog. Vet. J. 180, 290-303.

17

Exophthalmos associated to orbital zygomatic mucocele and complex maxillary malformation in a puppy

Alessandro Cirla[1,2,*], Marco Rondena[3], Giovanna Bertolini[1] and Giovanni Barsotti[2]

[1]San Marco Veterinary Clinic, via Sorio 114/c – 35141 Padova, Italy
[2]Department of Veterinary Science, University of Pisa, via Livornese Lato Monte – 56124 San Piero a Grado, Pisa, Italy
[3]San Marco Veterinary Laboratory, via Sorio 114/c – 35141 Padova, Italy

Abstract

A case of exophthalmos due to zygomatic mucocele in a puppy with ipsilateral segmental maxillary atrophy is reported. A 7-month-old, mixed breed, male dog suffered the sudden-onset of unilateral painful exophthalmos and a gradual swelling of the right temporal region. A compressing, right retrobulbar mass was observed by ultrasound. Computed tomography revealed a large multiloculated cyst-like lesion of the right zygomatic gland projecting into the orbital space, thus displacing the eyeball. The ipsilateral molar part of the maxillary bone was underdeveloped, besides showing crowded, abnormal, multiple, unerupted maxillary molar teeth in the caudal maxillary region. Modified lateral orbitotomy and a selective caudal maxillary bone access were performed. The cyst-like lesion was removed and the zygomatic gland and the wall was collected for histology, which confirmed the mucocele. Clinical and imaging examinations six months after surgery showed neither recurrence of the mucocele nor ocular abnormalities. A possible common pathogenic mechanism involving these two conditions could be hypothesized.
Keywords: Computed tomography, Dog, Exophthalmos, Maxillary atrophy, Zygomatic mucocele.

Introduction

The major salivary glands of the dog are the parotid, sublingual, mandibular and zygomatic glands. The zygomatic gland, in comparison with other salivary glands, is the least frequently involved in pathological conditions in dogs (Schmidt and Betts, 1978; Bellenger and Simpson, 1992; Cannon et al., 2011; Nemec et al., 2015). Salivary gland mucocele is a collection of saliva in a cavity lined by granulation tissue that occurs following disruption of a salivary gland or its ducts. The mucocele is the most common pathological condition of the salivary glands of the dog, most often involving the sublingual gland, although it can involve the other glands (Karbe and Nielsen, 1966; Bellenger and Simpson, 1992). Zygomatic mucocele is a condition rarely observed in veterinary medicine (Miller and Pickett, 1989; Bellenger and Simpson, 1992; Speakman et al., 1997; McGill et al., 2009), but it should be considered as a possible diagnosis in dogs presenting exophthalmos, protrusion of the third eyelid and a fluctuant, palpable, soft tissue mass around the zygomatic bone (Noghreyan et al., 1996). Since the zygomatic gland is located ventrally to the zygomatic arch, mild changes may not be detected in the early stages of the disease. Furthermore, clinical signs such as exophthalmos may be similar to the ones of other orbital diseases. Unilateral exophthalmos in dogs is observed in conjunction with a variety of diseases. The possible differential diagnoses for exophthalmos include primary or secondary orbital neoplasia, inflammatory orbital diseases, orbital varices, and cystic\exudative orbital diseases (zygomatic salivary gland mucocele, hematic cyst secondary to trauma or immune-mediated disease, dacryops, or orbital oedema) (Karbe and Nielsen, 1966; Harvey, 1971; Bellenger and Simpson, 1992; Guinan et al., 2007; Atkins et al., 2010; Adams et al., 2011; Cannon et al., 2011; Philp et al., 2012). Despite the variable underlying causes, the clinical signs of these various conditions are very similar to one another. Diagnostic imaging can be useful to differentiate a zygomatic gland disease from other orbital diseases (Penninck et al., 2001; Bartoe et al., 2007; Boston, 2010; Lee et al., 2014). Cases of zygomatic mucocele were reported in a cat and in a ferret (Miller and Pickett, 1989; Speakman et al., 1997).

The present report concerns the diagnostic and therapeutic management of a complex maxillary malformation and concurrent zygomatic mucocele in a puppy. To the authors' best knowledge, this is the first report on this condition in a dog

Case details

A 7-month-old, mongrel male dog was brought to our attention for further evaluation of an acute, painful, rapidly progressive enlargement of the right eye (OD). The dog's general condition was good, but facial

*Corresponding Author: Alessandro Cirla. San Marco Veterinary Clinic, via Sorio 114/c – 35141 Padova, Italy.
Email: alessandro.cirla@sanmarcovet.it

oedema was evident, mainly involving the temporal, frontal and zygomatic regions, as well as discomfort when opening the mouth. No palpable regional lymph nodes were detected. The dog's medical history was unremarkable, no history of trauma or previous ocular diseases were reported. Ophthalmic examination of the right eye revealed ocular discomfort, mucous secretion, protrusion of the nictitating membrane, chemosis and congestion of conjunctival vessels, moderate exophthalmos and lagophtalmos. The globe was substantially resistant to retropulsion, no visibile buccal lesions were detected. Complete ophthalmic examination of the OD was compromised by the nictitating membrane protrusion. However, the limited examination did not show any ocular lesions (Fig.1). No abnormalities were observed in the left eye.

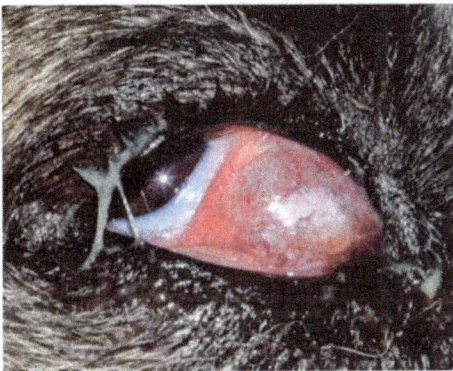

Fig. 1. Clinical appearance of OD. Note the mucous secretion, protrusion of the nictitating membrane, chemosis and congestion of conjunctival vessels.

A compressive orbital space-occupying lesion was clinically suspected and confirmed by ultrasonography (Logiq C5 Premium, 10 MHz linear probe, GE Healthcare). Orbital ultrasonographic examination revealed a 3,5 x 1,7 cm round echogenic structure with a large volume of anechoic content. Ocular ultrasound was normal (Fig.2).

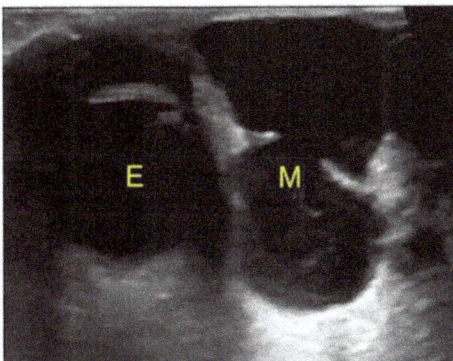

Fig. 2. Orbital ultrasound (10 MHz linear probe, transverse scan, temporal fossa approach) showing a large orbital fluid-filled space-occupying mass (M). The OD ocular examination (E) showed no abnormalities.

Ultrasound-guided fine-needle aspiration revealed a clear watery to viscous fluid highly suggestive of saliva collection.

Results of CBC analyses showed moderate leukocytosis (white blood cells: 26000/µl; reference interval 5450/ µl-12980/ µl). Serum biochemistry, coagulation test and urinalysis were unremarkable.

Computed tomography scan (CT) was scheduled to better define the extent and the origin of the lesion. After intramuscular premedication with 0.2 mg/kg methadone (Semfortan, Dechra Pharmaceuticals) and 2 µg/kg dexmedetomidine (Dexdomitor, Orino Pharma), general anesthesia was induced with 4 mg/kg propofol (Vetofol, Esteve) intravenously and maintained with isofluorane (IsoFlo; Halocarbon Laboratories) in oxygen. A 16 GA intravenous catheter was placed in the right cephalic vein for fluid administration throughout the anestethic period.

Computed tomography was performed using a second-generation dual-source CT scanner (SOMATOM Definition Flash, Siemens Healthcare, Milan Italy) with following parameters: single source, spiral mode, pitch 0.5, 128x0.6mm detector configuration, 120 KVp and 200 mAs and double reconstruction kernel for bone (H70) and soft tissue (B30) with 0.3 mm reconstruction interval.

Four CT series were obtained: a pre-contrast series, followed by two post-contrast series, in arterial and venous phase. Finally, a third late post-contrast series was obtained. Contrast medium (iodixanol 320mgI/mL) was injected at 37°C into a cephalic vein (640 mgI/kg) through the IV catheter, at 3,5 mL/s injection rate, followed by a saline flush with same injection rate via a dual-syringe injector system (Medrad, Stellant CT Injection System, Bayer, Milan, Italy).

CT images revealed a large multiloculated cyst-like lesion in the right orbital space, involving the zygomatic gland and displacing the eyeball dorso-laterally. The lesion had a thin wall and contained homogeneous, non-enhancing fluid. The molar part of the ipsilateral maxillary bone was underdeveloped. Crowded, abnormal, multiple, unerupted maxillary molar teeth were identified in the caudal maxillary region (Fig.3).

Differential diagnosis included odontogenic cyst (i.e. dentigerous cyst), maxillary bone cysts, and zygomatic mucocele associated to a maxillary bone defect.

Surgical exploration of the mass was recommended, with a view to its complete excision.

Modified lateral orbitotomy and selective caudal maxillary bone access were performed to provide ventral exposure of the orbit and dental extraction, while minimizing trauma to the globe and supporting structures.

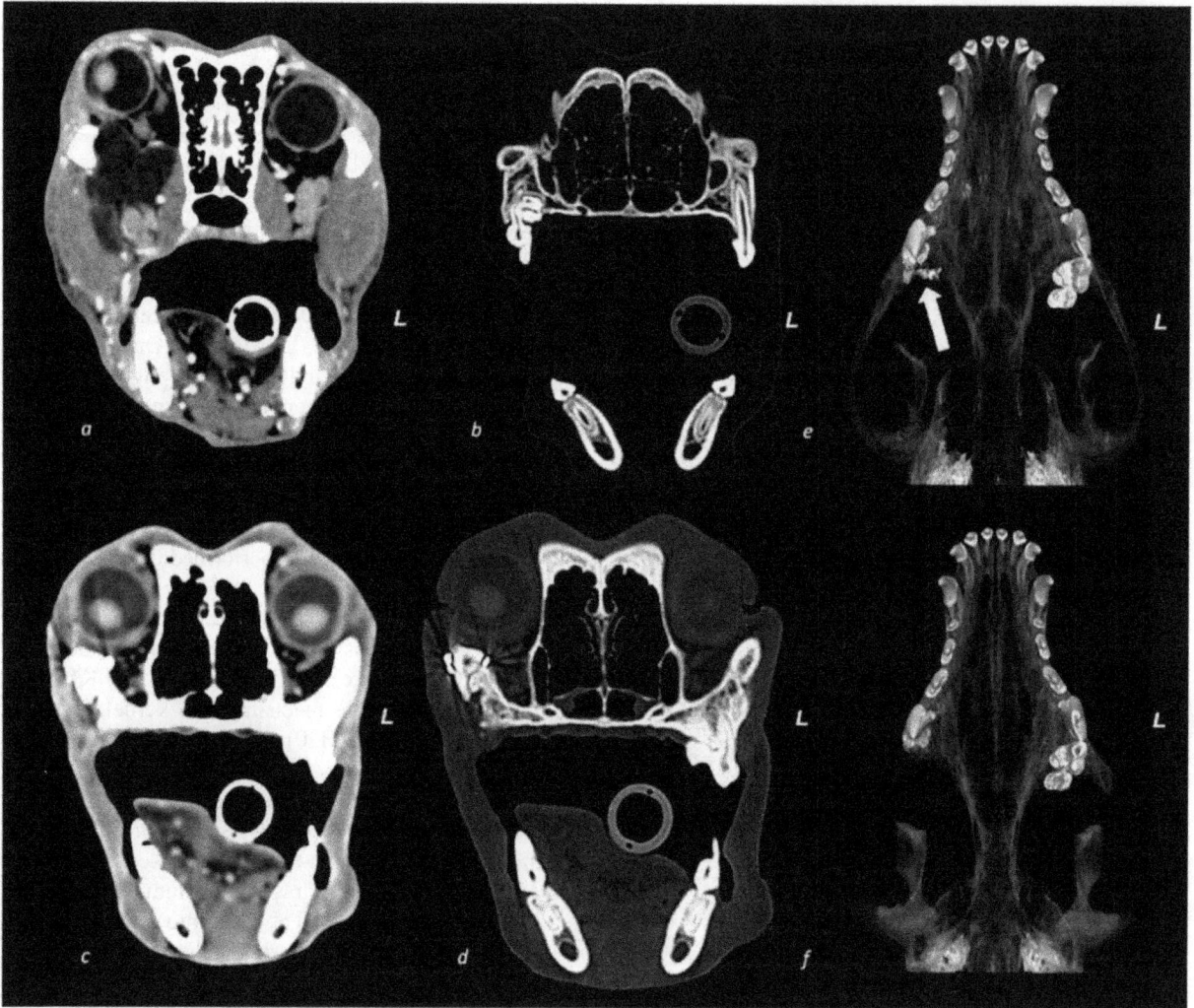

Fig. 3. Transverse plane through the orbit showing a large mass displacing the eyeball dorso-laterally (*a*) and crowded, multiple, abnormal, unerupted maxillary molars (*b*). Volume rendering, ventral view (*e*). Note the underdeveloped molar part of the right maxillary bone (arrow) and crowded, multiple, abnormal, unerupted maxillary molar teeth. Six month follow-up CT exam: transverse plane through the orbit (*c, d*) and volume rendering, ventral view showed no recurrence of the orbital pathology (*f*).

The dog was premedicated with 0.2 mg/kg methadone (Semfortan, Dechra Pharmaceuticals) and 2 µg/kg dexmedetomidine (Dexdomitor, Orino Pharma) intramuscularly. Anaesthesia was induced with 5 mg/kg propofol (Vetofol, Esteve) intravenously and maintained with a mixture of isofluorane (IsoFlo; Halocarbon Laboratories) and oxygen in a closed breathing circuit. Cefazolin (Cefazolina, Teva) was administered intravenously at the dosage of 22 mg/kg, 25 minutes before the anaesthetic induction. A curvilineal incision was made along the dorsal margin of the zygomatic arch. The palpebral nerve and the dorsal buccal branch of the facial nerve were identified through blunt dissection. These structures were delicately separated from the underlying tissues and retracted.

Prospective zygomatic osteotomy sites were identified, and 0.35 mm Kirschner wire placed in a hand-held orthopedic Jacobs chuck was used to drill sets of holes adjacent to each site.

Transection of the zygomatic arch was performed with a pneumatic saw between the previously drilled holes, and reflected dorsally without transection of the orbital ligament. The cystic structure was bluntly undermined from the surrounding tissues and its dorsal aspect was noted as connecting under the zygomatic arch to the ventral orbit. The mass and the zygomatic gland were removed as a whole and submitted for histopathological examination.

After saline irrigation, the transected zygomatic arch was replaced and fixed with a 22-gauge orthopedic wire. The surgical site was closed as normal. A posterior maxillary bone fenestration was then performed to allow the included teeth extraction. The bone cavity was thoroughly curetted and rinsed with sterile saline. A mucoperiosteal flap was raised buccally to close the surgical wound.

The dog recovered uneventfully from anesthesia and surgery, the exophthalmos resolved immediately postoperatively. At this time the patient received a complete ophthalmic examination of both eyes and showed no abnormalities. Complete ophthalmic examination included neuro-opthalmic examination, slit-lamp biomicroscopy and indirect ophthalmoscopy. Schirmer tear test I, retension of corneal sodium fluorescein dye and intraocular pressure estimation were performed.

The tissues submitted for histopathology were immediately fixed in 10 per cent neutral-buffered formalin, embedded in paraffin, sectioned at 4 μm and stained with haematoxylin and eosin. Microscopic evaluation of the biopsy tissues revealed numerous small acini of zygomatic gland embedded in a thick granulation tissue delineated in a border by abundant fibrin and amorphous hyaline homogeneous material (salivary secretion), partially infiltrated by macrophages consistent with mucocele (Fig. 4). There was no evidence of infection or malignant changes. Postoperatively, an Elizabethan collar prevented self-trauma at the surgical site.

The dog was placed on cephalexin orally at the dose of 22 mg/kg (IcfVet, Icf) for antibiotic prophylaxis. Methadone (Semfortan, Dechra) was given intravenously for the first 48 hours at the dose of 0.2 mg/kg for surgical pain management, and carprofen (Rimadyl, Pfizer Animal Health) was prescribed at a dose of 2.2 mg/kg to address inflammation.

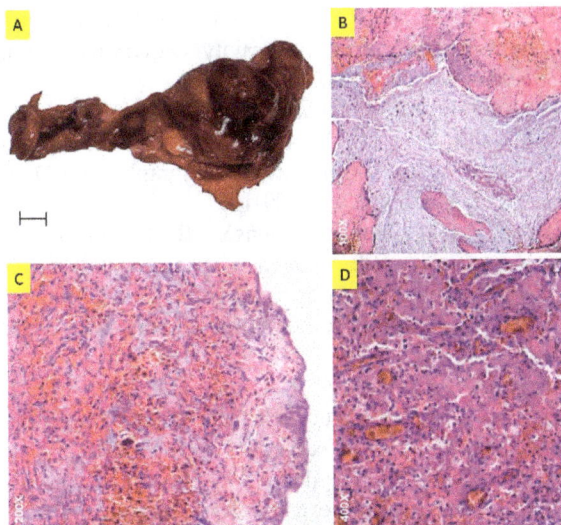

Fig. 4. Gross anatomy of the mass **(A)**. Histopathology of the mass haematoxylin and eosin x100 **(B)**, x200 **(C)** and x400 **(D)**. Note the granulation tissue embedding large, irregularly shaped lakes of clear amorphous material (mucous secretion/salivary secretion of zygomatic gland origin).

The dog was discharged from the hospital three days after surgery and re-evaluated 10 days postoperatively, at which time the skin sutures were removed. The incision was healing appropriately and there was no sign of orbital or periocular swelling. At this time, oral examination showed no abnormalities and the dog was eating well. No clinical signs of ocular complications secondary to the exophthalmia such as exposure keratitis or fundus lesions were detected. No orbital recurrence of the mucocele was present. At the 6-month clinical follow-up, the CT exam showed no recurrence (Fig. 3).

Discussion

We described a complex case of exophthalmos due to a zygomatic mucocele in a puppy with ipsilateral segmental maxillary malformation. A possible relationship between these two conditions could be hypothesized on the basis of advanced imaging features. Advanced imaging modalities play a key role in identifying the cause of exophthalmos. Both CT and MR imaging have been reported as useful diagnostic tools for the evaluation of canine mucocele (Boland et al., 2013; Torad and Hassan, 2013; Namsoon et al., 2014; Nemec et al., 2015).

Neoplasia, sialoliths, trauma, and foreign bodies invading the glandular structures have been identified as possible causes of mucocele in dogs (Harvey, 1971; Guinan et al., 2007; Atkins et al., 2010; Adams et al., 2011; Philp et al., 2012). Zygomatic mucocele in dogs has also been described as a postoperative complication secondary to caudal hemimaxillectomy or maxillary tooth extraction (Clarke and L'Eplattenier, 2010; Adams et al., 2011).

The puppy of the present report had no history of previous maxillary surgery or dental procedures. Furthermore in the present case, a trauma was not reported in the medical history and the CT examination allowed to exclude the presence of sialoliths and zygomatic foreign bodies.

The distinctive feature of our case was the concomitant malformation of the maxillary bone, lining the lateral part of the cystic formation. A maxillary epithelial cyst expanding into the orbital space was reported in a dog (Featherstone and Llabres Diaz, 2003) and was initially suspected also in the present case. Brachygnathia and other maxillary bone developmental defects were reported alone or in association with other craniofacial anomalies in dogs (Duncan et al., 1994; Nemec et al., 2015).

In humans, maxillary hypoplasia involving the dentoalveolar area is described as a complex disease associated to basal deformity (Jackson, 1989; Mueller and Callanan, 2007; Rege et al., 2012). This anomaly has been also described in a rare congenital disorder known as Crouzon syndrome (Padmanabhan et al., 2011).

The maxillary congenital hypoplasia somehow associated with the zygomatic mucocele cannot be ruled out. In general, the zygomatic mucocele clinically behaves as a progressively space-occupying lesion that can cause distortion of the surrounding bone (Mould, 1990; Featherstone and Llabres Diaz, 2003).

The focal, circular depression of the maxilla is uncommon for a benign lesion, although such presumed pressure necrosis of the bone has been previously described (Mould, 1990; Featherstone and Llabres Diaz, 2003). It is not unreasonable to assume that an expanding zygomatic mucocele might behave in a similar manner. In our case, the zygomatic mucocele might have created progressive pressure atrophy, causing the depression of the maxilla and its underdevelopment.

The combination of accurate clinical examination, interpretation of advanced cross-sectional imaging, including CT, and combined surgery was successful for the treatment of the zygomatic mucocele in our case associated to a maxillary malformation. Early diagnosis of the disease and its surgical management prevented later ocular complications.

Conflict of interest

The authors declare that there is no conflict of interests.

References

Adams, P., Halfacree, Z.J., Lamb, C.R., Smith, K.C. and Baines, S.J. 2011. Zygomatic salivary mucocoele in a Lhasa apso following maxillary tooth extraction. Vet. Rec. 168, 458-460.

Atkins, R.M., Hecht, S., Westermeyer, H.D. and McLean, N.J. 2010. What Is Your Diagnosis? J. Am. Vet. Med. Assoc. 237, 1375-1376.

Bartoe, J.T., Brightman, A.H. and Davidson, H.J. 2007. Modified lateral orbitotomy for vision-sparing excision of a zygomatic mucocele in a dog. Vet. Ophthalmol. 10, 127-131.

Bellenger, C.R. and Simpson, D.J. 1992. Canine sialocoeles - 60 clinical cases. J. Small Anim. Pract. 33, 376-380.

Boland, L., Gomes, E., Payen, G., Bouvy, B. and Poncet, C. 2013. Zygomatic salivary gland diseases in the dog: three cases diagnosed by MRI. J. Am. Anim. Hosp. Assoc. 49, 333-337.

Boston, S.E. 2010. Craniectomy and orbitectomy in dogs and cats. Can. Vet. J. 51, 537-540.

Cannon, M.S., Paglia, D., Zwingenberger, A.L., Boroffka, S.A., Hollingsworth, S.R. and Wisner, E.R. 2011. Clinical and diagnostic imaging findings in dogs with zygomatic sialadenitis: 11 cases (1990–2009). J. Am. Vet. Med. Assoc. 239, 1211-1218.

Clarke, B.S. and L'Eplattenier, H.F. 2010. Zygomatic salivary mucocoele as a postoperative complication following caudal hemimaxillectomy in a dog. J. Small Anim. Pract. 51, 495-498.

Duncan, W.K., Silberman, S.L., Trubman, A. and Meydrech, E.F. 1994. Prevalence and racial distribution of primary canine hypoplasia of the maxillary canine. Ped. Dent. 16, 365-367.

Featherstone, H. and Llabres Diaz, F. 2003. Maxillary bone epithelial cyst in a dog. J. Small Anim. Pract. 44, 541-545.

Guinan, J., Willis, A.M., Cullen, C.L. and Walshaw, R. 2007. Postenucleation orbital sialocele in a dog associated with prior parotid duct transposition. Vet. Ophthalmol. 10, 386-389.

Harvey, C.E. 1971. Traumatic frontal mucocoele in a dog: a case report. J. Small Anim. Pract. 12, 399-403.

Jackson, I.T. 1989. Maxillary hypoplasia. Clin. Plas. Surg. 16, 757-775.

Karbe, E. and Nielsen, S.W. 1966. Canine Ranulas, Salivary Mucoceles and Branchial Cysts. J. Small Anim. Pract. 7, 625-630.

Lee, N., Choi, M., Keh, S., Kim, T., Kim, H. And Yoon, J. 2014. Zygomatic Sialolithiasis Diagnosed with Computed Tomography in a dog. J. Vet. Med. Sci. 76, 1389-1391.

McGill, S., Lester, N., McLachlan, A. and Mansfield, C. 2009. Concurrent sialocoele and necrotising sialadenitis in a dog. J. Small Anim. Pract. 50, 151-156.

Miller, P.E. and Pickett, J.P. 1989. Zygomatic salivary gland mucocele in a ferret. J. Am. Vet. Med. Assoc. 194, 1437-1438.

Mould, J.R.B. 1990. Cholesterol granuloma of the maxilla in a dog. J. Small Anim. Pract. 31, 208-211.

Mueller, D.T. and Callanan, V.P. 2007. Congenital malformations of the oral cavity. Otolaryngol. Clin. North Am. 40, 141-160.

Namsoon, L., Mihyun, C., Seoyeon, K., Kim, T., Kim, H. and Yon, J. 2014. Zygomatic Sialolithiasis Diagnosed with Computed Tomography in a Dog. J. Vet. Med. Sci. 76, 1389-1391.

Nemec, A., Daniaux, L., Johnson, E., Peralta S. and Vertraete, F.J. 2015. Craniomaxillofacial abnormalities in dogs with congenital palatal defects: computed tomographic findings. Vet. Surg. 44, 417-422.

Noghreyan, A., Gatot, A., Hertzanu, Y. and Fliss, D.M. 1996. Zygomatic mucocele causing facial swelling. J. Oral Maxillofac. Surg. 54(12), 1469-1471.

Padmanabhan, V., Hegde, A.M. and Rai, K. 2011. Crouzon's syndrome: a review of literature and case report. Contemp. Clin. Dent. 2, 211-214.

Penninck, D., Daniel, G.B., Brawer, R. and Tidwell, A.S. 2001. Cross-sectional imaging techniques in veterinary ophthalmology. Clin. Tech. Small Anim.

Pract. 16, 22-39.

Philp, H.S., Rhodes, M., Parry, A. and Baines, S.J. 2012. Canine zygomatic salivary mucocoele following suspected oropharyngeal penetrating stick injury. Vet. Rec. 171, 402.

Rege, I.C., Sousa, T., Leles, C. and Mendonca, E.F. 2012. Occurrence of maxillary sinus abnormalities detected by cone beam CT in asymptomatic patients. BMC Oral Health 12, 30-37.

Schmidt, G.M. and Betts, C.W. 1978. Zygomatic salivary mucoceles in the dog. J. Am. Vet. Med. Assoc. 172, 940-942.

Speakman, A.J., Baines, S.J., Williams, J.M. and Kelly, D.F. 1997. Zygomatic salivary cyst with mucocele formation in a cat. J. Small Anim. Pract. 38, 468-470.

Torad, F.A. and Hassan, E.A. 2013. Clinical and ultrasonographic characteristics of salivary mucoceles in 13 dogs. Vet. Radiol. Ultrasound 54, 293-298.

18

Toxic effects of the administration of *Mikania glomerata* Sprengel during the gestational period of hypertensive rats

F.B. Fulanetti*, G.G.R. Camargo, M.C. Ferro and P. Randazzo-Moura

Pontifícia Universidade Católica de São Paulo. Rua Joubert Wey, 290 Sorocaba, SP. 18030-070, Brazil

Abstract

Herbal medicine is an ancient practice that has been gaining acceptance of the medical class through scientific studies that prove its effectiveness. However, its use should still be cautious. Medicinal plants have potential toxic effects not yet discovered, and may have unproven interactions with other medications. The use of drugs during pregnancy is still very dangerous and vigorously studied; however, there are few studies of herbal medicines in pregnant women. Existing studies prioritize on teratogenic or abortifacient effects. The aim of this study was to analyze the toxic effects of *Mikania glomerata* Sprengel administration, popularly known as "guaco" during the gestational period of hypertensive rats. For this experimental groups consisting of pregnant Wistar rats received treatments with guaco extract (1 to 2 mL). In order to analyze the possible toxic effects of guaco during pregnancy, weight gain of rats was assessed during pregnancy; reproductive performance of rats, morphological parameters, and fetal placental histology were compared. Although some parameters presented significant differences, we can conclude that changes prioritized by literature, such as toxicity, vasodilation and hypotension, have not been caused by guaco. The only fetal changes observed were due to the maternal hypertension. Some studies have reported vasodilator and hypotensive effects of guaco. However, only a few studies exist, and its actual effects remain unknown. Specific studies should be developed with higher doses of guaco for a definitive conclusion of its toxic and non-toxic effects.

Keywords: Guaco, Hypertensive pregnant rats, *Mikania glomerata*, Perinatal toxicity.

Introduction

Phytotherapic plants surpassed many barriers and obstacles in the present day. Many phytotherapic plants are sold in farmer's markets and fairs, they are present in some backyards, and are used as a therapeutic resource that is accessible to the population (Amorozo and Gely, 1988; Prance, 1992).

Pharmacological experiments provide a high level of medical acceptance. This acceptance is extremely important, because investing in drugs synthesized from natural products could be a center of growth for the chemical and pharmacological industry in Brazil, due to the country's great biodiversity of plants and medicinal raw materials (Cechinel-Filho and Yunes, 1998; Britto *et al.*, 2007).

Any medication used during pregnancy, including the use of medicinal plants, should always have its cost-effectiveness and benefit-harm considered in every situation. The scarcity of data of the use of medication during pregnancy makes it even more critical (Ferro, 1991).

Currently, other properties of the guaco extract were recognized, such as antimicrobial, anti-inflammatory, analgesic (Ferro, 1991), spasmodic, vasodilator, anti-ulcer, central nervous system depressant, anti-venom serum, anti-stress, insecticide, molluscicide, fungicide, anticoagulant and allergenic (Barreto and Hiruma-Lima, 2002). These effects are due to a component present in the leaves of *Mikania glomerata* Sprengel called coumarin (Ruppelt *et al.*, 1991). Coumarin is a volatile active ingredient found in several other plant species (Pereira *et al.*, 1994).

Mikania glomerata promotes relaxation of airways' smooth muscles, bronchi mainly, by improving the fluidization of exudates by tracheobronchial cough reflex, and exerts considerable diaphoretic effect on febrile cases (Oliveira *et al.*, 1984). The influence of the aqueous extract of guaco on acute inflammatory response was verified, showing that guaco inhibits the mobilization of leukocytes from the bone marrow into the blood (Vieira *et al.*, 2008).

By relaxing the smooth muscles, guaco could promote a decrease in blood pressure in patients with hypertension during pregnancy (Assis *et al.*, 2008; Ferrão *et al.*, 2006; Almeida *et al.*, 2008). Maternal hypertension may cause decreased placental blood flow. This condition results in low fetal and placental weight (Karlsson *et al.*, 1982; Kingdom and Kaufmann, 1999; Lieb *et al.*, 1981; Rudge *et al.*, 1999; Wallace *et al.*, 1999; Wigglesworth, 1964). It is suggested that, in hypertension, the oxygen deficiency is also decreased. This confirms that the oxygen saturation in the umbilical arteries and veins of the fetus of pregnant women with pre-eclampsia is decreased, leading to the conceptual commitment.

During hypertension, an accumulation of fibrin in the intima of the vessels occurs, which can lead to its

*Corresponding Author: Fernanda Bonet Fulanetti. Pontifícia Universidade Católica de São Paulo. Rua Joubert Wey, 290 Sorocaba, SP. 18030-070, Brazil. E-mail: fernandabonet@gmail.com

Toxic effects of the administration of Mikania glomerata Sprengel during the gestational period...

115

occlusion. The hyalinization and necrosis of the vessel wall deposits, coupled to macrophages, are present in two maternal conditions: high blood pressure associated with vasculitis or deciduous bacterial infection (Benirschke and Kaufmann, 2000; Janthanaphan *et al.*, 2006; Huppertz, 2008). Administration of guaco, with its active principle coumarin, can change this modification in the hypertensive placenta.

The pregnant rat is an important animal model for studies of reproductive toxicity. Until now, little information exists about the development of the placenta of pregnant rats (de Rijk *et al.*, 2002). Analysis of placentas submitted to other substances such as herbs, vitamins, minerals and bacteria have been reported (Hall, 1973; Lewis *et al.*, 2001; Kosif *et al.*, 2008; Graber *et al.*, 1971).

In this project, the effects of guaco were tested through macroscopic and histological examination of the placentas taken from normotensive and hypertensive rats, treated with guaco during pregnancy.

Materials and Methods

All the experiments were performed according to the standards established by the Brazilian Society of Laboratory Animal Science (SBCAL).

Normotense female and male Wistar rats, as well as spontaneously hypertensive female and male Wistar rats were used for the experiment, with a total of 15 females and 2 males. The spontaneously hypertensive rats presented tail blood pressure higher than 160 mmHg, and the females presented tail blood pressure higher than 150 mmHg, weighing 180-250 g. All the animals were kept in cages with water and food *ad libitum,* in an environment with controlled temperature and lighting (12 hours with light and 12 hours without light). The pregnancy was confirmed by the presence of spermatozoids in the vaginal lavage, which indicated the first day of pregnancy.

Dry extract of *Mikania glomerata* (guaco) resuspended in milli-Q water (20% solution) was administered by gavage to female spontaneously hypertensive rats, which received a volume of 1 mL (corresponding to 0.2 g of the extract guaco) or 2 mL (corresponding to 0.4 g of extract guaco) on the first, fifth, tenth and fifteenth day of gestation, at a fixed time. Control group of rats (normotensive and spontaneously hypertensive groups) received 1 mL of saline solution, with the same pattern of administration. Before the administration by gavage, the pregnant rats fasted for 3 hours, and the weighing of each animal was performed.

After 18 days of pregnancy, cesarean sections were performed. The ovaries and corpora lutea were carefully dissected and preserved, the fetuses were removed with their placentas. After macroscopic inspection, the fetuses were euthanized by halothane inhalation, weighted and fixed in Bouin solution for 48 hours, and later substituted with 70% alcohol. The placentas were kept in formaldehyde 10%.

During the macroscopic inspection, the following parameters were evaluated: number of corpora lutea and implants, number of living fetuses, weight of the fetuses and corresponding placenta. Anatomic measurements were performed using a caliper: anteroposterior skull, lateral-lateral skull, anteroposterior thorax, lateral-lateral thorax, skull-tail and tail.

The fertility rate of rats was assessed by the following equations:

Pre-implantation loss = (number of corpora lutea − number of deployments)/number of corpora lutea.

Post-implantation loss = (number of deployments − number of living fetuses)/number of deployments.

Index vitality was obtained using the following equation:

Number of living and lifeless _____ 100 %

Number of living fetuses _____ x %

For the placentas, macroscopic observation was performed. For histological evaluation, a minimum of six areas of the placenta were separated. Histological cuts were made using the paraffin inclusion protocol and rotary microtome, with 3 microns, and hematoxylin and eosin staining. A total of 168 slides were confectioned and visualized, considering the following patterns: measurement of the placenta fragment on the slide, measurement of the thickness of a vessel, presence of congestion under chorionic membrane, fibrin deposit, edema, and inflammation.

Results

Assessment of pregnancy

The rat's pregnancy was confirmed with the presence of sperm in the smear from the vaginal lavage of normotensive and/or hypertensive rats.

Weight gain of pregnant rats

Throughout the gestational period of rats, animal's weight was also held on the 1st, 5th, 10th, 15th and 18th day of gestation. It is observed that, in all protocols performed with hypertensive rats, weight gain was lower when compared to normotensive control group, suggesting that hypertension compromises the weight gain of pregnant rats (data not shown).

Evaluation of reproductive capacity

All cesarean sections were performed on the 18th day of gestation. The following parameters were observed: quantity and vitality of fetuses, presence or absence of fetal resorption, number of corpora lutea present in each ovary (Table 1).

During the evaluation of fetal vitality, it was observed that the fetuses of all groups were alive, i.e. vitality equal to 100%. It was noticed that all groups showed

Table 1. Morphological parameters and reproductive analysis (n=3-5).

Parameters	Treatments/Groups			
	Normotensive rats	Spontaneously hypertensive rats	Spontaneously hypertensive+ guaco (1 mL)	Spontaneously hypertensive+ guaco (2 mL)
Number of fetuses	56	26	28	36
Number of corpora lutea	58	39	40	50
Pre-implantation loss (%)	0.03±0.02	0.30±0.10	0.30±0.20	0.30±0.07
Post-implantation loss (%)	0.02±0.02	0.05±0.05	-	0.05±0.05
Index vitality (%)	100	100	100	100

pre-implantation loss, or found a greater number of corpora lutea than fetuses, but were not significantly different from the control groups of both normotensive rats and hypertensive rats, a fact physiologically normal in this experimental design. As for post-implantation losses, it is noteworthy that there was no significant difference between the experimental groups, although fetal resorption observed in control and treated groups. Fig. 1 shows the average weights of fetuses and placentas from different experimental groups, after the sacrifice of pregnant rats on day 18 of gestation. It is observed that fetuses and placentas with significantly lower weights predominated in the groups of hypertensive rats, this result was expected since this group had less weight gain during pregnancy; also note that the results were independent of the administration of guaco extract or saline solution, since there were no significant difference between spontaneously hypertensive group (saline solution) with spontaneously hypertensive + guaco (1 ml or 2 mL) group, due to the effect of hypertension.

Macroscopic analysis

All fetuses underwent fixation technique in Bouin's solution and then the macroscopic analysis was performed. All fetuses from hypertensive groups of rats (spontaneously hypertensive rats received saline solution, spontaneously hypertensive rats treated with 1 - 2 mL of guaco) presented measurements of external morphological parameters (antero-posterior and latero-lateral of cranium; antero-posterior and latero-lateral of thorax; cranium-caudal and tail) significantly lower when compared with the normotensive rats (control group), which was also expected since these fetuses were significantly lower when weighted at the time of cesarean section, effect also attributed to hypertension, as there was no significant difference between the groups treated with guaco (1 mL or 2 mL) (Fig. 2).

Microscopic analysis

In the normotensive rats control group, fragments of placentas averaged 0.30 cm, the largest fragment 0.60 cm and smaller 0.10 cm. The thickness of the vessels ranged from 0.01 to 0.05 mm, their average was 0.03 mm, for a total of 80 blades. Areas of congestion

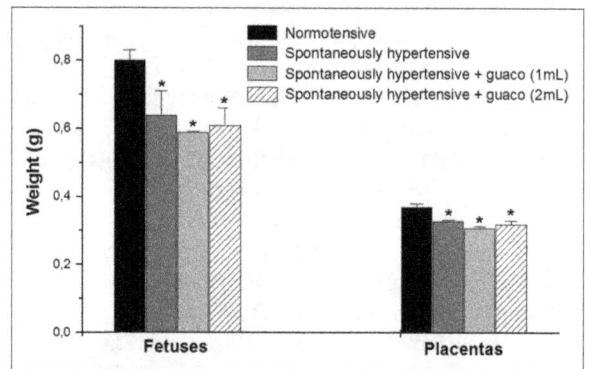

Fig. 1. Fetuses and placentas' weights (n=26-56).

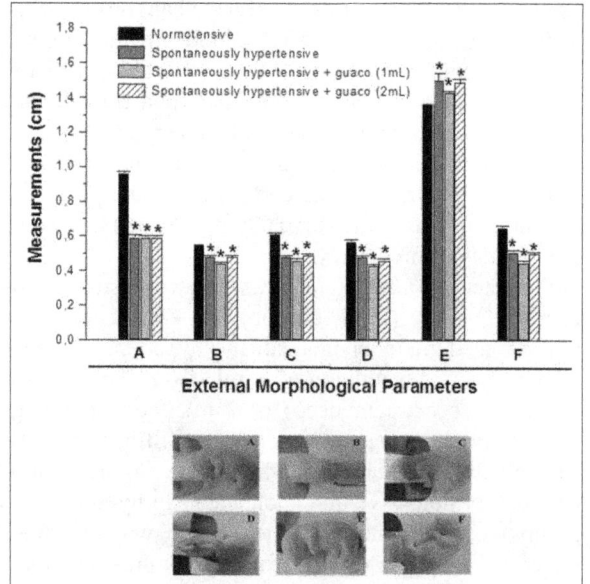

Fig. 2. External morphological parameters (cm) of fetuses of rats exposed to the following treatments: normotensive rats (n=56), spontaneous hypertensive rats (n = 26); spontaneously hypertensive rats treated with 1mL of guaco (n=28); spontaneously hypertensive rats treated with 2mL of guaco (n=36): antero-posterior (A) and latero-lateral (B) of cranium; antero-posterior (C) and latero-lateral (D) of thorax; cranium-caudal (E) and tail (F). Cesarean sections were performed on the 18th day of gestation. *p<0.05 when compared to the control group.

were found in 72 cases (90%), foci of hemorrhage in 61 cases (76.25%), inflammation in only one slide. The presence of fibrin was observed in seven placentas, and no areas with edema were observed in this group (Table 2).

In the group of spontaneously hypertensive rats (with saline solution), 45 slides were analyzed. Fragments measurement averaged 0.30 cm, the largest fragment of 0.4 cm and 0.2 cm from the smaller. The thickness of the vessels ranged from 0.02 to 0.04 mm, the average being 0,0266 mm. Congestion areas were observed in all cases, bleeding was found (86.66%), acute inflammation was observed in only one slide, and there no cases of edema and/or fibrin were observed in this group (Table 2).

In the spontaneously hypertensive rats group treated with 1 mL of guaco, consisting of 18 placentae, fragments averaged 0.3 cm, being the smallest in size of 0.2 cm. The thickness of the vessels ranged from 0.03 to 0.04 mm and average was 0.031 mm. Congestion was observed in 16 cases, corresponding to 88.80%. Bleeding was found in seven placentae (43.75%). Acute inflammation was observed in only one placenta, and no cases of edema and/or fibrin were observed in this group (Table 2).

In the spontaneously hypertensive rats group treated with 2 mL of guaco, 25 slides were analyzed. Fragments averaged 0.3 cm, the largest of 0.5 and smallest of 0.2 cm. Vessel thickness ranged from 0.01 to 0.04 mm and the mean value was 0.026 mm. Congestion was observed in 21 rats (84%). Inflammation was observed in only one placenta, and no cases of edema and/or fibrin were observed in this group (Table 2).

Foci of thrombosis were also found in a placenta in the hypertensive control group, suggesting the progression of maternal hypertension. Foci of lymphocytic infiltrate were observed in all groups of rats, which corroborate the findings of inflammation of some placentas, since lymphocytes are markers of inflammation (Fig. 3). Results are summarized in Table 2.

Discussion

Toxicology is a science which has greatly evolved, emerging reproductive toxicology, which studies the actions of toxic substances on various phases of the reproductive and developmental process (Gerenutti et al., 1992). Numerous plants are used as an alternative treatment for various diseases, but without proper evaluation of the toxicity of its components (Fraser and Nora, 1986). Most fetal changes are mainly due to maternal exposure to chemical agents (Gerenutti et al., 2006), which indicates the importance of this study to assess potential toxicities of guaco extract when administered during pregnancy in hypertensive rats.

The rat is an important animal model in reproductive toxicity testing. However, histopathological knowledge about development of the placenta, placental abnormalities, or inadequacies of the fetus and placenta is scarce and incomplete. An understanding of the development of normal placenta is required, in order to recognize the possible abnormalities, and there are few studies on morphometric changes during development of normal and hypertensive placenta.

Currently there are only two studies that reported the pregnant rat maternal blood parameters (Janthanaphan et al., 2006; Huppertz, 2008). Requirements related to maternal toxicity, required for current guidelines for registration of drugs, are limited mainly to food consumption and drug use (Hall, 1973). Drugs of herbal origin are not yet included in studies of maternal toxicity.

The use of spontaneously hypertensive rats is justified based on the results obtained in the literature, suggesting that guaco induces smooth muscle relaxing effect, vasodilator, and hypotensive effects that could promote reduction of blood pressure in hypertensive pregnant women, which have hypotensive reduced ability (Leite

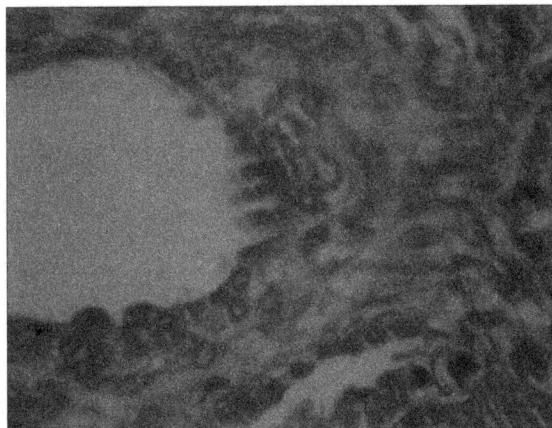

Fig. 3. Foci of lymphocytic infiltrate (H&E, 40x).

Table 2. Histological placental parameters analyzed during different treatments.

	Average vessel thickness (mm)	Congestion/ hemorrhage (%)	Fibrin (%)	Inflammation (%)	Total placentas (n)
Normotensive	0.03	83.7	8	1.25	80
Spontaneously hypertensive	0.02	100	0	2.2	45
Spontaneously hypertensive+guaco (1 mL)	0.03	33.3	0	5.5	18
Spontaneously hypertensive+guaco (2 mL)	0.02	84	0	4	25

et al., 1992; Santos *et al.*, 1996), indicating this plant as a promising pharmacological tool in complementary therapy for pregnancy-related hypertension.

Maternal hypertension may cause decreased placental blood flow, reducing the transfer of specific nutrients such as glucose and amino acids. This condition results in low fetal and placental weight (Karlsson *et al.*, 1982; Kingdom and Kaufmann, 1999; Lieb *et al.*, 1981; Rudge *et al.*, 1999; Wallace *et al.*, 1999; Wigglesworth, 1964), data corroborated when pregnant hypertensive rats, treated or not with guaco extract, exhibited reduced weight of fetuses and placentas. According to some authors, in cases of hypertension there is a decreased placental perfusion (Wallace *et al.*, 1999). In the opinion of others, this decrease is caused by changes in placental spiral arterioles, which leads to insufficient placental flow and, consequently, the intrauterine growth retardation (Low and Galbraith, 1974; Kingdom and Kaufmann, 1999; Scott and Jordan, 1972). Small placentas are associated with factors such as low pre-pregnancy weight, high levels of maternal hemoglobin during pregnancy, hypertension, among others (Naeye, 1987).

In hypertension, the ability to vasodilate is reduced. The guaco extract has the active ingredient coumarin, which triggers various biological effects, including vasodilation - an important change to reduce the effects of hypertension on offspring (Schenkel *et al.*, 2001). This effect was not observed in this study with the concentrations studied, since the restriction of the blood supply was maintained during pregnancy, as confirmed by the decrease in weight of fetuses and placentas when compared to normotensive rats. The methodology used in this study was similar to other studies that have observed acute toxicity (Pérez-Guerrero *et al.*, 2001) and reproductive capacity (Gerenutti *et al.*, 2006).

The pre-implantation and post-implantation of blastocysts undergo differential physiological effects under the actions of chemicals, serving to distinguish embryotoxicity and direct toxic effects on uterine function. The rate of pre-implantation losses establishes the relationship between two variables: number of corpora lutea and number of implantation (Ford, 1982). The results of this study showed no change in number of deployments in relation to number of corpora lutea. In relation to post-implantation losses, the finding of resorptions present in both control and hypertensive groups can be justified, since the placenta is exposed to the same influences of intrauterine environment, and other countless extra-uterine aggressions of various kinds (Beebe *et al.*, 1996; Albuquerque, 2009).

In fetuses subjected to macroscopic analysis, anatomical abnormalities were not seen in any of the experimental groups (Damasceno *et al.*, 2008). But the measures of external morphological parameters (anteroposterior and lateral-lateral skull, anteroposterior and lateral-lateral

thorax, cranial-caudal and tail) were significantly lower when compared with the normotensive control group, which was also proved, since these fetuses were significantly lower when weighted at the time of cesarean section, effect attributed to hypertension.

In conclusion, the results obtained in this study show that the *Mikania glomerata* extract did not show the possibility of teratogenicity, and also did not determine control over the vasoconstrictor effect in hypertensive rats, with the studied concentrations. The histological analysis concluded that no significant alterations between the analyzed groups occurred; all the groups presented congestion, whereas inflammation, edema and fibrin deposits were found in an insignificant number of placentas, independent of control or treated group. The weight reduction of the hypertensive rats, fetuses and their respective placentas were determined by hypertension, not by the administration of the plant extract, data confirmed when compared to the spontaneously hypertensive rats (saline solution).

Therefore, new complementary studies about the plant extract are necessary, in order to determine the toxic and vasodilatation potential, which will indicate a safe use for pregnant women, who use the commercialized *Mikania glomerata* extract as an alternative treatment for superior airway problems, especially to fluidize tracheobronchial exudates and for its significant effect of relaxing the smooth muscles of the bronchi.

Acknowledgments

The authors thank PIBIC/CNPq and CEPE/CNPq for financial support.

Conflict of interest

The authors declare that there is no conflict of interest.

References

Albuquerque, L.B.L. 2009. Estudos in vitro e in vivo de Plathymenia reticulata Benth [dissertação]. São Paulo: Programa de Pós-Graduação em Ciências Farmacêuticas, Universidade de Sorocaba.

Almeida, M.F.B., Guinsburg, R., Martinez, F.E., Procianoy, R.S., Leone, C.R., Marba, S.T.M., Rugolo, L.M.S.S., Luz, J.H. and Lopes, J.M.A. 2008. Perinatal factors associated with early deaths of preterm infants born in Brazilian Network on Neonatal Research centers. Jornal de Pediatria da Sociedade Brasileira de Pediatria 84(4), 300-307.

Amorozo, M.C.M. and Gely, A. 1988. Uso de Plantas Medicinais por Caboclos do Baixo Amazonas; Barcarena: PA; Museu Paraense Emílio Goeldi 4, 47.

Assis, T.R., Viana, F.P. and Rassi, S. 2008. Estudo dos Principais Fatores de Risco Maternos nas Síndromes Hipertensivas da Gestação. Universidade Federal de Goiás1, Universidade Católica de Goiás2, Goiânia, GO, Brasil.

Barreto, T.E. and Hiruma-Lima, C.A. 2002. Potencial

farmacológico de um Fragmento de Mata de Galeria, Fisionomia do Bioma Cerrado, denominado Mata do Butignoli – Botucatu – SP. Estudo monográfico – Instituto de Biociências, Universidade Estadual Paulista, Botucatu.

Beebe, L.A., Cowan, L.D. and Altshuler, G. 1996. The epidemiology of placental features: associations with gestacional age and neonatal outcome. Obstet. Gynecol. 87, 771-778.

Benirschke, K. and Kaufmann, P. 2000. Pathology of the human placenta. 4th ed. New York: Springer.

Britto, V.L.M.Q., Resende, R.F., Gouveia, N.M., Amaral, F.C., Teixeira, E.H., Pereira, W.F. and Espíndola, F.S. 2007. Plantas medicinais e fitoterápicos no contexto da academia, governo e organizações da sociedade civil: exemplo de iniciativas populares no município de Uberlândia-MG. Rev. Ed. Popular, Uberlândia 6, 93-101.

Cechinel-Filho, V. and Yunes, R.A. 1998. Estratégias para a obtenção de compostos farmacologicamente ativos a partir de plantas medicinais: conceitos sobre modificação estrutural para otimização da atividade. *Química Nova*, São Paulo 21(1), 99-105.

Damasceno, D.C., Kempinas, W.G., Volpato, G.T., Consoni, M., Rudge, M.V.C. and Paumgartten, F.J.R. 2008. *Anomalias Congênitas - Estudos Experimentais*. Editora Coopmed, Belo Horizonte-MG, pp: 1-99.

de Rijk, E.P.C.T., Esch, E.V. and Flik, G. 2002. Pregnancy Dating in the Rat: Placental Morphology and Maternal Blood Parameters. Toxicol. Pathol. 30(2), 271-282.

Ferrão, M.H.L., Pereira, A.C.L., Gersgorin, H.C.T.S., Paula, T.A.A., Corrêa, R.R.M. and Castro, E.C.C. 2006. Efetividade do tratamento de gestantes hipertensas. Departamento de Ciências Biológicas da Universidade Federal do Triângulo Mineiro, MG, Brasil.

Ferro, V.O. 1991. Aspectos Farmacognósticos de Mikania smilacina DC. Curso de Pós-Graduação em Ciências Farmacêuticas da USP, Tese de Doutorado.

Ford, W.C. 1982. The effect of deoxy-6-fluoroglucose on the fertility of male rats and mice. Contraception 25(5), 535-545.

Fraser, F.C. and Nora, J.J. 1986. Genética Humana. 2nd Ed. Guanabara, Rio de Janeiro.

Gerenutti, M., Del Fiol, F. and Groppo, F.C. 2006. Performance reprodutiva de ratas grávidas e efeitos embriotóxicos da ciprofloxacina. Pharmazie 61(1), 79-80.

Gerenutti, M., Spinosa, H.deS. and Bernardi, M.M. 1992. Effects of bracken fern (Pteridium aquilinum L Kuhn) feeding during the development of female rats and their offspring. Vet. Hum. Toxicol. 34(4), 307-310.

Graber, S.E., Scheffel, U., Hodkinson, B. and McIntyre, P.A. 1971. Placental transport of vitamin B12 in the pregnant rat. J. Clin. Invest. 50(5), 1000-1004.

Hall, G.A. 1973. Changes in the Rat Placenta Following Inoculation with Salmonella Dublin. Am. J. Pathol. 72(1), 103-118.

Huppertz, B. 2008. Placental origins of preeclampsia: challenging the current hypothesis. Hypertension 51(4), 970-975.

Janthanaphan, M., Kor-anantakul, O. and Geater, A. 2006. Placental weight and its ratio to birth weight in normal pregnancy at Songkhlanagarind Hospital. J. Med. Assoc. Thai. 89(2), 130-137.

Karlsson, K., Ljungblad, U. and Lundgren, Y. 1982. Blood flow of the reproductive system in renal hypertensive rats during pregnancy. Am. J. Obstet. Gynecol. 142, 1039-1044.

Kingdom, J.C. and Kaufmann, P. 1999. Oxigen and placental vascular development. Adv. Exp. Med. Biol. 474, 259-275.

Kosif, R., Akta, G. and Öztekin, A. 2008. Microscopic Examination of Placente of Rats Prenatally Exposed to Aloe barbadensis: A Preliminary Study. Int. J. Morphol. 26(2), 275-281.

Leite, M.G.R., Silva, M.A.M., Lino, C.S., Viana, G.S.B. and Matos, F.J.A. 1992. Atividade broncodilatadora em *Mikania glomerata*, Justicia pectoralis e Torresca cearensis. Anais do XII Simpósio de Plantas Medicinais do Brasil 1, 21.

Lewis, R.M., Doherty, C.B., James, L.A., Burton, G.J. and Hales, C.N. 2001. Effects of Maternal Iron Restriction on Placental Vascularization in the Rat. Placenta 22(6), 534-539.

Lieb, S.M., Zugaib, M., Nuwayhid, B., Tabsh, K., Erkkola, R., Ushioda, E., Brinkmann III, C.R. and Assali, N.S. 1981. Nitroprusside induced hemodynamic alterations in normotensive and hypertensive pregnant sheep. Am. J. Obstet. Gynecol. 139, 925-931.

Low, J.A. and Galbraith, R.S. 1974. Pregnancy characteristics of intrauterine growth retardation. Obstet. Gynecol. 44, 122-126.

Naeye, R.L. 1987. Functionally important disorders of the placenta, umbilical cord, and fetal membranes. Hum. Pathol. 18, 680-691.

Oliveira, F., Alvarenga, M.A., Akisue, G. and Akisue, M.K. 1984. Isolamento e identificação de componentes químicos de *Mikania glomerata* Sprengel e de Mikania laevigata Schultz Bip. ex Baker. Rev. Farm. Bioq USP, São Paulo 20(2), 169-183.

Pereira, N.A., Pereira, B.M., do Nascimento, M.C., Parente, J.P. and Mors, W.B. 1994. Pharmacological screening of plants recommended by folk medicine as anti-snake venom; IV. Protection against jararaca venom by isolated constituents. Planta Med. 60, 99-100.

Pérez-Guerrero, C., Herrera, M.D., Ortiz, R., Alvarez de Sotomayor, M. and Fernández, M.A. 2001. A pharmacological study of Cecropia obtusifolia Bertol aqueous extract. J. Ethnopharmacol. 76, 279-284.

Prance, G.T. 1992. *Out of the Amazon*; HMSO: London, pp: 83.

Rudge, M.V., Gomes, C.M., Calderon Ide, M., Ramos, M.D., Abbade, J.F., de Oliveira, M.G. and da Silva, M.G. 1999. Study of the evolution of the placenta and fetal pancreas in the pathophysiology of intrauterine growth retardation due to restricted maternal diet. São Paulo Med. J. 117, 49-56.

Ruppelt, B.M., Pereira, E.F., Gonçalves, L.C. and Pereira, N.A. 1991. Pharmacological screening of plants recommended by folk medicine as anti-snake venom I. Analgesic and anti-inflammatory activities. Memórias do Instituto Oswaldo Cruz 86(Suppl. II), 203-205.

Santos, T.C., Tomassini, C.B., Sanchez, E. and Cabral, L.M. 1996. Anais do XII Simpósio de Plantas Medicinais do Brasil, pp:149.

Schenkel, E.P., Zaninnin, M., Mentz, L.A., Bordignon, S.A.L. and Irgang, B. 2001. Plantas Tóxicas. In: Simões, C.M.O., Schenkel, E.P., Gossmann, G., Mello, J.C.P., Mentz, L.A. and Petrovick, P.R. Farmacognosia: da planta ao medicamento. UFSC/UFRGS, Porto Alegre 1, pp: 755-788.

Scott, J.M. and Jordan, J.M. 1972. Placental insufficiency and small-for-dates baby. Am. J. Obstet. Gynecol. 113, 823-832.

Vieira, R.B., Macedo, S.M.D. and Schwanz, M. 2008. Inibição do recrutamento celular pelo extrato aquoso de Mikania laevigata Schultz Bip. ex. Baker e cumarina em ratos submetidos à peritonite. Departamento de Ciências da Saúde, Curso de Farmácia, Universidade Regional Integrada do Alto Uruguai e das Missões. URI – Campus de Erechim.

Wallace, J.M., Bourke, D.A. and Aitken, P.P. 1999. Nutrition and fetal growth: paradoxical effects in the overnourished adolescent sheep. J. Reprod. Fertil. Suppl. 54, 385-399.

Wigglesworth, J.S. 1964. Experimental growth retardation in fetal rat. J. Pathol. Bacteriol. 88, 1-13.

19

Baseline values of immunologic parameters in the lizard *Salvator merianae* (*Teiidae*, Squamata)

Ana Paula Mestre[1,2,3,*], Patricia Susana Amavet[2,3] and Pablo Ariel Siroski[1,2,4]

[1]*Laboratorio de Zoología Aplicada: Anexo Vertebrados, Facultad de Humanidades y Ciencias, Universidad Nacional del Litoral, (FHUC-UNL/MMA), Argentina*
[2]*Consejo Nacional de Investigaciones Científicas y Técnicas (CONICET), Santa Fe, Argentina*
[3]*Laboratorio de Genética, Departamento de Ciencias Naturales (FHUC-UNL), Santa Fe, Argentina*
[4]*Laboratorio de Biología Celular y Molecular Aplicada, Instituto de Ciencias Veterinarias del Litoral (ICiVet-Litoral-UNL-CONICET), Esperanza, Santa Fe, Argentina*

Abstract

The genus *Salvator* is widely distributed throughout South America. In Argentina, the species most abundant widely distributed is *Salvator merianae*. Particularly in Santa Fe province, the area occupied by populations of these lizards overlaps with areas where agriculture was extended. With the aim of established baseline values for four immunologic biomarkers widely used, 36 tegu lizards were evaluated tacking into account different age classes and both sexes. Total leukocyte counts were not different between age classes. Of the leucocytes count, eosinophils levels were higher in neonates compared with juvenile and adults; nevertheless, the heterophils group was the most prevalent leukocyte in the peripheral blood in all age classes. Lymphocytes, monocytes, heterophils, azurophils and basophils levels did not differ with age. Natural antibodies titres were higher in the adults compared with neonates and juveniles lizards. Lastly, complement system activity was low in neonates compared with juveniles and adults. Statistical analysis within each age group showed that gender was not a factor in the outcomes. Based on the results, we concluded that *S. merianae* demonstrated age (but not gender) related differences in the immune parameters analyzed. Having established baseline values for these four widely-used immunologic biomarkers, ongoing studies will seek to optimize the use of the *S. merianae* model in future research.

Keywords: Biomarkers, Immune system, Reptilian, *Salvator merianae*, Sentinel model.

Introduction

The genus *Salvator* (previously *Tupinambis*; Harvey *et al.*, 2012) belongs to the order Squamata, and is widely distributed throughout South America. In Argentina, the most abundant and widely distributed species is the "iguana overa (Spanish) or tegu lizard (English)" (*Salvator merianae*) (Ávila-Pires, 1995; Harvey *et al.*, 2012). This lizard is a diet generalist that feeds on a wide range of animals and fruits (de Castro and Galetti, 2004) and whose daily and seasonal activity cycles are strongly related to temperature (Winck *et al.*, 2011). From April-June (colder months), their metabolism decreases until environmental temperature increases. From October-December (warmer months), the annual reproductive cycles takes place. In those times, nests are built in caves in the ground or tree roots that are isolated from the climate changes to ensure a proper incubation temperature and humidity for the development of embryos (Yanosky and Mercolli, 1992). Since 1982 *S. merianae* has been included in Appendix II of CITES (Convention on International Trade in Endangered Species of Wild Fauna and Flora) and it is considered of "Least Concern" for

conservation status by the IUCN (International Union for Conservation of Nature) (Embert *et al.*, 2009). In addition, this species has been under management on a sustainable use program in Santa Fe province (Argentina), known as Iguana Project (PI - Secretary of State for Environment and Sustainable Development of the Province of Santa Fe. Resolution Number 0031/07). This program is based on the ranching technique, which implies the collection of eggs from natural environment, subsequent artificial incubation, birth and breeding of the animals under controlled conditions until they reach an appropriate size to be released into the wild and to avoid predation or influence of low temperatures (Schaumburg *et al.*, 2012).

In recent years, the habitats of this species have been negatively impacted by expansion of agriculture, especially soybean monocultures. The implementation of a system that combines the use of new technologies includes use/application of chemicals in bulk. The effects of these agents, combined with environmental factors (i.e., habitat fragmentation/degradation, draining of wetlands) have produced a decline in the populations of various wild species, among them

*Corresponding Author: Ana P. Mestre. Laboratorio de Zoología Aplicada: Anexo Vertebrados, Facultad de Humanidades y Ciencias, Universidad Nacional del Litoral, (FHUC-UNL/MMA), Santa Fe, Argentina. Email: anapaulamestre@yahoo.com

several types of reptiles (Gibbons *et al.*, 2000; Santos and Llorente, 2009; Weir *et al.*, 2015). In particular, tegu lizard populations have plummeted in areas where agricultural activity has advanced.

As with any endangered host species, it is essential to monitor their health status and ability to defend from infections, as a result of changes in their external environments. Immunity to infection is mediated by two general systems, innate (or natural) and acquired (or adaptive). Components of the natural immune system are markedly conserved between insects and mammals, indicating a common ancestral origin for this branch of immunity (Hoffmann *et al.*, 1999). Only vertebrates have the adaptive immune system, which play an important role when innate immunity is not precise enough to a particular challenge or in response to recurrence of a given challenge (Collado *et al.*, 2008). Exposure of native animals to certain pesticides, whether acute or chronic, could affect both their innate and acquired immune responses (Burns *et al.*, 1996). Previous studies have shown some pesticides have effects on immunity; they can alter structures of some components of the immune system (IS), and in some cases also reduce host resistance to antigens and infectious agents (Hernández Coronado, 2007; Modesto and Martinez, 2010; Ray *et al.*, 2015). Studies in broad-snouted caiman (*Caiman latirostris*), another native reptile, demonstrated alterations in the IS of hatchlings and neonates that had been exposed to glyphosate, endosulfan, or cypermethrin formulations (Siroski, 2011; Harvey *et al.*, 2012; Latorre *et al.*, 2013; Siroski *et al.*, 2016).

White blood cells (WBC) are involved in a significant amount of processes in the IS. In certain situations, increases or decreases in values of select blood components can be used as markers to diagnose disease or changes in host nutritional status (González Fernández, 2003). The innate immune system can be monitored through assessments of two humoral components: levels of natural antibodies (NAb) and the functionality of the complement system (CS). Natural antibodies are encoded directly by the germline genome (Avrameas, 1991) and do not require somatic hyper mutation and recombination during ontogenesis as occurs with the adaptive antibody repertoire. The CS is an important part of the innate immune system and can be sequentially activated in a cascade type reaction by numerous routes (Siroski *et al.*, 2016).

The aim of this study was to evaluate four widely-used immune biomarkers, e.g., total and differential leukocyte count, NAb levels, and CS activity, in order to determine baseline values for *S. merianae* of varying ages. This data would, in turn, allow for the potential implementation of this species as a model for use in evaluating exposures of environmentally relevant species to different environmental stressors.

Materials and Methods

Animals

This research was approved by the Ethics Committee and Security (ECAS) of Facultad de Ciencias Veterinarias, Universidad Nacional del Litoral (#258/16, Santa Fe, Argentina). All animals were treated in accord with the Reference Ethical Framework for Biomedical Research: Ethical Principles for Research with Laboratory, Farm, and Wild Animals (NSTRC, 2005).

In this study were used 36 specimens of tegu lizards: 12 neonates (NE; 2-days-old), 12 juveniles (JUV; 6-mo-old) and 12 adults (AD; > 4-yr-old; 6 males, 6 females). The NE and JUV animals came from eggs collected in the Managed Natural Reserve "El Fisco" located in Santa Fe Province, Argentina; corresponding to a Protected Natural Area (Law 12.930, 2008) situated at least 20 km away from possible pesticide application area or other industrial contaminant activity (Siroski *et al.*, 2016). As part of the ranching program "PI", the eggs were artificially incubated under controlled conditions of temperature (29-32°C) and relative humidity (< 20%). Adult lizards were taken out from the breeding stock in captivity in the "PI". All lizards were fed *ad libitum* three times a week. The NE and JUV could be sexed when they were below 20 cm in snout-vent length (SVL) (Yanosky and Mercolli, 1992). Therefore, gender determination was performed using the mound scale method as well as through observations of hypertrophy of the jaw muscles in males (Hall, 1978; Yanosky and Mercolli, 1992).

Blood samples

Peripheral blood samples were obtained from the caudal vein (Olson *et al.*, 1977) with heparinized syringes (25 G × 5/8″ needles for NE lizards and 1″ needles (21G) for JUV and AD lizards). Aliquots of the collected blood were used for measures of WBC and for differential leukocyte population counts. The remaining sample was centrifuged at 2500 × g for 15 min and stored at -80°C until used for the determination of NAb levels and CS activity (Siroski *et al.*, 2016).

Total white blood cells and differential leukocyte population counts

WBC counts were performed using a Neubauer chamber. An aliquot of whole blood was diluted 1:200 with a solution of 0.6% NaCl and then examined under microscope at 400X. All results were expressed as total cells/mm^3 blood (Lewis *et al.*, 2008). For the differential counts, two smears were prepared/animal, fixed with ethanol, and then stained with May-Grunwald-Giemsa solution. The preparations were then coded to achieve maximum objectivity during the analysis. Amounts of each leukocyte subtype (e.g., heterophil, basophil, eosinophil, lymphocyte, monocyte, azurophil)/100 WBC analyzed were determined manually using an optical microscope.

Each subtype was expressed in relation to WBC count recorded beforehand. Also, lobularity index was calculated (LI = number of counted lobes / number of heterophils counted) from the classification of heterophilic granulocytes according to Arneth (Charipper, 1928) to evaluate the degree of leukocyte maturity (García *et al.*, 1997).

Natural antibodies titres

Determination of agglutinating NAb titres was conducted using a hemagglutination assay described by Matson *et al.* (2005). This assay is based on agglutination between NAb from lizard plasma samples and rabbit red blood cells (RRBC) obtained from a breeding stock maintained at the Universidad Nacional del Litoral. Here, whole rabbit blood was centrifuged at $2500 \times g$ for 15 min to separate the plasma. A buffer solution was then prepared with phosphate-buffered saline (PBS, pH 7.4) containing rabbit plasma (1%) (Sigma, St. Louis, MO). The pelleted RRBC were then washed with PBS several times until the supernatant was clear, and then a 1% RRBC (v/v) solution in PBS was prepared. For the assay itself, to 96-well round (U)-bottom plates (Corning Costar, Corning, NY), 25 µl (PBS with rabbit plasma) was added into wells in Columns 1-12. Thereafter, 25 µl test plasma was added to wells in the first column. Samples were then serially diluted to a final dilution of 1:2048 (Column 11). As a negative control, no lizard plasma was placed into the Column 12 (i.e., well contained only PBS). Finally, 25 µl RRBC solution was added into wells in all columns (1-12). After incubation at 25°C for 1 hr, NAb titres were determined. Titres were assigned as the inverse of the highest dilution yielding a button; in cases where an individual had negative hemagglutination in all wells, a titre of 0 was assigned. From the average of all titres in a given age group, a mean titre for each group was calculated.

Complement System (CS) activity

Lizard CS activity was determined via assessment of sheep red blood cell (SRBC) hemolysis (Siroski *et al.*, 2010). The SRBC were collected from Merino sheep (*Ovis aries*) with heparinized syringes. The blood was washed with PBS several times until the supernatant was clear, and then a 2% SRBC (v/v) solution in PBS was prepared. In the assay, lizard plasma was incubated with an equal volume of 2% SRBC for 30 min at 25°C and then centrifuged at 2500 x g for 5 min. Thereafter, 300 µl of the resultant supernatant was transferred to a microplate for measure of optical density [at 540 nm] in a Multiskan RC microplate reader (Multiskan Labsystem, Helsinki, Finland). As a positive control, 2 µl Triton X-100 was added to 1 ml of 2% SRBC and the mixture shaken until complete hemolysis was attained. The level of SRBC hemolysis in each sample was divided by the absorbance of the positive control

to obtain the maximum percentage of hemolysis (% MH). All results were expressed as mean % MH [± SE].

Statistical analysis

Data were tested for homogeneity using a Levene test, and for normality using a Kolmogorov-Smirnov test. To determine differences among the groups, data were analyzed using a one-way analysis of variance (ANOVA) followed by a Tukey test. When the data did not meet the assumptions of normality and / or homogeneity of variances, it were analyzed using a non-parametric Kruskal-Wallis test followed by a Mann-Whitney test. Comparisons of variables analyzed as a function of gender were done using a Student *t*-test except for eosinophil data that were analyzed using a non-parametric Mann-Whitney test. Differences were considered significant with $p < 0.05$. All data are reported as means ± SE.

Results

Because the morphological characterization of the leukocytes of this lizard has not yet been reported, we include images of all leucocytes types (Fig. 1).

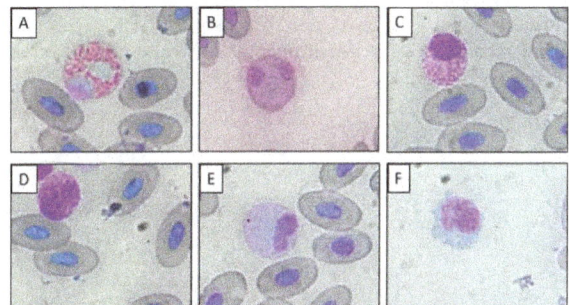

Fig. 1. Leukocytes of *S. merianae*. **(A, B):** Heterophils with cytoplasm full of rod granules **(A)** and of little round granules **(B)**. **(C):** Eosinophil with cytoplasm full of round granules. **(D):** Basophil with big round granules. **(E):** Monocyte and **(F):** Big lymphocyte. In the last two, low nucleus/cytoplasm ratio and low concentration of heterochromatin.

The results for the total WBC counts showed there were no differences among the age classes of *S. merianae*. Nevertheless levels of eosinophils were higher in NE compared with JUV and AD groups (Fig. 2). With respect to the others leucocyte types no differences were observed among age classes. When the mean of all cell types in the three age classes were compared, it was found that the heterophils group was the most prevalent leukocyte in the peripheral blood in all age classes. In this type of leucocyte the nucleus was rounded, with one or two lobes, being infrequent the presence of three or more lobes, determining an IL of 1.76 ± 0.10 for NE, 1.65 ± 0.58 for JUV and 1.61 ± 0.92 for AD. The comparison among age classes was not different. Natural antibody titres differed among the groups. Values associated with AD were higher compared with those for NE and JUV (Fig. 3).

This clearly indicated that the levels of NAb in younger lizards were very low (in many cases, there were titres of 0). With regard to CS activity, the data indicated there were also differences among the age classes. Neonate blood imparted a low value of maximum hemolysis compared with the blood from JUV or AD (Fig. 4). Lastly, comparisons performed for each parameter examined here showed there were no gender-related differences.

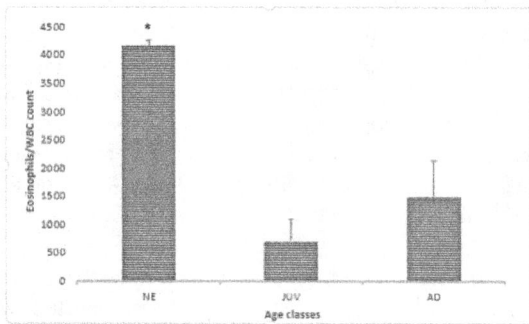

Fig. 2. Eosinophils level in relation with total number of WBC in each age class. NE (neonate), JUV (juvenile), AD (adult). Values shown are means (± SE) from 12 lizards/group. *Value significantly different from other groups (p < 0.05).

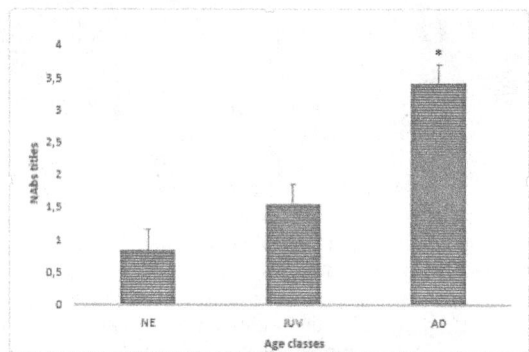

Fig. 3. NAb titres in each age class. NE (neonate), JUV (juvenile), AD (adult). Values shown are mean (±SE) from 12 lizards/group. *Value significantly different from other groups (p < 0.05).

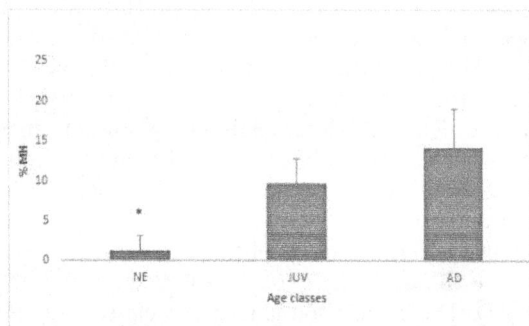

Fig. 4. Maximum percentage hemolysis (%MH) in each age class. NE (neonate), JUV (juvenile), AD (adult). Values shown are means (± SE) from 12 lizards/group. *Value significantly different from other groups (p < 0.05).

Discussion

Reptile immunology involves cell-mediated and humoral components; however, knowledge about immune function in reptiles remains limited. Several characteristics of *S. merianae* suggest it could potentially be useful as a sentinel organism for monitoring of environmental agent impact on their habitat (Schaumburg *et al.*, 2016).

The present study sought to establish some baseline parameters for such use; in particular, information on the IS of these hosts. Similar results were obtained for other authors who did not find differences in levels of WBC among different age classes in reptiles. Studies on *Chelonoidis chilensis chilensis* (Troiano and Silva, 1998), from captive *Caiman latirostris* and *C. yacare* (Mussart *et al.*, 2006) and *Iguana iguana* (Novoa-Fajardo *et al.*, 2008) have reported an absence of influence from age on this hematologic parameter. However, Barboza *et al.* (2008) reported values significantly lower in adult than in both juvenile and sub–adult of *C. latirostris*. Further, the present study showed lower WBC counts compared to Novoa-Fajardo *et al.* (2008) results, and higher values in relation to that seen in other studies (Mussart *et al.*, 2006; Barboza *et al.*, 2008; Silvestre, 2014).

Regarding the endpoint of differential leukocyte counts, here we have considered azurophils as a variation of normal monocytes, as well as some authors (Montali, 1988; Huber and, 1998; Claver and Quaglia, 2009). In contrast, others researches consider them as a distinct cell type (Troiano *et al.*, 1996; Kanchanapangka *et al.*, 1999; Salakij *et al.*, 2002; Maceda-Veiga *et al.*, 2015).

Similar to the one reported by Rios *et al.* (2003) for *Lama guanicoe*, in this study a higher level of eosinophils was seen in neonates compared to juveniles and adult lizards. This could be a consequence of some exposures to allergens present in the nest material in contact with neonates. This result contrast with findings by Barboza *et al.* (2008) who observed an age-related increase in eosinophil levels in *C. latirostris*. Overall, the means levels of eosinophils in adult *S. merianae* were generally higher than those reported by Silvestre (2014).

Similar to what was seen by Troiano *et al.* (1996), Troiano and Silva (1998) and and Rios *et al.* (2003), this study did not reveal any differences among age classes in regard to other leukocyte types, while Stacy *et al.* (2011) described age related changes in lymphocyte and heterophils percentages in *Caretta caretta* turtles. The lobularity index here observed was similar to the ones reported by Cabagna Zenklusen *et al.* (2011) in *Rhinella fernandezae* and Salinas *et al.* (2015) in *Rhinella arenarum*. With regard to NAb levels, our analysis of titres showed the highest values in the adults compared with juveniles and neonate lizards. This increase in NAb with age has been also reported in mammals, birds, and others reptiles (Parmentier *et al.*, 2004; Benatuil *et al.*, 2008; Sparkman and Palacios, 2009; Ujvari and Madsen, 2011; Zimmerman *et al.*, 2013). In reptiles of all ages, the specific antibody response is slower and less robust than in mammalian counterparts (Zimmerman *et al.*, 2010). This thus implies that the increase in NAb tires with age might be viewed as a "positive" change in immunity with age in these reptiles (Ujvari and Madsen, 2011). Studies about complement-system activity have been reported with a variety of reptiles. In *Alligator mississippiensis* (Merchant *et al.*, 2005), *Crocodylus porosus* and *C. johnstoni* (Merchant and Britton, 2006), and *Caiman latirostris* (Siroski, 2011), potent CS were reported; this suggested a strong physiological importance for this system in terms of protection against various pathogens (Siroski, 2011). In the present study, a low percentage of maximum hemolysis was detected in *S. merianae* compared to the above-mentioned species. This could be a trait of the *S. merianae* itself. On the other hand, differences in CS activity were noted among the *S. merianae* age classes, indicating activity of this system increased with age. Strasser *et al.* (2000) reported similar results in relation to age in mammals. Thus, future studies must consider that results of this technique are likely to be variable with age. According with findings in other studies on sentinel species, the comparisons between sexes revealed no differences in the endpoints assessed here. Khan *et al.* (2016) found no gender-related differences in WBC levels, differential leukocyte counts, or other biochemical/hematological parameters in dogs in Bangladesh. Latorre *et al.* (2015) noted no differences between males and female *Phrynops hilarii* (a side-necked turtle) in any of the variables that were analyzed, including WBC levels and differential leukocyte counts. In contrast, Barboza *et al.* (2008) found that male *C. latirostris* had total leukocyte, eosinophil, heterophil, and monocytes levels greater than those of females. Similarly, Stacy and Whitaker (2000) found mean WBC count and mean heterophil counts were significantly greater in adult male *C. palustris* than in adult females. Troiano *et al.* (1996) found inter-sex differences too, both in total count and differential leukocyte in other caiman species. Considering the results obtained in this study, sex, unlike age, should not be considered a key variable in studies that may use *S. merianae* as a model. In conclusion, the baseline values obtained in this study contributed to knowledge of IS of the *Salvator merianane*. Thus, of these four immunologic biomarkers studied, three showed differences among age classes, unlike sexes, in the analyzed species. These variations among age classes should be considered in future studies that may use *S. merianae* as sentinel model.

Acknowledgements

This study was supported by ANPCyT (GLP PICT 2011-1349, Argentina) y ANPCyT (PSA PICT 2013-1402, Argentina) y Proyecto Iguana (PI- Secretary of State for Environment and Sustainable Development of the Province of Santa Fe. Resolution Number 0031/07). This study is part of APM research as a Doctoral Fellow at the Consejo Nacional de Investigaciones Científicas y técnicas (CONICET). The authors would like to thank especially Mariana Cabagna for hers help in the identification of leukocyte population, Gisela Poletta, Pamela Burella and María Agustina Latorre for their contributions in improving the manuscript and Gisela Ríos with the figure design.

Conflict of interest

The authors declare that there is no conflict of interest.

References

Ávila-Pires, T. (Ed.). 1995. Lizards of *Brazilian Amazonia* (Reptilia: Squamata) Leiden: Zoologische. Verhandelinger, pp: 706-710.

Avrameas, S. 1991. Natural autoantibodies: from 'horror autotoxicus' to 'gnothi seauton'. Immunol. Today 12, 154-159.

Barboza, N., Mussart, N., Coppo, J., Fioranelli, S. and Koza, G. 2008. Internal medium of *Caiman latirostris* in captivity. Influence of sex, growth, and season. Res. Vet. 19, 33-41.

Benatuil, L., Kaye, J., Cretin, N., Godwin, J., Cariappa, A., Pillai, S. and Iacomini, J. 2008. Ig knock in mice producing anti-carbohydrate antibodies: Breakthrough of B-cells producing low affinity anti-self antibodies. J. Immunol. 180, 3839-3848.

Burns, L., Meade, B. and Munson, A. 1996. Toxic Responses of the Immune System. In: Casarett & Doull's Toxicology: Basic Science of Poisons. 5th Edition. (Klaassen C, Ed.). New York: McGraw Hill, pp: 355-402.

Cabagna Zenklusen, M., Lajmanovich, R., Attademo, A., Peltzer, P., Junges, C., Fiorenza Biancucci, G. and Bassó, A. 2011. Hematología y citoquímica de las células sanguíneas de *Rhinella fernandezae* (Anura: Bufonidae) en Espinal y Delta-Islas del río Paraná, Argentina. Rev. Biol. Trop. 59, 17-28.

Chariper, H. 1928. Studies on the Arneth count. -XII.The effect of the injection of thyroid extract on the polynuclear count in a perennibranchiate amphibian (*Necturus maculosus*). Exp. Physiol. 19, 109-113.

Claver, J. and Quaglia, A. 2009. Comparative morphology, development, and function of blood cells in non-mammalian vertebrates. J. Exp. Pet Med. 18, 87-97.

Collado, V., Porras, R., de Simón, M. and Lucía, E. 2008. The innate immune system: Mechanisms. Rev. Comp. Vet. 2, 1-16.

de Castro, E. and Galetti, M. 2004. Numbers of blood cells and their variation. In: Biology of Reptiles (Gans C, and Parsons T, Eds.). New York: Academic Press, pp: 93-109.

Embert, D., Fitzgerald, L. and Waldez, F. 2009. *Tupinambis merianae*. In: IUCN 2010. IUCN Red List of Threatened Species; Version 2010.4. [Accessed: May 2015]. At: www.iucnredlist.org.

García, B., Rubio, F. and Carrasco, M. 1997. Hematología. Citología, fisiología y Patología de hematíes y leucocitos. Paraninfo, Madrid, España.

Gibbons, J., Scott, D., Ryan, T., Buhlmann, K., Tuberville, T., Metts, B., Greene, J., Mills, T., Leiden, Y., Poppy, S. and Winne, C.T. 2000. The global decline of reptiles, déjà vu amphibians. Biosci. 50, 653-666.

González Fernández, A. 2003. Phylogeny of the Immune System. In: Immunology Online Chapter 16. Madrid: Universidad de Córdoba & Sweden Diagnostics. [Accessed: April 2016]. At: http://www.vi.cl/foro/topic/5698-capitulos-de-inmunologa-apuntes/page_st_100.

Hall, B. 1978. Note on the husbandry, behavior, and breeding of captive tegu lizards *Tupinambis teguixin*. Intl. Zoo Yearbook 1978, 91-101.

Harvey, M., Ugueto, G. and Gutberlet, R. 2012. Review of Teiid morphology with a revised taxonomy and phylogeny of the Teiidae (Lepidosauria: Squamata). Zootaxa. 34, 1-156.

Hernández Coronado, M. 2007. Evaluación de la Intoxicación Aguda de Atrazina Sobre la Respuesta Inmune de Tilapia (*Oreochromis niloticus*). Centro Universitario de Ciencias Biológicas y Agropecuarias. Universidad de Guadalajara. Doctoral Thesis.

Hoffmann, J., Kafatos, F., Janeway, C. and Ezekowitz, R. 1999. Phylogenetic perspectives in innate immunity. Sci. 284, 1313-1318.

Huber, T. and Zon, L. 1998. Transcriptional regulation of blood formation during Xenopus development. Semin. Immunol. 10, 103-109.

Kanchanapangka, S., Youngprapakorn, P., Pipatpanukul, K., Krobpan, S. and Kongthaworn, N. 1999. Differentiation of crocodilian granulocytes via histochemical techniques. 4th symposium Diseases in Asian Aquaculture, Cebu City. Philippines. #43.

Khan, S., Epstein, J., Olival, K., Hassan, M., Hossain, M., Rahman, K. and Desmond, J. 2016. Hematology and serum chemistry reference values of stray dogs in Bangladesh. Open Vet. J. 1, 13-20.

Latorre, M., López González, E., Larriera, A., Poletta, G. and Siroski, P. 2013. Effects of in vivo exposure to Roundup® on immune system of *Caiman latirostris*. J. Inmunotoxicol. 10, 349-354.

Latorre, M., López González, E., Siroski, P. and Poletta, G. 2015. Basal frequency of micronuclei and hematological parameters in the side-necked turtle, *Phrynops hilarii*. Acta Herpet. 10, 31-37.

Lewis, S., Bates, I. and Bain, B. 2008. Hematología Práctica. 10th Edition. Madrid, Elsevier.

Maceda-Veiga, A., Figuerola, J., Martínez-Silvestre, A., Viscor, G., Ferrari, N. and Pacheco, M. 2015. Inside the red-box: Applications of hematology in wildlife monitoring and ecosystem health assessment. Sci. Total Environ. 514, 322-332.

Matson, K., Ricklefs, R. and Klasing, K. 2005. A hemolysis-hemagglutination assay for characterizing constitutive innate humoral immunity in wild and domestic birds. Dev. Comp. Immunol. 29, 275-286.

Merchant, M., Pallansch, M., Paulman, R., Wells, J., Nalca, A. and Ptak, R. 2005. Antiviral activity of serum from the American alligator (*Alligator mississippiensis*). Antiviral Res. 66, 35-38.

Merchant, M. and Britton, A. 2006. Characterization of serum complement activity of saltwater (*Crocodylus porosus*) and freshwater (*Crocodylus johnstoni*) crocodiles. Comp. Biochem. Physiol. A. Mol. Integr. Physiol. 143, 488-493.

Modesto, K. and Martinez, C. 2010. Effects of Roundup Transorb on fish: Hematology, anti-oxidant defenses and acetylcholinesterase activity. Chemosphere 81, 781-787.

Montali, R. 1988. Comparative pathology of inflammation in the higher vertebrates (reptiles, birds and mammals). J. Comp. Pathol. 99, 1-20.

Mussart, N., Barboza, N., Fioranelli, S., Koza, G., Prado, W. and Coppo, J. 2006. Age, sex, year season, and handling system modify the leukocytal parameters from captive *Caiman latirostris* and *Caiman yacare* (Crocodylia: Alligatoridae). Res. Vet. 17, 3-10.

Novoa-Fajardo, D., Benítez-Tumay, I., Corredor-Matus, J. and Rodríguez-Pulido, J. 2008. Hallazgos hematológicos en iguana verde suramericana (*Iguana iguana*), de ejemplares ubicados en zona urbana y suburbana de Villavicencio (Meta). Orinoquia. 12, 67-79.

NSTRC (National Scientific and Technical Research Council). 2005. Reference Ethical Framework for Biomedics Research: Ethical Principles for Research with Laboratory, Farm, and Wild Animals, #1047. Anexo II, Buenos Aires, Argentina: CONICET.

Olson, G.A., Hessler, J.R and Faith, R.E. 1977. Techniques for the blood collection and intravascular infusion of reptiles. Lab. Anim. Sci. 25, 783-786.

Parmentier, H., Lammers, A., Hoekman, J., de Vries Reilingh, G., Zaanen, I. and Savelkoul, H. 2004. Different levels of natural antibodies in chickens divergently selected for specific antibody responses. Dev. Comp. Immunol. 28, 39-49.

Ray, S., Mukherjee, S., Bhunia, N., Bhunia, A. and Ray, M. 2015. Immunotoxicological threats of pollutants in aquatic invertebrates. Emerging pollutants in the environment -Current and further implications. InTech. 6, 149-167.

Rios, C., Zapata, B., Marín, M. P., Pacheco, S., Rivera, K., González, B.A. and Bas, F. 2003. Cambios hematológicos, bioquímica sanguínea y cortisol sérico en crías de guanaco (lama guanicoe) en cautiverio desde el nacimiento al destete. Av. Cienc. Vet. 18, 1-2.

Salakij, C., Salakij, J., Apibal, S., Narkkong, N., Chanhome, L. and Rochanapat, N. 2002. Hematology, morphology, cytochemical staining, and ultrastructural characteristics of blood cells in king cobras (Ophiophagus hannah). Vet. Clin. Pathol. 31, 116-126.

Salinas, Z., Salas, N., Baraquet, M. and Martino, A. 2015. Biomarcadores hematológicos del sapo común Bufo arenarum en ecosistemas alterados de la provincia de Córdoba. Acta toxicol. Argent. 23, 25-35.

Santos, X. and Llorente, G. 2009. Decline of a common reptile: Case study of the viperine snake Natrix maura in a Mediterranean wetland. Acta Herpet. 4(2), 161-169.

Schaumburg, L., Poletta, G., Siroski, P. and Mudry, M. 2012. Baseline values of micronuclei and Comet assay in lizard Tupinambis merianae (Teiidae, Squamata). Ecotoxicol. Environ. Saf. 84, 99-103.

Schaumburg, L., Siroski, P., Poletta, G. and Mudry, M. 2016. Genotoxity induced by Roundup® (Glyphosate) in tegu lizard (Salvator merianae) embryos. Pesticide Biochem. Physiol. 130, 71-78.

Silvestre, A. 2014. Hematología y bioquímica en reptiles. EN PORTADA. Barcelona–Espanha, pp: 32-35.

Siroski, P. 2011. Caracterización del Sistema de Complemento e Identificación de Componentes del Sistema Inmune Innato del Yacaré Overo (Caiman latirostris). Doctoral Thesis.

Siroski, P., Merchant, M., Parachu Marco, V., Piña, C. and Ortega, H. 2010. Characterization of serum complement activity of broad snouted caiman (Caiman latirostris, Crocodilia: Alligatori-dae). Zool. Stud. 49, 64-70.

Siroski, P., Poletta, G., Latorre, M., Merchant, M.,

Ortega, H. and Mudry, M. 2016. Immunotoxicity of commercial-mixed glyphosate in broad snouted caiman (Caiman latirostris). Chem-Biol. Interact. 244, 64-70.

Sparkman, A. and Palacios, M. 2009. A test of life-history theories of immune defense in two ecotypes of the garter snake, Thamnophis elegans. J. Anim. Ecol. 78, 1242-1248.

Stacy, B. and Whitaker, N. 2000. Hematology and blood biochemistry of captive mugger crocodiles (Crocodylus palustris). J. Zoo Wild. Med. 31, 339-347.

Stacy, N., Alleman, A. and Sayler, K. 2011. Diagnostic hematology of reptiles. Clin. Lab. Med. 1, 87-108.

Strasser, A., Teltscher, A., May, B., Sanders, C. and Niedermüller, H. 2000. Age-associated changes in the immune system of German shepherd dogs. J. Vet. Med. A. Physiol. Pathol. Clin. Med. 47(3), 181-192.

Troiano, J., Silva, M., Esarte, M., Márquez, A. and Mira, G. 1996. Valores hematológicos de las especies argentinas del genero Caiman (Crocodylia-Alligatoridae). Rev. Facena. 12, 111-117.

Troiano, J. and Silva, M. 1998. Valores hematológicos de referencia en tortuga terrestre argentina (Chelonoidis chilensis chilensis). Anal Vet. 18, 47-51.

Ujvari, B. and Madsen, T. 2011. Do natural antibodies compensate for humoral immuno-senescence in tropical pythons? Func. Ecol. 25, 813-817.

Weir, S., Yu, S., Talent, L., Maul, J., Anderson, T. and Salice, C. 2015. Improving reptile ecological risk assessment: oral and dermal toxicity of pesticides to a common lizard species (Sceloporus occidentalis). Environ. Toxicol. Chem. 34, 1778-1786.

Winck, G., Blanco, C. and Cechin, S. 2011. Population ecology of Tupinambis merianae (Squamata, Teiidae): Home-range, activity and space use. Anim. Biol. 61, 493-510.

Yanosky, A. and Mercolli, C. 1992. Tegu lizard (Tupinambis teguixin) management in captivity at El Bagual Ecological Reserve. Argentina Arch. Zootec. 41, 41-51.

Zimmerman, L., Vogel, L. and Bowden, R. 2010. Understanding the vertebrate immune system: Insights from the reptilian perspective. J. Exp. Biol. 213, 661-671.

Zimmerman, L., Clairardin, S., Paitz, R., Hicke, J., LaMagdeleine, K., Vogel, L. and Bowden, R. 2013. Humoral immune responses are maintained with age in a long-lived ectotherm, the red-eared slider turtle. J. Exp. Biol. 216, 633-640.

20

Doppler ultrasonography of the *pectinis oculi* artery in harpy eagles (*Harpia harpyja*)

Wanderlei de Moraes[1,2], Thiago A.C. Ferreira[1], André T. Somma[1], Zalmir S. Cubas[2], Bret A. Moore[3] and Fabiano Montiani-Ferreira[1,*]

[1]*Universidade Federal do Paraná (UFPR), Departamento de Medicina Veterinária, Rua dos Funcionários, 1540, 80035-050, Curitiba - PR, Brazil*
[2]*ITAIPU Binacional, Diretoria de Coordenação, Departamento de Áreas Protegidas, Refúgio Biológico Bela Vista, Rua Teresina, 62, Vila C,85870-280, Foz do Iguaçu - PR, Brazil*
[3]*University of California-Davis, School of Veterinary Medicine, Ophthalmology, 1 Garrod Drive, Davis, CA, 95695, USA*

Abstract

Twenty harpy eagles (*Harpia harpyja*) without systemic or ocular diseases were examined to measure blood velocity parameters of the *pectinis oculi* artery using Doppler ultrasonography. Pectinate artery resistive index (RI) and pulsatility index (PI) were investigated using ocular Doppler ultrasonography. The mean RI and PI values across all eyes were 0.44±0.10 and 0.62±0.20 respectively. Low RI and PI values found in the harpy eagle´s *pectinis oculi* artery compared with the American pekin ducks one and other tissue suggest indeed a high metabolic activity in *pecten oculi* and corroborates the hypothesis of a nutritional function and/or intraocular pressure regulation.

Keywords: Avian posterior segment, Pulsatility index, Raptors, Resistive index.

Introduction

The harpy eagle (*Harpia harpyja*) is the largest and most powerful neotropical raptor. They primarily inhabit the Amazon rainforest, but can be found extending from Mexico to South of Brazil (Banhos *et al.*, 2016). They are considered a vulnerable species according to the Brazilian list of endangered fauna (Brazil, 2014) due to deforestation, given their dependency on rainforest habitat, where they builds nests within the canopy and hunts tree-dwelling mammals like sloths (Banhos *et al.*, 2016). As are all eagles, they are primarily visual hunters, with eyes that contain many adaptations for increased visual acuity, including large globes (Güntürkün, 2000; Jones *et al.*, 2007), accommodation by corneal and lenticular measures (Samuelson, 2007), bifoveate retinae (Tucker, 2000), and an anangiotic (avascular) retina (Ruggeri *et al.*, 2010).

As with all avian species, an anangiotic retina leaves the inner retinal layers without a direct blood supply, therefore limiting delivery of nutrients and rapid removal of wastes. However, a vascular structure called the *pecten oculi* is found projecting anteriorly from the optic disc into the vitreous body of all birds (class Aves or clade Avialae) (Brach, 1977; Kern, 2006; Kiama *et al.*, 2006; Rahman *et al.*, 2010; Micali *et al.*, 2012; Mustafa and Ozaydjn, 2013). *Pecten oculi* are pigmented, vascularized, and are traditionally classified into one of three morphologies: 1) conical (e.g. as found in kiwis); 2) vaned (e.g. as found in ostriches, rheas, and tinamous), or 3) pleated (e.g. as found in all the other avian species) (Brach, 1977; Baumel, 1993; Montiani-Ferreira, 2001; Kern, 2006; Kiama *et al.*, 2006; Rahman *et al.*, 2010; Micali *et al.*, 2012; Mustafa and Ozaydjn, 2013).

Other than a structure providing nutritional support for the anangiotic retina (Rodriguez-Peralta, 1975), the *pecten oculi* has been hypothesized to function in intraocular pH and pressure regulation (Brach, 1975), stabilization of the vitreous body (Tucker, 1975), reduction of intraocular glare and maintenance of intraocular pressure (Seaman and Himelfarb, 1963), and in maintenance of the blood ocular barrier for the retina and vitreous body (Barlow and Ostwald, 1972).

Color and pulsed Doppler ultrasonography have been used to further investigate the function of *pecten oculi* by measuring blood velocity parameters (BVPs) such as peak systolic velocity (Vmax), end diastolic velocity (Vmin), pulsatility index (PI), resistive index (RI) and time-averaged maximum frequency (TAmax) (Ferreira *et al.*, 2015). These parameters may assist to evaluate vascular integrity in many organs and tissues (Carvalho and Chammas, 2011; Ferreira *et al.*, 2015). Moreover, it is known that RI and PI values are directly related to the level of metabolism within a particular tissue or organ. When diastolic velocity increases relative to systolic velocity, RI and PI values decrease (Carvalho and Chammas, 2011). High diastolic velocity suggests

***Corresponding Author:** Fabiano Montiani-Ferreira. Universidade Federal do Paraná (UFPR), Departamento de Medicina Veterinária, Rua dos Funcionários, 1540, 80035-050, Curitiba - PR, Brazil. Email: montiani@ufpr.br*

a high metabolic rate due to a demand for continuous blood flow (Carvalho and Chammas, 2011). Consequently, knowledge of BVPs provides information that is suggestive of the metabolic activity of the *pecten oculi* and may offer insight to its function within the eye (Greenfield *et al.*, 1995; Gellat-Nicholson *et al.*, 1999; Carvalho and Chammas, 2011; Ferreira *et al.*, 2015). To the authors' knowledge, only one study applying this concept using Doppler imaging ultrasonography of the *pecten oculi* was previously performed on American pekin ducks (*Anas platyrhynchos domestica*) (Ferreira *et al.*, 2015).

The objective of this investigation was to evaluate the BVPs in the *pectinis oculi* artery of harpy eagles in order to make conjectures about the metabolic activity of the *pecten oculi* and its function. A second objective was to verify these earlier findings and help establish repeatability and validity of using Doppler imaging ultrasonography as a reliable method to assess metabolic activity of ocular tissues.

Materials and Methods

This study was approved by the Federal University of Paraná's Animal Welfare Committee and was conducted according to the ARVO Statement for the Use of Animals in Ophthalmic and Vision Research.

Animals

Twenty harpy eagles, born and raised in captivity, consisting of 13 males and seven females (confirmed by cytogenetics) where evaluated. All of the birds were born and belonged to the ITAIPU BINACIONAL's Biological Sanctuary, located on the border between Brazil and Paraguay, in the State of Paraná, Brazil. The birds had a mean weight of 5.85± 1.2kg, and a mean age of 41.94 months (ranging from 12 to 88 months). Only individuals with no evidence of ocular abnormalities following slit lamp biomicroscope (Hawk Eye; Dioptrix, L'Union, France) and indirect ophthalmoscope (EyeTech; São Paulo, Brazil) evaluation were included in the study. All ophthalmic examinations were performed by the same veterinary ophthalmologist (TF).

Ocular Doppler Ultrasonography

All animals in this study are handled and manually restrained regularly as part of their husbandry and management program. This practice conditions them to handling, thus facilitating veterinary examinations and treatments, and reduces the overall stress of the birds. For all procedures described herein, all animals were physically restrained by experienced and well-trained personnel wearing adequate protective equipment (leather gloves and aprons). All birds were hooded just prior to having measurements taken, with claws closed with adhesive tape and beak closed manually by the examiner.

Blood velocity parameters in the *pecten oculi* were evaluated using an ultrasound system (Logiq 5 GE;

Chicago, United States) coupled with a high-frequency 12 MHz ultrasound transducer in both eyes. After instillation of one drop of a topical analgesic solution (proximetacaine 0.5% - Anestalcon - Alcon do Brasil, São Paulo, Brazil), ultrasonic gel (Carbogel, São Paulo, Brazil) was applied over the corneal surface. The ultrasound transducer was perpendicularly positioned in a horizontal plane, from 4 to 10 o'clock. The long axis of the transducer was placed on top of the corneal surface (transcorneal technique), with the marker pointing nasally and inclined 45°. First the base of the pecten was observed by B-mode ultrasound, near the optic nerve. Doppler settings used were: frequency (5.0 MHz), gain (24.5 dB), pulse repetition frequency (1.4 KHz) and wall filter (89 Hz). The *pectinis oculi* artery was located on the more nasal portion using the power Doppler mode to inspect the blood flow. The formulas to determine the resistive index and pulsatility index for the *pectinis oculi* artery were RI=(Vmax-Vmin)/Vmax and PI=(Vmax-Vmin)/TMAX, respectively (Greenfield *et al.*, 1995; Gellat-Nicholson *et al.*, 1999; Carvalho and Chammas, 2011; Ferreira *et al.*, 2015), where RI= resistance index; Vmax= the maximum, peak systolic velocity of the *pectinis oculi* artery; Vmin= the minimum, end diastolic velocity of the *pectinis oculi* artery; PI= pulsatility index; and; TAMAX= is the time-averaged mean of the maximum velocity. RI values can vary from 0 to 1 (Nelson and Pretorius, 1988; Martinoli *et al.*, 1998; Gellat-Nicholson *et al.*, 1999; Brooks *et al.*, 2007).

Statistical Analysis

Descriptive statistics of blood flow parameters is presented. The normality of the distribution of residuals was tested graphically and confirmed by a p value > 0.05 on the Shapiro-Wilk test. T-tests were performed to compare values obtained on right and left eyes and on males and females. Differences were considered significant when $P<0.05$. Statistical analysis was performed using StatView (StatView, Mountain View, CA).

Results

Doppler ultrasonography was successfully performed in 39/40 eyes (one eye had a severe corneal lesion at the time of the Doppler investigation and was excluded from the study). During ultrasonography the pecten was easily located in the posterior segment of each eye as a hyperechoic structure emerging directly anteriorly from the optic nerve. The *pectinins oculi* artery was identified directly underneath the most nasal portion of the *pecten oculi* and Doppler blood velocity parameters were determined. Ocular Doppler ultrasonography examination allowed images to be obtained of the *pectinis oculi* artery in spectral Doppler mode (Fig. 1A). The artery was located directly underneath the nasal portion of the *pecten* and was clearly identified for all BVP measurements (Fig. 1B).

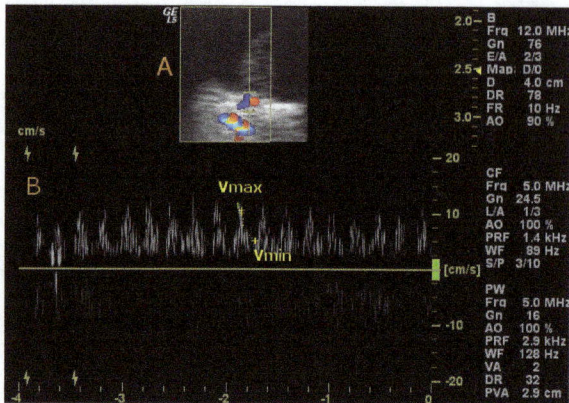

Fig. 1. Spectral (Pulsed) Doppler images. (A): Detection of *pectinis oculi* artery in the most nasal portion of *pecten oculi*; (B): Doppler waves indicated as Vmax (peak systolic velocity) and Vmin (end diastolic velocity).

All blood velocity parameters are described in Table 1. No significant differences between right and left eyes were found, and no significant differences were found between sex and age of the harpy eagles (*P*>0.05).

Table 1. *Pectinis oculi* artery blood velocity parameters of twenty harpy eagles (*Harpia harpyja*).

Both eyes (*n*=39)	Mean	Variance	Std. Dev.	Std. Err
Vmax	15.34	30.457	5.519	0.884
Vmin	2.912	17.87	4.227	0.677
RI	0.44	0.011	0.103	0.017
PI	0.618	0.042	0.204	0.033
TAmax	11.174	23.129	4.809	0.77

Vmax - peak systolic velocity; Vmin - end diastolic velocity; RI - pectinate artery resistive index; PI - pulsatilityindex;TAmax- time-averaged maximum frequency.

Discussion

Investigations of BVPs have been made in many organs and tissues in different species such as cat (Carvalho, 2009; Reis *et al.*, 2014), chicken (Barua *et al.*, 2007), dog (Lamb *et al.*, 1999; Lee *et al.* 2014; Souza *et al.*, 2014), rabbit (Abdallah *et al.*, 2010), crab-eating foxes (Silva *et al.*, 2014) and more recently, in ducks (Ferreira *et al.*, 2015). Assumptions about a tissue's metabolism can be made from its blood supply's Vmax, Vmin, RI and PI parameters (Carvalho and Chammas, 2011). Higher metabolism is signified by lower RI and PI values, whereas low or slower metabolism is signified by higher RI and PI values (Carvalho and Chammas, 2011).

For the purpose of comparison, the anterior ciliary artery and short posterior ciliary artery in dogs have been shown to have RI values of 0.53 and 0.44 respectively, the first supplies blood to the ciliary body whereas the second to the choroid and retina that have higher metabolism than ciliary body (Gellat-Nicholson *et al.*, 1999).

RI values of the long posterior ciliary artery (LPCA) have been demonstrated in the rabbit and the dog as a means to evaluate the importance of the LPCA as a vascular supply to the retina, which is a very highly metabolic tissue (Gellat-Nicholson *et al.*, 1999; Abdallah *et al.*, 2010; Ferreira *et al.*, 2015). The rabbit has been shown to have a very low RI (0.09±0.05) compared to the dog (0.51±0.006), suggesting that the LPCA is of greater importance as a vascular supply to the non-central region of the merangiotic rabbit retina than in the holangiotic retina of dogs (Tokoro, 1972; Bill, 1985; Gellat-Nicholson *et al.*, 1999; Samuelson, 2007; Abdallah *et al.*, 2010; Yang *et al.*, 2011; Ferreira *et al.*, 2015).

A previous study of the RI and PI values of the *pectinis oculi* artery in American pekin ducks showed similar RI and PI values of the short posterior ciliary artery that supplies the ciliary body in the dog (Gellat-Nicholson *et al.*, 1999; Abdallah *et al.*, 2010; Ferreira *et al.*, 2015). The RI and PI values of the *pectinis oculi* artery in harpy eagles found in the present study were also similar. Considering these findings, perhaps there are similarities between the function of the *pecten oculi* and ciliary body, as suggested by the previous theory that the *pecten oculi* could be used for maintenance of IOP through fluid production/excretion into the eye (Seaman and Himelfarb, 1963).

However, another investigation contradicts this theory, as they found several structures that would suggest otherwise: choroidal lacunas within the endothelium, absence of well-delimited basal lamina muscular tunica, innervation and acellular material filling their lumens, and the same characteristic of lymphatic vessels (De Stefano and Mugnaini, 1997). Furthermore, the choroidal lacunae become smaller and less numerous near the optic nerve, *pecten oculi,* and iridotrabecular angle, and therefore are not a part of a Schlemm's canal (De Stefano and Mugnaini, 1997). Several other observations made on the *pecten oculi* also give support to the hypothesis of a secretory function, including 1) extrusion of dye from the pecten accompanying each heart beat during fluorescein angiography (Bellhorn and Bellhorn, 1975), 2) the pecten's high content of carbonic anhydrase and alkaline phosphatase (Bawa and YashRoy, 1972; Amemiya, 1982), 3) evidence that the pecten acts as an agitator to propel perfusate towards the central retina (Pettigrew *et al.*, 1990), and 4) evidence of the pecten having a crucial role in maintaining retinal health (appearance of retinal damage after *pectin oculi* ablation (Wingstrand and Munk, 1965).

In this study, we showed that Doppler imaging is capable of successfully enabling characterization of the main hemodynamic features of the *pectinis oculi* artery in harpy eagles.

Based on the evidence provided here, i.e. high BVP results, as similarly reported in American pekin ducks, we provide indirect evidence for a potential secretory function of the *pecten oculi*. Future studies should also specifically evaluate the *pecten oculi* using other methods of investigation and in other species of birds.

Acknowledgements
The authors thank ITAIPU Binacional for allowing this research and the staff of the Departament of Protected Areas for all of the technical and logistical support provided.

Conflict of Interest
The authors declare that there is no conflict of interest.

References

Abdallah, W., Fawzi, A., Patel, H., Dagliyan, G., Matsuoka, N., Grant, E. and Humayun, M. 2010. Blood velocity measurement in the posterior segment of the rabbit eye using combined spectral Doppler and power Doppler ultrasound. Graefes Arc. Clin. Exp. Ophthalmol. 248(1), 93-101.

Amemiya, T. 1982. Electron histochemical study of alkaline phosphatase activity in the pecten oculi of the Chick. Graefes Arch. Clin. Exp. Ophthalmol. 219(1), 11-14.

Banhos, A., Hrbek, T., Sanaiotti, T.M. and Farias, I.P. 2016. Reduction of Genetic Diversity of the Harpy eagle in Brazilian Tropical Forests. PLoS One. 2016; 11(2), e0148902.

Barlow, H.B. and Ostwald, T.J. 1972. Pecten of the pigeon's eye as an intra-ocular eye shade. Nature 236(64), 88-90.

Barua, A., Abramowicz, J.S., Bahr, J.M., Bitterman, P., Dirks, A., Holub, K.A., Sheiner, E., Bradaric, M.J., Edassery, S.L. and Luborsky, J.L. 2007. Detection of ovarian tumors in chicken by sonography: a step toward early diagnosis in humans? J. Ultrasound Med. 26(7), 909-919.

Baumel, J. 1993. Handbook of Avian Anatomy: NominaAnatomica Avium. 2nd ed. Cambridge, MA: Nuttall Ornithological Club, pp: 179-190.

Bawa, S.R. and YashRoy, R.C. 1972. Effect of dark and light adaptation on the retina and pecten of chicken. Exp. Eye Res. 13(1), 92-97.

Bellhorn, R.W. and Bellhorn, M.S. 1975. The avian pecten. I. Fluorescein permeability. Ophthalmic Res. 7, 1-7.

Bill, A. 1985. Some aspects of the ocular circulation. Invest. Ophthalmol. Vis. Sci. 26, 410-424.

Brach, V. 1975. The effect of intraocular ablation of the pecten oculi of the chicken. Invest. Ophthalmol. Vis. Sci. 14, 166-168.

Brach, V. 1977. The functional significance of the avian pecten: a review. Condor. 79(3), 321-327.

Brazil. 2014. Enviroment Ministry (Ministério do Meio Ambiente) - MMA, Instituto Chico Mendes de Conservação da Biodiversidade - ICMBio. Lista brasileira da fauna ameaçada de extinção. Brasília:MMA/ ICMBio. Available from: http://www.icmbio.gov.br/portal/biodiversidade/fa una-brasileira/lista-de-especies/5607-especie-5607.html. Accessed on: 28 Jun. 2015.

Brooks, D.E., Komaromy, A.M., Kallberg, M.E., Miyabachi, T., Olliver, F.J. and Lambrou, G.N. 2007. Blood flow velocity response of the ophthalmic artery and anterior optic nerve head capillaries to carbogen gas in the rhesus monkey model of optic nerve head ischemia. Vet. Ophthalmol. 10(1), 20-27.

Carvalho, C.F. 2009. Ultrassonografia Doppler em pequenos animais, Eds., Roca. São Paulo, pp: 200-274.

Carvalho, C.F. and Chammas, M.C. 2011. Normal Doppler velocimetry of renal vasculature in Persian cats. J. Feline Med. Surg. 13, 399-404.

De Stefano, M.E. and Mugnaini, E. 1997. Fine structure of the choroidal coat of the avian eye: lymphatic vessels. Invest. Ophthalmol. Vis. Sci. 38, 1241-1260.

Ferreira, T.A., Turner, A.G. and Montiani-Ferreira, F. 2015. Hemodynamics of the pectinis oculi artery in American Pekin Duck (Anas platyrhynchos domestica). Vet. Ophthalmol. 19, 409-413.

Gellat-Nicholson, K.J., Gellat, K.N., MacKay, E., Brooks, D.E. and Newell, S.M. 1999. Doppler imaging of ophthalmic vasculature of the normal dog: blood velocity measurements and reproducibility. Vet. Ophthalmol. 2, 87-96.

Greenfield, D.S., Heggerick, P.A. and Hedges, T.R. 1995. Color Doppler imaging of normal orbital vasculature. Ophthalmol. 102, 1598-1605.

Güntürkün, O. 2000. Sensory physiology: vision. In: Sturkie's Avian Physiology, Eds., Whittow, G.C. New York, NY: Academic Press, pp: 1-19.

Jones, M.P., Pierce, K.E. and Ward, D. 2007. Avian vision: A review of form and function with special consideration to birds of prey. J. Exotic Pet Med. 16, 69-87.

Kern, T.J. 2006. Exotic Animal Ophthalmology. In Veterinary Ophthalmology, Eds., Gelatt, K.K.Gainsville, FL: Blackwell, pp: 1370-1405.

Kiama, S.G., Mainac, J.N., Bhattacharjeed, J., Mwangia, D.K., Macheriae, R.G. and Weyrauch, K.D. 2006. The morphology of the pecten oculi of the ostrich, Struthiocamelus. Ann. Anat. 188(6), 519-528.

Lamb, C.R., Burton, C.A. and Carlis, C.H. 1999. Doppler measurement of hepatic arterial flow in dogs: technique and preliminary findings. Vet. Radiol. Ultrasound 40(2), 77-81.

Lee, S., Park, N., Kim, J. and Eom, K.D. 2014. Doppler ultrasonographic evaluation of renal arterial resistive and pulsatility indices inoverhydrated Beagles. Am. J. Vet. Res. 75, 344-348.

Martinoli, C., Derchi, L.E., Rizzato, G. and Solbiati, L. 1998. Power Doppler sonography: general principles, clinical applications, and future prospects. Eur. Radiol. 8(7), 1224-1235.

Micali, A., Pisani, A., Ventrici, C., Puzzolo, D., Roszkowska, A.M., Spinella, R. and Aragona, P. 2012. Morphological and Morphometric Study of the Pecten Oculi in the budgerigar (Melopsittacusundulatus). Anat. Rec. 295, 540-550.

Montiani-Ferreira, F. 2001. Ophthalmology. In Biology, Medicine and Surgery of South American Wild Animals, Eds., Fowler M. E., Cubas Z. Ames, IA: Iowa State Press, pp: 437-456.

Mustafa, O.D. and Ozaydjn, T.A. 2013. Comparative morphometrical study of the pecten oculi in different avian species. Sci. W. J. Article ID 968652.

Nelson, T.R. and Pretorius, D.H. 1988. The Doppler signal: where does it and what does it mean? Am. J. Roentgenol. 151(3), 439-447.

Pettigrew, J.D., Wallman, J. and Wildsoet, C.F. 1990. Saccadic oscillations facilitate ocular perfusion from the avian pecten. Nature 25, 362-363.

Rahman, M.L., Lee, E., Aoyama, M. and Sugita, S. 2010. Light and electron microscopy study of the pecten oculi of the jungle crow (Corvus macrorhynchos). Okajimas Folia Anat. Jpn. 87, 75-83.

Reis, G.F., Nogueira, R.B., Silva, A.C., Oberlender, G., Muzzi, R.A. and Mantovani, M.M. 2014. Spectral analysis of femoral artery blood flow waveforms of conscious domestic cats. J. Feline Med. Surg. 16(12), 972-978.

Rodriguez-Peralta, L.A. 1975. Hematic and fluids barriers of the retina and vitreous body. J. Comp. Neurol. 132(1), 109-124.

Ruggeri, M., Major, Jr,J.C., McKeown, C., Knighton, R.W., Puliafito, C.A. and Jiao, S. 2010. Retinal Structure of Birds of Prey Revealed by Ultra-High Resolution Spectral-Domain Optical Coherence Tomography. Invest Ophthalmol. Vis. Sci. 51, 5789-5795.

Samuelson, D.A. 2007. Ophthalmic anatomy. In Veterinary Ophthalmology, Eds., Gelatt, K.K. Gainsville, FL: Blackwell, pp: 37-148.

Seaman, A.R. and Himelfarb, T.M. 1963. Correlated ultrafine structural changes of the avian pecten oculi and ciliary body of Gallus domesticus. Am. J. Ophthalmol. 56, 278-296.

Silva, A.S., Feliciano, M.A., Motheo, T.F., Oliveira, J.P., Kawanani, A.E., Werther, K., Palha, M.D. and Vicente, W.R. 2014. Mode B ultrasonography and abdominal Doppler in crab-eating-foxes (Cerdocyonthous). Pesq. Vet. Bras. 34, 23-28.

Souza, M.B., Barbosa, C.C., Pereira, B.S., Monteiro, C.L., Pinto, J.N., Linhares, J.C. and Silva, L.D. 2014. Doppler velocimetric parameters of the testicular artery in healthy dogs. Res. Vet. Sci. 96(3), 533-536.

Tokoro, T. 1972. Relationship between the blood flow velocity in the ciliary body and the intraocular pressure of rabbit eyes. Invest. Ophthalmol. 11(11), 945-954.

Tucker, R. 1975. The surface of the pecten oculi in the pigeon. Cell Tissue Res. 157, 457-465.

Tucker, V.A. 2000. The deep fovea, sideways vision and spiral flight paths in raptors. J. Exp. Biol. 203(24), 3745-3754.

Wingstrand, K.G. and Munk, O. 1965. The pecten oculi of the pigeon with particular regard to its function. Det K. D. Vidensk. Selskab. 14, 5-90.

Yang, Q., Shen, J., Guo, W., Wen, J., Wang, Z. and Yu, D. 2011. Effect of acute intraocular pressure elevation on blood flow velocity and resistance in the rabbit ophthalmic artery. Vet. Ophthalmol. 14(6), 353-357.

21

Laboratory reference intervals for systolic blood pressure, rectal temperature, haematology, biochemistry and venous blood gas and electrolytes in healthy pet rabbits

Miguel Gallego[*]

Centro Veterinario Madrid Exóticos, Madrid, Spain

Abstract

Prospective data from 86 healthy pet rabbits were evaluated to establish reference intervals for hematology, biochemistry, urinalysis, venous blood gas and electrolytes, rectal temperature and systolic blood pressure. Reference intervals for rectal temperature (37.4-39.6 °C) and systolic blood pressure (75-134 mm/Hg) were previously unreported in pet rabbits. Differences by more than 30% with reference intervals present in the bibliography were observed in the blood biochemistry and urinalysis, being attributed to the variability in methodological factors with the present study.

Keywords: Biochemistry, Hematology, Rabbits, Rectal temperature, Systolic blood pressure.

Introduction

In the veterinary literature that covers pet rabbit medicine, many of the laboratory reference values come from studies in laboratory rabbits. These studies are carried out on breeds (mostly on the New Zealand White rabbit) of rabbits that not correspond with the constellation of breeds and mixed-breeds of pet rabbits that come to the daily clinic, samples are obtained by methods that differ from methods employed in the pet clinic practice, and husbandry between laboratory and pet rabbits is far different. It is known that laboratory values in rabbits and other species differ according to the breed, sampling method, stress, immobilizing agents, haemolysis, husbandry, etc (Fox *et al.*, 1970; McLaughlin and Fish, 1994).

According to the sampling method there are several venipuncture collection sites in rabbits that have been used in laboratory animals but many of these sites are not routinely employed in the daily clinic for various reasons. Venipuncture of the jugular vein usually requires sedation and the dewlap may interfere in the extraction. The marginal veins of the ear and the cephalic vein are often good options for inserting an intravenous catheter (the author prefers the marginal veins of the ear because it is more difficult for the rabbit to remove it without an elizabethan collar), but blood extractions are difficult due to the restraint of the animal and to the small vein size, except in large breeds. Although avascular necrosis of the pinna has been described widely in the literature after puncturing the central artery of the ear (Melillo, 2007; Graham and Mader, 2012) it has only been observed by the author on rare occasions and is a good collection site for arterial blood gas analysis in pet rabbits (Ardiaca *et al.*,

2013). Blood extraction from the cranial vena cava and cardiocentesis may be dangerous to the rabbit and requires deep sedation, so the author only recommends this sites for euthanasia or in emergency situations in which the risk / benefit for the animal has been weighed.

In the author's opinion, as well as of other authors (Melillo, 2007; Graham and Mader, 2012), the lateral saphenous vein is the most easily accessible venipuncture site in non-sedated rabbits, allowing to extract a sufficient blood volume for routine blood tests with an adequate restraint of the rabbit.

In some difficult cases, such as animals in critical condition, it would be helpful to warm the area over the vessel to promote vasodilation, facilitating successful venipuncture and collection of blood. In some cases, especially in the case of the central artery of the ear, the author employs a local anesthetic cream[a] prior to the venipuncture (Cooke, 2000) because it prevents a sudden movement of the member at the moment of introducing the needle through the skin.

The importance of this work lies in the scarcity of bibliography concerning laboratory references taken in healthy pet rabbits.

Materials and Methods

Animals

In the first part of the study, prospective data from 86 healthy pet rabbits were employed to establish reference intervals for urinalysis, blood biochemistry, hematology, venous gasometry, rectal temperature and systolic blood pressure (SBP). Rabbits were included in the study when an informed client consent was obtained, the rabbits had undergone an unremarkable full physical examination, the medical history had no

*Corresponding Author: Miguel Gallego. Centro Veterinario Madrid Exóticos, Calle Meléndez Valdés 17, 28015, Madrid, Spain. Email: *miguel.galego@gmail.com*

reportable health problems, and, if there were other complementary tests that did not reveal evident alterations. The study animals consisted of 8 sexually intact females, 31 neutered females, 20 sexually intact males and 27 neutered males. The ages ranged from 5 months to 10 years.

The reference intervals for urinalysis were obtained from 40 rabbits, from 60 for blood biochemistry, from 54 for hematology, from 47 for gasometry and rectal temperature, and from 38 for SBP.

Blood data, rectal temperature and systolic blood pressure collection

Blood samples for hematology and blood biochemistry were obtained from one saphenous vein in awake rabbits employing a little amount of alcohol 70% over the site of venipuncture. Lipemic, hemolyzed or clotted blood samples were discarded. The amount of blood extracted never exceeded 0.5% of the animal weight in grams, expressed in milliliters, i.e. 0.5 ml per 100 g of body weight, which has been considered a safe amount in a healthy rabbit (Cooke, 2000; Melillo, 2007; Wesche, 2014).

For hematology, blood in EDTA tubes was analyzed in a cell counter (MS4 Vet; Melet Schloesing) in less than 30 minutes after extraction. For biochemistry, blood in lithium heparin tubes was centrifuged immediately after extraction and analyzed in less than two hours with an automated analyzer (Chemray 120; Rayto).

For venous gasometry, a sample of at least 70 µl of blood from the other saphenous vein was obtained with a gasometry syringe (1 ml / 25 IU dry balanced heparin; Westmed) and analyzed in a gasometer (ABL80Basic FLEX; Radiometer) immediately. Rectal temperature was measured in all rabbits that undergone a venous gasometry analysis with a digital thermometer (Thermoval rapid flex; Hartmann) as follows; the owner or an operator supported the rabbit standing with its four legs on the exploration table and a second operator inserted the thermometer into the rectum to a distance of approximately 3 cm.

To assess the SBP, the mean value of at least 3 measurements by doppler ultrasonography (Vettex Uni, 8 mhz flat probe; Huntleigh) in the forearm were obtained using a cuff with a width of 40% of the circumference of the limb, located proximally to the elbow, and shaving the palmar zone proximal to the first phalanx to place the probe.

Urinalysis performance

Urine samples were collected by manual expression of the urinary bladder (Fig. 1) on a surface cleaned without quaternary ammonium disinfectants nor chlorhexidine, as the dipstick manufacturer recommends.

Urine samples (n = 43) were centrifuged at 9,800 rpm for 45 seconds (StatSpin® VT, Iris Sample Processing).

In the supernatant, a dipstick (10 Combur UX® test; Roche) was processed with an automatic device (Urisys®; Roche). Urinary sediment was evaluated by light microscopy (40X) without stain it (Fig. 2). Urine samples with active sediment were discarded. Urine sand-like crystals were analyzed by infrared spectroscopy in three sediment samples in which no other crystals were observed, because they could not be classified according to their appearance.

Statistical analysis

Reference intervals with 90% confidence were obtained employing the software Reference Value Advisor (Geffré et al., 2011). The reference intervals obtained were compared with some present in the bibliography. Due to the lack of information concerning the laboratory methods used in many of the evaluations present in the bibliography that were compared with the results obtained in the present study, the comparison between reference values was considered complex; values that differ by more than 30% from the value of the reference interval obtained in the present work were noticed.

Results and Discussion

Values that differ by more than 30% with all the reference intervals evaluated in the bibliography are alkaline phosphatase (ALP), aspartate aminotransferase (AST), gamma-glutamyl transferase (GGT) and glucose.

Urine sand-like crystals were classified as amorphous calcium carbonate (Fig. 2).

Laboratory reference intervals were established in a group of 86 healthy rabbits (Tables 1 and 2). The results of the present study show that differences of more than 30% with reference intervals present in the bibliography were observed only in the blood biochemistry and urinalysis. The disparity between published reference values is well known, therefore it is generally recommended to establish a reference interval for each laboratory (Tvedten and Thomas, 2012).

The reference interval obtained for the glucose value in this work (112-231 mg/dL (6.22-12.82 mmol/L)) is higher than in the literature evaluated. Glucose can increase artifactually in stressful situations in rabbits. The stress that a rabbit undergoes during the trip to the veterinary clinic and by management necessary for the extraction of blood could explain this result and that of lactate dehydrogenase (LDH) value (53-239 IU/L), which is elevated with respect to Wesche (2014). However, other indicators of stress such as total white blood cell count, creatine kinase and AST (McLaughlin and Fish, 1994) did not showed elevations known to be produced by stress in the present work if this values are compared with some published reference intervals (Table 1).

Table 1. Reference interval obtained for hematology (n = 54), biochemistry (n = 60) and systolic blood pressure (n = 38) in healthy rabbits.

BIOCHEMISTRY	Reference interval (90% Confidence)	Varga, 2014	Wesche, 2014	Melillo, 2007
Magnesium mg/dL (mmol/L)	1.9-3.2 (0.95-1.6)	0.8-1.2 (a)	-	-
ALP (IU/L)	42-120	10-70*	-	12-96
ALT (IU/L)	19-68	25-65	27-72	45-80
AST (IU/L)	6-38	10-98*	10-78*	35-130*
CPK (IU/L)	93-473	-	59-175*	140-372
GGT (IU/L)	8-21	0-7*	0-5*	0-7*
LDH (IU/L)	53-239	-	28-102*	-
Bile acids (µmol/L)	26-34	< 40	-	<40
Total bilirubin mg/dL (µmol/L)	0-0.4 (0-6.84)	0.2-0.5 (3.4-8.5)	0.2-1 (2.6-17.1)*	0-0.7 (0-11.97)*
Glucose mg/dL (mmol/L)	112-231 (6.22-12.82)	76-141 (4.2-7.8)*	99-148 (5.5-8.2)*	75-155 (4.16-8.6)*
Total protein g/dL (g/L)	6-7.6 (60-76)	5.4-7.5 (54-75)	4.9-7.1 (49-71)	5.4-7.5 (54-75)
Albumin g/dL (g/L)	3.1-4.3 (31-43)	2.7-5 (27-50)	2.7-5 (27-50)	2.7-5 (27-50)
Globulin (g/L)	2.1-3.7 (21-37)	1.5-2.7 (15-27)	1.5-3.3 (15-33)	1.5-2.7 (15-27)
Cholesterol mg/dL (mmol/L)	6-65 (0.16-1.68)	12-116 (0.3-3)*	4-77 (0.1-2)	10-80 (0.26-2.07)
Triglycerides mg/dL (mmol/L)	22-188 (0.25-2.12)	124-156 (1.4-1.76)	124-156 (1.4-1.76)	-
Amylase (IU/L)	82-343	200-500*	212-424	200-400
Lipase (IU/L)	38-210	-	-	-
HAEMATOLOGY	Reference interval (90% Confidence)	Varga, 2014	Wesche, 2014	Graham and Mader, 2012
Hematocrit (%)	33-46	33-48	30-40	33-55
RBC (x106/ul)	4.6-7.4	4-7	5.1-7.6	5.1-7.9
WBC (x103/ul)	4.1-10.8	5-12	5.2-12.5	5.2-12.5
Haemoglobin (g/dL)	10.1-15.1	10-15	10-15	10-17.4
MCV (fl)	59.5-69.3	60-75	60-69	57.8-66.5
MCHC (g/dL)	29.3-37.9	34.5	30-35	29-37
MCH (pg)	18.5-24.5	19-23	19-22	17.1-23.5
Platelets (x103/ul)	134-567	250-600	250-650	250-650
SBP (mmHg)	75-134	-	-	-

(ALP): alkaline phosphatase; (ALT): alanine aminotransferase; (AST): aspartate aminotransferase; (CPK): creatine phosphokinase; (GGT): gamma-glutamyl transferase; (LDH): lactate dehydrogenase; (MCH): mean corpuscular hemoglobin; (MGHC): mean corpuscular hemoglobin concentration; (MCV): mean corpuscular volume; (RBC): red blood cell count; (WBC): white blood cell count; (SBP): systolic blood pressure. (*) Value that differs by more than 30% from the value of the reference interval obtained in the present work; (a): Cooke, 2000.

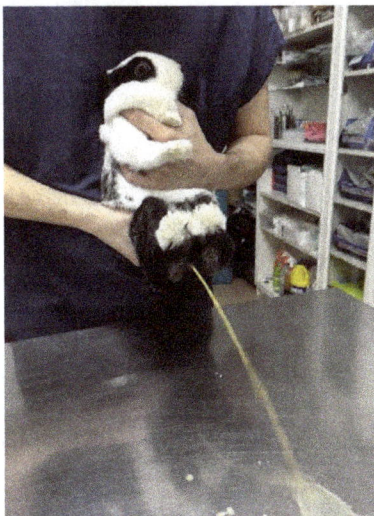

Fig. 1. Urine sample collection from a rabbit by manual expression of the urinary bladder.

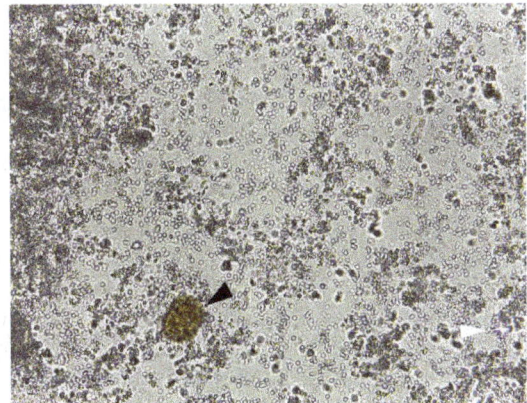

Fig. 2. Normal sediment of the rabbit urine (40X). The sand-like material are amorphous crystals of calcium carbonate (analyzed by infrared spectroscopy). In the urinary sediment of rabbits we can also find a moderate amount of calcium carbonate dihydrate crystals (black arrowhead) and, occasionally, calcium oxalate crystals (white arrowhead).

Table 2. Reference range obtained for urinalysis (n = 43) and acid-base balance (n = 47) in healthy rabbits and comparison with other reference values present in the literature.

URINALYSIS	Reference interval (90% confidence)	Varga, 2014	Wesche, 2014	Melillo, 2007
pH (strip)	8-9	7.6-8.8	7.5-9	7.5-9
USG (strip)	1010-1015	-	-	-
Leucocytes (strip) (uL)	0-25	-	0	-
Nitrites (strip)	neg	-	-	-
Proteins (strip) mg/dL (g//L)	0-30 (0-3)	0-traces*	0-traces*	-
Glucose (strip) mg/dL (mmol/L)	0	0-traces	0-traces	-
Ketones (strip) (mg/dL)	0-15	-	0	0
Urobilinogen (strip) mg/dL (mmol/L)	0-1 (0-1.7)	-	-	-
Bilirubin (strip) mg/dL (mmol/L)	0	-	0	-
Erythrocytes (strip) (uL)	0	-	0	-
Sediment	ACC, CCD, CO	CC, CO, STR	CCM, AnCC, STR	-
GASOMETRY (venous blood)	Reference interval	Ardiaca *et al.*, 2013	Wesche, 2014	Melillo, 2007
pH	7.23-7.56	7.25-7.53	-	-
pCO2 (mmHg)	28.5-50.7	28.9-52.9	-	-
pO2 (mm/Hg)	18-48.3	-	-	-
HCO3- (mmol/L)	15.8-30.2	17-32.5	16-32	-
Base excess (mmol/L)	-8.8-5.7	-10-8	-	-
Anion gap (mmol/L)	8.8-26.4	11-26	-	-
Sodium (mmol/L)	139-149	136-147	130-155	138-150
Potassium (mmol/L)	3.8-6.1	3.4-5.7	3.3-5.7	3.5-6.9
Chloride (mmol/L)	96-113	93-113	92-120	-
Lactate (mmol/L)	2-10 (a)	2.1-15.2 (b)	-	-
Rectal temperature (°C)	37.4-39.6	-	-	-

(ACC): amorphous calcium carbonate; (AnCC): anhydrous calcium carbonate; (CC): calcium carbonate; (CCD): calcium carbonate dihydrate; (CCM): calcium carbonate monohydrate; (CO): calcium oxalate; (HCO3-): bicarbonate; (STR): struvite; (pCO2): partial pressure of carbon dioxide; (pO2): partial pressure of oxygen.
(*): Value that differs by more than 30% from the value of the reference interval obtained in the present work; (a): The upper limit of detection for lactate employing the gasometer ABL80Basic FLEX; Radiometer, is 10 mmol/L; (b): Ardiaca *et al.*, 2016.

In the author's opinion stress may have caused minimal changes in the value of glucose and LDH, but these values can be assumed as normal if the same methodology is employed.

The reference interval obtained for the ALP value in this work (42-120 IU/L) is higher than in the literature evaluated. It is possible that the wide range of ages of the animals included in the study (5 months to 9 years) explains this fact because the ALP value is known to be higher in young rabbits (Melillo, 2007; Varga, 2014; Wesche, 2014) and the results have not been evaluated by ages.

The reference interval obtained for the GGT value in this work (8-21 IU/L) is higher than in the literature evaluated. Elevated GGT in pet rabbits has been associated with hepatic lipidosis, hepatic coccidiosis and could be an indicator of biliary stasis as in other species (Melillo, 2007; Wesche, 2014). In the present work the rabbits were considered healthy for meeting the inclusion criteria and a literature search failed to find causes by which the GGT value can be elevated artefactually in rabbits, so the reference interval obtained for the GGT value in the present work can be considered as valid if the same methodology is used.

The reference interval obtained for the AST value in this work (6-38 IU/L) is lower than in the literature evaluated. A literature search failed to find causes by which the AST value can be artefactually low in rabbits, so the reference interval obtained for the AST value in the present work can be considered as valid if the same methodology is used. A literature search failed to find references for rectal temperature (37.4-39.6 °C) and systolic blood pressure (75-134 mmHg) values in healthy unanesthetized pet rabbits.

Conclusion

Laboratory reference intervals of importance in the daily clinical practice of pet rabbits were reported, including rectal temperature (37.4-39.6 °C) and systolic blood pressure (75-134 mm/Hg), previously unreported in pet rabbits.

Conflict of interest

The authors declare that there is no conflict of interests.

References

Ardiaca, M., Bonvehí, C. and Montesinos, A. 2013. Point-of-Care Blood Gas and Electrolyte Analysis in Rabbits. Vet. Clin. North Am. Exot. Anim. Pract. 16, 175-195.

Ardiaca, M., Dias, S., Montesinos, A., Bonvehi, C., Barrera, S. and Cuesta, M. 2016. Plasmatic l-lactate in pet rabbits: association with morbidity and mortality at 14 days. Vet. Clin. Pathol. 45(1), 116-123.

Cooke, S.W. 2000. Clinical chemistry. In: Manual of rabbit medicine and surgery. 1st edn. Eds P.A. Flecknell. British Small Animal Veterinary Association, Gloucester, pp: 25-32.

Fox, R.R., Laird, C.W., Blau, E.M., Schultz, H.S. and Mitchell, B.P. 1970. Biochemical parameters of clinical significance in rabbits. I. Strain variations. J. Hered. 61, 261-265.

Geffré, A., Concordet, D., Braun, J.P. and Trumel, C. 2011. Reference Value Advisor: a new freeware set of macroinstructions to calculate reference intervals with Microsoft Excel. Vet. Clin. Pathol. 40(1), 107-112.

Graham, J.E. and Mader, D.R. 2012. Basic approach to veterinary care. In: Ferrets, rabbits and rodents. Clinical medicine and surgery. 3rd edn. Eds K.E. Quesenberry and J.W. Carpenter. Elsevier, Missouri, pp: 174-182.

McLaughlin, M.R. and Fish, R.E. 1994. Clinical biochemistry and hematology. Sources of variation. In: The biology of the laboratory rabbit. 2nd edn. Eds P.J. Manning, D.H. Ringler and C.E. Newcomer. Academic Press, San Diego, pp: 112.

Melillo, A. 2007. Rabbit Clinical Pathology. J. Exot. Pet Med. 16, 135-145.

Tvedten, H. and Thomas, J.T. 2012. General laboratory concepts. In: Small animal clinical diagnosis by laboratory methods. 5th ed. Eds M.D. Willard and H. Tvedten. Elsevier Saunders, Missouri, pp: 1-11.

Varga, M. 2014. Clinical pathology. In: Textbook of rabbit medicine. 2nd ed. Eds M. Varga. Butterworth-Heinemann, Edinburg, pp: 111-136.

Wesche, P. 2014. Clinical pathology. In: BSAVA manual of rabbit medicine. 1st edn. Eds Meredith, A. and Lord, B. British Small Animal Veterinary Association, Gloucester, pp: 124-137.

22

Malignant renal schwannoma in a cat

Monier Sharif[1], Adel Mohamed[1,*] and Manfred Reinacher[2]

[1]Department of Pathology and Anatomy, Faculty of Veterinary Medicine, University of Omar Al-Mukhtar, Al-Beida, Libya
[2]Institute for Veterinary Pathology, Justus-Liebig-University, Frankfurter Str. 96, 35392 Giessen, Germany

Abstract

A nine-year-old male European shorthair cat with rapidly enlarging mass at the left kidney doubted to be malignant was presented. The purpose of this study is to present the clinical, radiological and pathological findings of a primary renal tumor in the cat. Grossly, the mass mostly encapsulated the kidney. Histologically, excisional biopsy showed worrying histological features. A sarcoma-like tumor composed mainly of neoplastic spindle-shaped cells. Neoplastic nodules of aggregations of fusiform cells arranged in multidirectional bundles. Immunohistochemically, several immunohistochemical satins (melan-A, S-100, vimentin, actin, desmin, cytokeratin, neurofilament, melan-A, NSE, synaptophysin, chromogranin, Glial Fibrillary Acidic Protein GFAP, Collagen IV and CD99) were used to differentially diagnose the mass. The stained neoplastic sections positively tested to S-100, but negative to the other aforementioned immunohistochemical stains. Immunohistochemistry with S-100 antibody staining showed an unusually strong positive reaction throughout the tumor cells. Based on our comparative diagnosis relative to other tumors, in addition to the progressive clinical signs, histopathological and immunohistochemical results, this case was presumptively diagnosis as a malignant schwannoma. According to our investigation of the relevant literature, this study of malignant renal Schwannoma (malignant peripheral nerve sheath tumor) is a highly rare case not previously characterized in a cat.

Keywords: Cat, Immunohistochemistry, Kidney, Schwannoma, Tumor.

Introduction

There are a few reports of schwannomas in cats: in the oral cavity (Boonsriroj et al., 2014), in the head (Watrous et al., 1999), in the forelimb (Tremblay et al., 2005), and in the eye (Evans et al., 2010). Primary renal tumors are uncommon in domestic animals, so that only 12% of renal tumors are primary, while 88% are secondary. In general, 99% of renal tumors are malignant, 77% of which are epithelial and 23% mesenchymal in origin. Renal tumors of neural origin are extremely rare (Meuten, 2002). According to our survey, only one case of renal tumor from neural origin has been reported in a cat (Jones et al., 1995).

Schwannoma is a tumor that arises from the Schwann's cells that are present among the cell types that form the nerve sheath. Malignant Schwannoma is part of a larger group of rare malignant peripheral nerve sheath tumors (MPNSTs) which are also called soft tissue sarcomas or neurofibrosarcomas (Rapini et al., 2007).

Case details

A 9-year-old male European shorthair male, castrated, cat was referred for clinical investigation. Initial diagnosis showed that the cat suffered from loss of appetite and low water intake with abdominal distension. Radiography and ultrasonography investigations revealed a mass approximately 15 cm in diameter within the left kidney. The cat was admitted for nephrectomy and the excised specimen was submitted for histopathology investigation at the Institute for Veterinary Pathology, Justus-Liebig-University, Giessen, Germany. No information on the cat after performing surgery.

The kidney together with the tumor mass were fixed in neutral buffered 10% formalin solution. A specimen from the tissue was processed, embedded in paraffin, sectioned at 4 μm thickness and stained with Haematoxylin and Eosin (H&E). Other sections were stained with Periodic Acid Schiff Stain (PAS), Azan trichrome stain and Warthin-Starry (WS) stain.

Immunohistochemistry was performed using polyclonal rabbit anti-S-100 antibody (Z0311 DAKO Co.). Anti-S-100 has strong tendency to positively react with most melanocytic tumors, Schwannomas, ependymomas, astrogliomas and glioblastomas, and sometimes with salivary gland tumors (Kawahara et al., 1988). Along with anti-S-100, and for differential diagnosis, the sample was stained with other antibodies for Neurofilaments, Glial fibrillary acidic protein (GFAP), Melan-A, NSE, Synaptophysin, Chromogranin (using the ABC method) and CD99 (monoclonal antibody 12E7 raised against the MIC2 protein).

Corresponding Author: Adel Mohamed. Department of Pathology and Anatomy, Faculty of Veterinary Medicine, University of Omar Al-Mukhtar, Al-Beida, Libya. Email: *adel.mohamed@omu.edu.ly*

The gross examination, of formalin fixed kidney, showed a singular, roughly spherical encapsulated tumor mass in the left kidney. The mass was about 5.5 x 4.5 x 4 cm superficially nodular, greyish-white in color, and greasy in texture. The tumor was detected at one pole of the kidney.

The tumor is well demarcated and distinguished from the normal renal tissue; it encapsulates the outside of the kidney and infiltrates inside the renal pelvis but it does not expand to the renal parenchyma (Fig. 1). The left adrenal gland could not be located. Right kidney was normal. Based on mass location and size, this tumor might be a primary tumor.

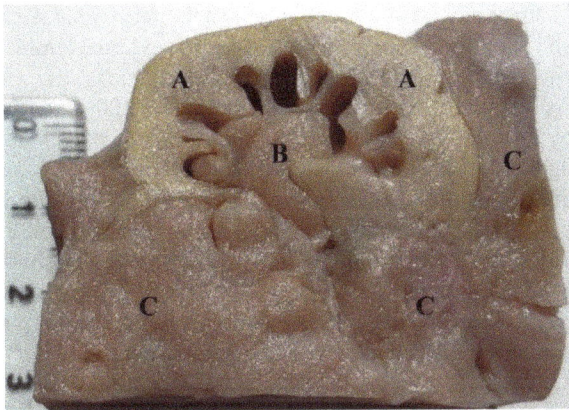

Fig. 1. Growth of tumor mass around and inside the hemisected kidney; tumor mass, in light brownish color, is encapsulating most of the kidney (C), infiltrating inside the pelvis (B) without reaching the yellowish medulla and cortex (A).

Excised specimen was sent for histopathological examination which demonstrates thick capsules with loose tissues in some parts. Most of the neoplastic cells were arranged in dense bundles with increased cellularity like Antoni A areas of a classic schwannoma, and some in loosely arranged streams of cells like Antoni B (Fig .2).

In other parts of the tumor, single-cell groups were distributed as a fibro-vascular stroma which appeared to be mostly myxomatous.

The neoplastic cells appeared spindle-like or oval in shape with indistinct borders. The cytoplasm was eosinophilic with a moderate amount of PAS-positive fine granules. The nuclei, which appeared at the center as oval, elongated or spindle-like in shape, were hyperchromatic and finely stippled. The nucleoli were mostly singular and basophilic. Mitotic activity ranged from 3 to 5 per high power field (HPF). WS stain showed no evidence of external lamina to confirm the diagnosis of Schwannoma. The Azan stain showed a low to moderate amount of collagen fibres between the tumor cells. Renal tissue invasion, necrosis and hemorrhaging were evidence of malignancy.

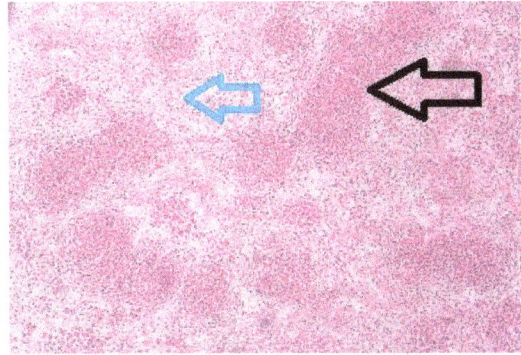

Fig. 2. Hematoxylin and eosin stained kidney tissue section reveals Neoplastic cells arranged in bundles and in streams (100x). The black arrow points at a dense area (Antoni A) and the blue arrow points at a looser area (Antoni B).

There were heterologous elements in form of cartilaginous islets (Fig. 3). Additionally, a mild multifocal lymphocytic interstitial nephritis was noted. Immunostaining showed that all tumor cells were strongly positive for anti-S-100 polyclonal antibodies (Fig. 4) and negative for Melan-A, Vimentin, actin, desmin, cytokeratin, neurofilament, melan-A, NSE, synaptophysin, chromogranin, Glial Fibrillary Acidic Protein GFAP, Collagen IV and CD99.

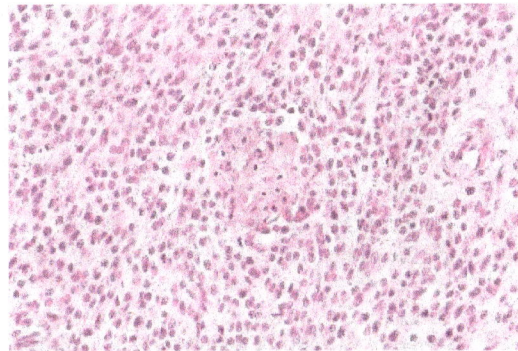

Fig. 3. Hematoxylin and eosin stained kidney tissue section shows spindle and oval Neoplastic cells with cartilaginous islets at the middle (400x).

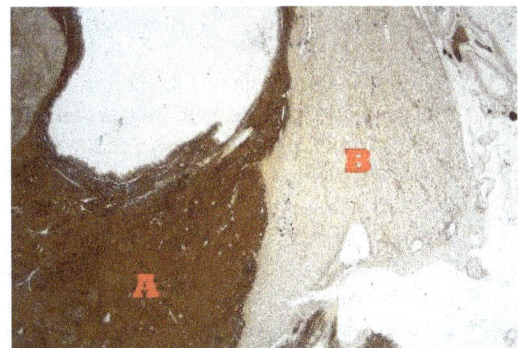

Fig. 4. Immunohistochemistry (IHC) shows tumor cells are diffusely immunoreactive for S-100 antibody (dark brown). (40x). The dark brown area is an indication for a positive reaction for S-100 antibody (A), where (B) indicates the negative reaction.

Discussion

In such cases, morphological appearance might point at carcinoma as the primary suspect. Histological examination as well as immunohistochemistry, however, opposed this indication. Negative reaction with cytokeratin in particular excluded epithelial origin for this tumor. On the other hand, S-100 protein is normally expressed in cells originating from the neural crest (Schwann's cells, and melanocytes), as well as myoepithelial cells, chondrocytes, macrophages, adipocytes, keratinocytes, Langerhans cells, (Wilson *et al.*, 1991; Coppola *et al.*, 1998), dendritic cells, and some breast epithelial cells (Shinzato *et al.*, 1995).

According to the literature, the expression of S-100 proteins varies between tumor types: 100% of Schwannomas and 100% of neurofibromas (with considerably lower stain intensity in neurofibromas than in schwannomas) 70-90% of melanomas and 50% of malignant peripheral nerve sheath tumors, paraganglioma stromal cells, histiocytoma and clear cell sarcomas (Nonaka *et al.*, 2008).

Immunohistochemistry showed negative reaction with antibodies to Melan-A, which is normally expressed by melanocytes. The negative expression of Melan-A excluded melanoma as a candidate and limited the diagnosis to a tumor of neural origin. In using anti-S-100 as an antibody indicator of neural origin, it is important to note that antibodies to S-100 family proteins react with many neural tumors outside the central nervous system, such as:

1- Schwannomas (Sabel and Teepen, 1995; Sarlomo-Rikala *et al.*, 1998).
2- Neurofibroma (Karvonen *et al.*, 2000).
3- Perineurioma: Fletcher (2007) stated that a small minority of perineuriomas show focal S-100 positivity. However, Weidenheim and Campbell (1986), Kleihues and Sobin (2000), Rankine *et al.* (2004) and Boyanton *et al.* (2007) reported that perineuriomas were negative for S-100 proteins.
4- Melanocytic tumors (Gaynor *et al.*, 1981; Orchard, 2000).
5- Adrenal Oncocytic Pheochromocytoma: Fletcher (2007) stated that only sustentacular cells within pheochromocytomas showed positive reaction with antibodies to S-100 proteins. However, Lin *et al.* (1998) and Mearini *et al.* (2012) reported that Pheochromocytomas showed negative reaction with antibodies to S-100 proteins.
6- Liposarcomas (Andrion *et al.*, 1991; McDonald *et al.*, 2011).
7- Synovial sarcomas (Olsen *et al.*, 2006).
8- Chondrosarcomas (rarely, and express cytokeratin) had positive reaction with antibodies to S-100 according to Oakley *et al.*

(2008), but negative reaction according to Swanson *et al.* (1990).
9- Ossifying fibromyxoid tumor of soft parts (Miettinen *et al.*, 2008).

According to the WHO classification of neural origin tumors, Schwannomas diffusely, strongly and uniformly react with antibodies to S-100 protein, vimentin, and GFAP (Koestner, 1999). In this particular case, S-100 staining was strongly and diffusely positive but vimentin and GFAP staining were negative.

Ultrastructure of external lamina usually persists, in an attenuated and interrupted form, adjacent to cells of malignant Schwannomas (Ghadially, 2013). External lamina tends to be absent in Schwannomas (Erlandson and Woodruff, 1982). In this tumor, the external lamina was not clear and contained sporadic remnants.

As a result of the mutual expression of S-100 proteins by a variety of neural tumors to different degrees, and due to the absence of conclusive evidence, differential diagnosis was conducted to investigate and compare potential candidates with Schwannoma mainly based on the expression of S-100 and distinctive histopathological features:

Neurofibromas exhibit less reactivity (40%) with S-100 antibody in comparison with Schwannomas, which react 100% with S-100 antibody. Neurofibromas were categorized into neuro and fibroblastic sub-tumor regions. Neuro components express only 40% of the tissue stained with S-100 antibody whereas the fibroblastic component does not express S-100 and reacts with antibodies to vimentin (Anton *et al.*, 1994). In our study, cells were 100% S-100 positive. Microscopically, neurofibroma cells are elongated and arranged in interlacing bundles. Based on differential histological test and S-100 immune reaction, neurofibroma was a weak candidate for this case study. Perineurioma is an uncommon nerve sheath tumor expressing epithelial membrane antigen (EMA). Therefore, most Perineuriomas stain positively for EMA, Claudin-1, vimentin and collagen (Kleihues and Sobin, 2000) but negatively for S-100 protein and cytokeratin (Giannini *et al.*, 1997; van Roggen *et al.*, 2001). Although some other previously mentioned research studies stated that perineurioma cells do not express S-100 proteins, Fletcher (2007) reported that a small minority of cases may show positive reaction with S-100.

Histologically, perineurioma has been categorized into two types: intraneural and soft tissue perineuroma. Perineurioma cells appear well-differentiated and spindle-like in shape with stretched nuclei and eosinophilic cytoplasm. Perineuriomas are characterized by parallel cell arrangement to form concentric whorls known as onion bulbs (Hornick *et al.*, 2009).

This feature does not appear in the histological examination for this case. Both differences in histological appearance and the controversial reaction with S-100 antibody gave considerable reason for eliminating Perineurioma tumor in this case.

Malignant melanoma was initially a strong suspect due to the positivity of the tumor for S-100. For specificity, we applied immune staining using an antibody to Melan-A, which is a melanoma-specific marker (Smith et al., 2002) for which more than 67% of feline melanomas are cytoplasmatic positive (Ramos-Vara et al., 2002). Our case was negative for expression of Melan-A.

Ossifying fibromyxoid tumor of soft parts (OFMT) is an extremely rare tumor of bone and soft tissue (Graham et al., 2011). Although our survey of the literature showed no previous report of OFMT in domestic animals, previous studies in human revealed different expression levels of S-100 by ossifying fibromyxoid tumor cells: 73% (Graham et al., 2011), 60% (Folpe and Weiss, 2003) and 53% (Gebre-Medhin et al., 2012). These expression levels were considerably lower in comparison with our study, in which the degree of expression of S-100 was unusually high, with almost 100%.

Furthermore, our IHC results showed no expression of desmin which had been reported 38% in (Graham et al., 2011), 13% (Folpe and Weiss, 2003) and 82% in OFMT (Gebre-Medhin et al., 2012).

Histologically, OFMT presents as a multi lobular growth consisting of nests of spherical-to-ovoid cells embedded in fibromyxoid stroma (Gebre-Medhin et al., 2012). It is also characterized by atypical necrosis and mitosis with high cellular activity rates >2 MF/50 HPF (Folpe and Weiss, 2003).

According to the known histological features of OFMT and the IHC results (S-100 and desmin) obtained in this study, OFMT was likely not the correct tumor in this case. However, theoretically, OFMT could not be completely excluded from the comparison with Schwann's cell tumors.

Adrenal oncocytic pheochromocytoma positively expresses chromogranin, synaptophysin, neuron-specific enolase, neurofilament, serotonin, bombesin, ACTH, vimentin, desmin, S-100 protein, and cytokeratins including AE1/3, CAM 5.2, cytokeratin 7, and cytokeratin 20. (Li and Wenig, 2000). Gross appearance examination of our case showed that the tumor originated from the kidney pelvis whereas Pheochromocytoma originates from the medulla of the adrenal gland. In addition, according to our observations, Oncocytic pheochromocytoma usually stains with yellow in formalin fixation. This phenomenon was not observed in our case.

Liposarcomas express S-100 in fat cells and lipoblasts. PAS positive elements might be seen as well in some adipocytes and lipoblasts, which positively react with anti-vimentin but vary in intensity and might not react in poorly differentiated lesions due to lack of expression. Transition from low to high grade non-lipogenic morphology can occur within a well-differentiated liposarcoma. Heterologous elements occur in 5-10% of cases with myogenic, osteo/chondrosarcomatous, or rarely angiosarcomatous elements. Myxoid liposarcoma (Van Roggen and Fletcher, 1999) and spindle cell liposarcoma (Dei Tos et al., 1994) were both reported as S-100 positive. In our case, no adipose cell differentiation was observed, and the diagnosis of liposarcoma can be easily excluded based on the histological appearance.

Diagnosis of schwannomas is based on presence of some features, including: (1) Antoni Type A or B histologic feature (Cordy, 1978). (2) Round cells with few cytoplasmic components, enclosed by a basal lamina (Erlandson and Woodruff, 1982). (3) Positive immunohistochemical staining to S-100 of neuronal origin (Wechsler et al., 1973; Vinores et al., 1984).

Generally, discrimination between benign and malignant schwannoma is sometimes challenging; since both kinds have comparable morphological features (Boonsriroj et al., 2014). Malignant schwannoma is usually densely packed arranged in patterns with high mitotic range (Pumarola et al., 1996). Whereas, benign schwannoma usually is small in size, grows superficially with low mitotic activities (Kindblom et al., 1998).

Although positive immunoreactivity for S-100 is an indication of benign and most malignant Schwannomas (Matsunou et al., 1985), cells in this tumor showed malignant characteristics in histological examination, e.g. Antoni A and B patterns and neoplastic cells with different sizes and shapes.

Conclusion

From these comparisons, which were conducted based on the strong expression of S-100 and from the exclusion of the aforementioned tumors, the findings of our investigation matched malignant schwannoma as the most likely diagnosis in this case. Unlike these malignant tumors, cellular schwannoma reveals a strong and diffuse reactivity for S-100. Figure 2 clearly shows two different groups of cells (Antoni patterns A and B); a looser area with low density of cells and interwoven dense cells with clear myxoid changes. Antoni patterns, in this case, may be a good indicator for malignant schwannoma versus benign schwannoma.

In addition, and in comparison with similar studies (Mandrioli et al., 2005; Cho et al., 2006; Boonsriroj et al., 2014; Duke et al., 2015), histomorphological and immunohistochemical means helped in reaching that malignant schwannoma is the final diagnosis in our case.

Conflict of interest
The authors declare that there is no conflict of interests.

References

Andrion, A., Gaglio, A., Dogliani, N., Bosco, E. and Mazzucco, G. 1991. Liposarcoma of the thyroid gland. Fine-needle aspiration cytology, immunohistology, and ultrastructure. Am. J. Clin. Pathol. 95(5), 675-679.

Anton, E.S., Weskamp, G., Reichardt, L.F. and Matthew, W.D. 1994. Nerve growth factor and its low-affinity receptor promote Schwann cell migration. Nat. Acad. Sci. 91(7), 2795-2799.

Boonsriroj, H., Kimitsuki, K., Akagi, T. and Chun-Ho, P.A.R.K. 2014. Malignant epithelioid schwannoma of the oral cavity in a cat. J. Vet. Med. Sci. 76(6), 927-930.

Boyanton Jr, B.L., Jones, J.K., Shenaq, S.M., Hicks, M.J. and Bhattacharjee, M.B. 2007. Intraneural perineurioma: a systematic review with illustrative cases. Arch. Pathol. Lab. Med. 131(9), 1382-1392.

Cho, H.S., Kim, Y.S., Choi, C., Lee, J.H., Masangkay, J.S. and Park, N.Y. 2006. Malignant schwannoma in an American buffalo (Bison bison bison). J. Vet. Med. A. Physiol. Pathol. Clin. Med. 53(8), 432-434.

Coppola, D., Fu, L., Nicosia, S.V., Kounelis, S. and Jones, M. 1998. Prognostic significance of p53, bcl-2, vimentin, and S 100 protein-positive langerhans cells in endometrial carcinoma. Hum. Pathol. 29(5), 455-462.

Cordy, D.R. 1978. Nervous system and eye. Tumors in Domestic Animals. Moulton, J.C. Ed. 2nd ed., University of California Press, Berkeley, pp: 654-660.

Dei Tos, A.P., Mentzel, T., Newman, P.L. and Fletcher, C.D. 1994. Spindle Cell Liposarcoma, A Hitherto Unrecognized Variant of Liposarcoma Analysis of Six Cases. Am. J. Surg. Pathol. 18(9), 913-921.

Duke, F.D., Teixeira, L.B.C., Galle, L.E., Green, N. and Dubielzig, R.R. 2015. Malignant uveal schwannoma with peripheral nerve extension in a 12-week-old color-dilute Labrador Retriever. Vet. Pthol. 52(1), 181-185.

Erlandson, R.A. and Woodruff, J.M. 1982. Peripheral nerve sheath tumors: an electron microscopic study of 43 cases. Cancer 49(2), 273-287.

Evans, P.M., Lynch, G.L. and Dubielzig, R.R. 2010. Anterior uveal spindle cell tumor in a cat. Vet. Ophthalmol. 13(6), 387-390.

Fletcher, C.D. 2007. Diagnostic Histopathology of Tumors, 3rd ed. 1883 pp. in 2 volumes with 2 CD-ROMs. Churchill Livingstone Elsevier Limited, Philadelphia, PA, USA.

Folpe, A.L. and Weiss, S.W. 2003. Ossifying fibromyxoid tumor of soft parts: a clinicopathologic study of 70 cases with emphasis on atypical and malignant variants. Am. J. Sur. Pathol. 27, 421-431.

Gaynor, R., Irie, R., Morton, D., Herschman, H., Jones, P. and Cochran, A. 1981. S100 protein: a marker for human malignant melanomas? Lancet, 1(8225), 869-871.

Gebre-Medhin, S., Nord, K.H., Möller, E., Mandahl, N., Magnusson, L., Nilsson, J., Jo, V.Y., von Steyern, F.V., Brosjö, O., Larsson, O. and Domanski, H.A. 2012. Recurrent rearrangement of the PHF1 gene in ossifying fibromyxoid tumors. Am. J. Pathol. 181(3), 1069-1077.

Ghadially, F.N. 2013. Ultrastructural pathology of the cell and matrix: a text and atlas of physiological and pathological alterations in the fine structure of cellular and extracellular components. 3rd Ed. Butterworth-Heinemann.

Giannini, C., Scheithauer, B.W., Jenkins, R.B., Erlandson, R.A., Perry, A., Borell, T.J., Hoda, R.S. and Woodruff, J.M. 1997. Soft-tissue perineurioma: evidence for an abnormality of chromosome 22, criteria for diagnosis, and review of the literature. Am. J. Surg. Pathol. 21(2), 164-173.

Graham, R.P., Dry, S., Li, X., Binder, S., Bahrami, A., Raimondi, S.C., Dogan, A., Chakraborty, S., Souchek, J.J. and Folpe, A.L. 2011. Ossifying fibromyxoid tumor of soft parts: a clinicopathologic, proteomic and genomic study. Am. J. Surg. Pathol. 35(11), 1615-1625.

Hornick, J.L., Bundock, E.A. and Fletcher, C.D. 2009. Hybrid schwannoma/perineurioma: clinicopathologic analysis of 42 distinctive benign nerve sheath tumors. Am. J. Surg. Pathol. 33(10), 1554-1561.

Jones, B.R., Alley, M.R., Johnstone, A.C., Jones, J.M., Cahill, J.I. and McPherson, C. 1995. Nerve sheath tumours in the dog and cat. N. Z. Vet. J. 43(5), 190-196.

Karvonen, S.L., Kallioinen, M., Ylä-Outinen, H., Pöyhönen, M., Oikarinen, A. and Peltonen, J. 2000. Occult neurofibroma and increased S100 protein in the skin of patients with neurofibromatosis type 1: new insight to the etiopathomechanism of neurofibromas. Arch. Dermatol. 136(10), 1207-1209.

Kawahara, E., Oda, Y., Ooi, A., Katsuda, S., Nakanishi, I. and Umeda, S. 1988. Expression of Glial Fibrillary Acidic Protein (GFAP) in Peripheral Nerve Sheath Tumors: A Comparative Study of Immunoreactivity of GFAP, Vimentin, S-100 Protein, and Neurofilament in 38 Schwannomas and 18 Neurofibromas. Am. J. Surg. Pathol. 12(2), 115-120.

Kindblom, L. G., Meis-Kindblom, J. M., Havel, G. and Busch, C. 1998. Benign epithelioid schwannoma. Am. J. Surg. Pathol. 22, 762-770.

Kleihues, P. and Sobin, L.H. 2000. World Health Organization classification of tumors. Cancer 88(12), 2887.

Koestner, A. 1999. Histological classification of tumors of the nervous system of domestic animals. Armed Forces Institute of Pathology: American Registry of Pathology: World Health Organization Collaborating Center for Comparative Oncology.

Li, M. and Wenig, B.M. 2000. Adrenal oncocytic pheochromocytoma. Am. J. Surg. Pathol. 24(11), 1552-1557.

Lin, B.T.Y., Bonsib, S.M., Mierau, G.W., Weiss, L.M. and Medeiros, L.J. 1998. Oncocytic adrenocortical neoplasms: a report of seven cases and review of the literature. Am. J. Surg. Pathol. 22(5), 603-614.

Mandrioli, L., Gentile, A., Morini, M., Bettini, G. and Marcato, P.S. 2005. Malignant, solitary, nasopharyngeal schwannoma in a cow. Vet. Rec. 156(17), 552-553.

Matsunou, H., Shimoda, T., Kakimoto, S., Yamashita, H., Ishikawa, E. and Mukai, M. 1985. Histopathologic and immunohistochemical study of malignant tumors of peripheral nerve sheath (malignant Schwannoma). Cancer 56(9), 2269-2279.

McDonald, A.G., Dal Cin, P., Ganguly, A., Campbell, S., Imai, Y., Rosenberg, A.E. and Oliva, E. 2011. Liposarcoma arising in uterine lipoleiomyoma: a report of 3 cases and review of the literature. Am. J. Surg. Pathol. 35(2), 221-227.

Mearini, L., Del Sordo, R., Costantini, E., Nunzi, E. and Porena, M. 2012. Adrenal oncocytic neoplasm: a systematic review. Urol. Intern. 91(2), pp.125-133.

Meuten, D.J. 2002. Tumors of the urinary system. Tumors in Domestic Animals, 4th Edition, pp: 509-546.

Miettinen, M., Finnell, V. and Fetsch, J.F. 2008. Ossifying fibromyxoid tumor of soft part--a clinicopathologic and immunohistochemical study of 104 cases with long-term follow-up and a critical review of the literature. Am. J. Surg. Pathol. 32(7), 996-1005.

Nonaka, D., Chiriboga, L. and Rubin, B.P. 2008. Differential expression of S100 protein subtypes in malignant melanoma, and benign and malignant peripheral nerve sheath tumors. J. Cutan. Pathol. 35(11), 1014-1019.

Oakley, G.J., Fuhrer, K. and Seethala, R.R. 2008. Brachyury, SOX-9, and podoplanin, new markers in the skull base chordoma vs chondrosarcoma differential: a tissue microarray-based comparative analysis. Mod. Pathol. 21(12), 1461-1469.

Olsen, S.H., Thomas, D.G. and Lucas, D.R. 2006. Cluster analysis of immunohistochemical profiles in synovial sarcoma, malignant peripheral nerve sheath tumor, and Ewing sarcoma. Mod. Pathol. 19(5), 659-668.

Orchard, G.E. 2000. Comparison of immunohistochemical labelling of melanocyte differentiation antibodies melan-A, tyrosinase and HMB 45 with NKIC3 and S100 protein in the evaluation of benign naevi and malignant melanoma. Histochem. J. 32(8), 475-481.

Pumarola, M., Anor, S., Borras, D. and Ferrer, I. 1996. Malignant epithelioid schwannoma affecting the trigeminal nerve of a dog. Vet. Pathol. 33, 434-436.

Ramos-Vara, J.A., Miller, M.A., Johnson, G.C., Turnquist, S.E., Kreeger, J.M. and Watson, G.L. 2002. Melan A and S100 protein immunohistochemistry in feline melanomas: 48 cases. Vet. Pathol. 39(1), 127-132.

Rankine, A.J., Filion, P.R., Platten, M.A. and Spagnolo, D.V. 2004. Perineurioma: a clinicopathological study of eight cases. Pathology 36(4), 309-315.

Rapini, R.P., Bolognia, J.L. and Jorizzo, J.L. 2007. Dermatology: 2-Volume Set. St. Louis: Mosby.

Sabel, L.H.W. and Teepen, J.L.J.M. 1995. The enigmatic origin of olfactory schwannoma. Clin. Neurol. Neurosurg. 97(2), 187-191.

Sarlomo-Rikala, M., Lahtinen, T., Andersson, L.C., Mieltinen, M. and Knuutila, S. 1998. Different patterns of DNA copy number changes in gastrointestinal stromal tumors, lelomyomas, and schwannomas. Hum. Pathol. 29(5), 476-481.

Shinzato, M., Shamoto, M., Hosokawa, S., Kaneko, C., Osada, A., Shimizu, M. and Yoshida, A. 1995. Differentiation of Langerhans cells from interdigitating cells using CD1a and S-100 protein antibodies. Biotech. Histochem. 70(3), 114-118.

Smith, S.H., Goldschmidt, M.H. and McManus, P.M. 2002. A comparative review of melanocytic neoplasms. Vet. Pathol. 39(6), 651-678.

Swanson, P.E., Lillemoe, T.J., Manivel, J.C. and Wick, M.R. 1990. Mesenchymal chondrosarcoma. An immunohistochemical study. Arch. Pathol. Lab. Med. 114(9), 943-948.

Tremblay, N., Lanevschi, A., Doré, M., Lanthier, I. and Desnoyers, M. 2005. Of all the nerve! A subcutaneous forelimb mass on a cat. Vet. Clin. Pathol. 34(4), 417-420.

Van Roggen, G. and Fletcher, M. 1999. Myxoid tumours of soft tissue. Histopathol. 35(4), 291-312.

Van Roggen, J.F.G., McMenamin, M.E., Belchis, D.A., Nielsen, G.P., Rosenberg, A.E. and Fletcher, C.D. 2001. Reticular perineurioma: a distinctive variant of soft tissue perineurioma. Am. J. Surg. Pathol. 25(4), 485-493.

Vinores, S.A., Bonnin, J.M., Rubinstein, L.J. and Marangos, P.J. 1984. Immunohistochemical demonstration of neuron-specific enolase in neoplasms of the CNS and other tissues. Arch. Pathol. Lab. Med. 108(7), 536-540.

Watrous, B.J., Lipscomb, T.P., Heidel, J.R. and Normal, L.M. 1999. Malignant peripheral nerve sheath tumor in a cat. Vet. Radiol. Ultrsound 40(6), 638-640.

Wechsler, W., Pfeiffer, S.E., Swenberg, J.A. and Koestner, A. 1973. S-100 protein in methyl-and ethylnitrosourea induced tumors of the rat nervous system. Acta Neuropathol. 24(4), 287-303.

Weidenheim, K.M. and Campbell, Jr, W.G. 1986. Perineurial cell tumor. Virchows Arch. A. Pathol. Anat. Histopathol. 408(4), 375-383.

Wilson, A.J., Maddox, P.H. and Jenkins, D. 1991. CD1a and S100 antigen expression in skin Langerhans cells in patients with breast cancer. J. Pathol. 163(1), 25-30.

23

Cystolithiasis in a Syrian hamster: a different outcome

D. Petrini[1], M. Di Giuseppe[2,]*, G. Deli[3] and C. De Caro Carella[4]

[1]*Freelance Veterinarian, Pisa, Italy*
[2]*Centro Veterinario per Animali Esotici, Viale Regione Siciliana Sud – Est 422-426, 90129 Palermo, Italy*
[3]*Freelance Veterinarian, Roma, Italy*
[4]*School of Veterinary Medicine, Louisiana State University, USA*

Abstract

A 14-month-old intact male Syrian hamster was admitted for lethargy and hematuria. A total body radiographic image and abdominal ultrasonography showed the presence of a vesical calculus. During cystotomy, a sterile urine sample was obtained and sent to the diagnostic laboratory along with the urolith for analysis. Urine culture was found negative for bacterial growth, and the urolith was identified as a calcium-oxalate stone. Diet supplementation with palmitoylethanolamide, glucosamine and hesperidin was adopted the day after discharge. One year follow up revealed no presence of vesical calculi. Although this is the report of a single clinical case, this outcome differs from the results reported in the literature characterized by recurrences after few months. Considering the positive outcome and the beneficial properties of palmitoylethanolamide, glucosamine, and hesperidin, these nutritional elements in Syrian hamsters, are recommended to reduce recurrence after surgical treatment of urolithiasis.

Keywords: Glucosamine, Hamster, Hesperidin, PEA, Urolithiasis.

Introduction

Urolithiasis is a common disease in hamsters and it is associated with a high incidence of short -term recurrence after surgical treatment. The etiology of this pathology remains unknown, although dry food diet has been suggested as a possible predisposing factor. This case report describes diagnostic and surgical approaches, as well as dietary management, and successful long-term management of urolithiasis in a Syrian hamster.

Case details

A 14-month old intact male Syrian hamster was admitted for signs of lethargy and hematuria. The subject was housed in a 60x30 cm clear plastic cage lacking a cover. Specific recycled paper litter was used in the cage as substrate. Diet was constituted of a mix of several seeds, daily fresh greens, and fruits. Canine dry food in appropriate amounts was integrated once a week in order to increase protein intake. No sunflower seeds were included in the described diet.

During clinical examination, urine scald in the perineal area and weight loss were detected (-18.6% reduction of body weight since the last annual health check, occurred six months prior to presentation). Anesthesia of the subject was induced with isoflurane (Isoflo®, Esteve, Spain) (5%) in oxygen, delivered at 2 L/min into an induction chamber and maintained via face mask with isoflurane (2%) in oxygen (0.5 L/min) to allow diagnostic procedures. A ventro-dorsal and a latero-lateral radiographic projection showed the presence of a radio-opaque area in the caudal abdomen, compatible with the diagnosis of urolithiasis (Fig. 1). Abdominal ultrasonography showed an irregular, hyper-echoic urolith (3x3 mm) producing a black acoustic shadow inside the empty bladder (Fig. 2). Neither hydro-nephrosis nor hydro-ureter were detected during the study.

Since the size of the urolith would not allow its passage through the urethra, surgical removal via cystotomy was elected right away. The subject was sedated with midazolam (Midazolam®, Bioindustria L.I.M, Italy) 0.3 mg/kg, and buprenorphine (Buprenodale®, Dechra, Spain) 0.06 mg/kg. Anesthesia was induced and maintained with isoflurane (Isoflo®, Esteve, Spain) delivered in oxygen, via customized face mask. After aseptic preparation of the surgical site, laparotomy was approached via ventral midline using a #11 surgical blade. Once the bladder was exposed, it was isolated with gauze moistened with warm sterile saline (Fig. 3). Sterile cotton swabs were used to manipulate soft tissues during surgery to avoid damage with standard-sized surgical instruments. Incision of the bladder was made at the ventral aspect, close to the apex to avoid damage of the ureters. After removal of the stone, the bladder was irrigated with warm sterile saline and sutured using a single layer of continuous inverted suture pattern with a 6/0 poliglecaprone (Monocryl®, Ethicon, USA) as previously described1,2,3 Abdominal wall and skin were sutured with 4/0 poliglecaprone (Monocryl®, Ethicon, USA), using a continuos pattern suture. A sterile urine sample, as well as the urolith (Fig. 4), were submitted to a diagnostic laboratory for

*****Corresponding Author:** Marco Di Giuseppe. Centro Veterinario per Animali Esotici, Viale Regione Siciliana Sud-Est 422-426, 90129 Palermo, Italy. E-mail: *marcodigiuseppe@yahoo.com*

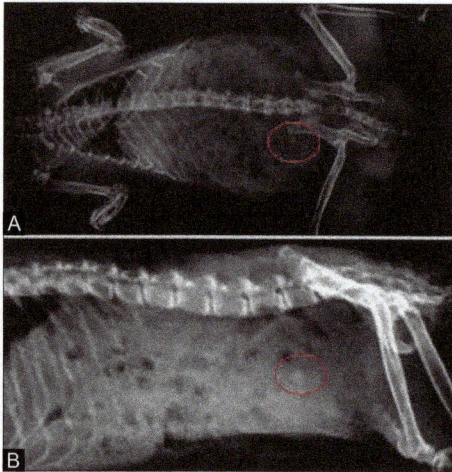

Fig. 1. Radiographic ventro-dorsal (A) and radiographic latero-lateral (B) projections of a 14 months old intact male Syrian hamster under general anesthesia showing a radio-opaque urolith (red circle).

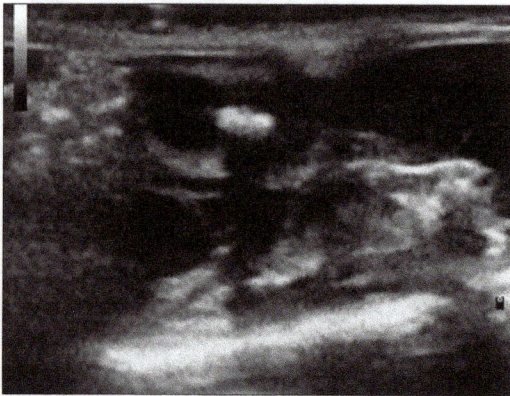

Fig. 2. Abdominal ultrasonographic image showing the empty bladder with a 3x3 mm hyper-echoic urolith, producing a black acoustic shadow.

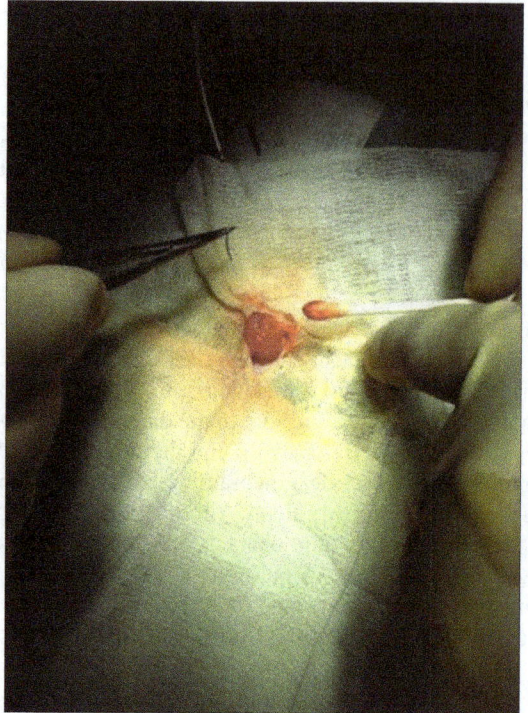

Fig. 3. Surgical view of the cystotomy. The Syrian hamster was positioned in dorsal recumbency, and the bladder was isolated with moistened gauzes.

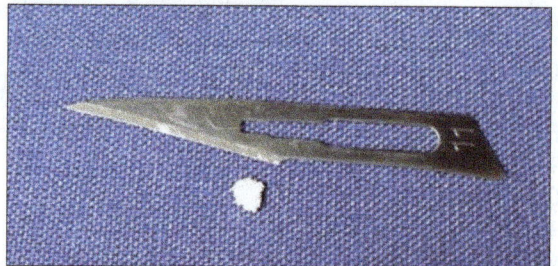

Fig. 4. Particular of the urolith in relationship to a #11 surgical blade.

culture and sensitivity, and composition of the stone. The animal recovered uneventfully from anesthesia and surgery, and spontaneous urination began within a few minutes after complete recovery. On the same day, it was discharged with meloxicam (Metacam®, Boehringer Ingelheim, Germany) 0.2 mg/kg to be administered orally every twelve hours) and tramadol (Altadol®, Formevet, Italy) 5 mg/kg to be administered orally every twelve hours for five days for pain management, as well as with enrofloxacin (Baytril®, Bayer, Germany) 10 mg/kg to be administered orally every twenty-four hours. Lactated Ringer's solution was administered subcutaneously once per day at a dose of 57 ml/kg/day for five days. Urine culture was negative for bacterial growth, and urolith was identified as composed by calcium oxalate and ammonium.

After proper informed consent was obtained from the owner, a diet supplement for canine and feline species containing palmitoylethanolamide (PEA), glucosamine and hesperidin was added to the animal's regular diet. These three active ingredients are present in one single veterinary capsule, commercially available in Italy (Urys®, Innovet, Italy). The manufacturer's recommendation is to administer the liquid contained in one capsule for every ten kilograms of body weight for dogs and cats, and the indications for this product include preservation of the physiologic protective mechanisms of the urinary tract, protection from inflammation and oxidative damage, as well as preserving normal mucosal function. The content of one capsule was aspirated with a disposable 1 ml syringe, and one drop (about 0.025 ml) was given once a day orally to the animal, after the needle was removed from the syringe. The administered dose is equivalent to 3.75 mg of PEA, 5 mg of glucosamine, and 3 mg of hesperidin per day equivalent approximately to 107 mg/kg of PEA, 143 mg/kg of glucosamine and 85.7 of hesperidin.

The animal was admitted to the hospital a year later for follow up. Physical examination and radiographic studies were repeated. No evidence of reoccurrence of urolithiasis was found, which was consistent with clinical signs and history of the past year.

Discussion

Available literature reports only two previous cases of cystoliths in hamster and in both cases recurrences were reported within a few months post-surgery (Bauck and Hagan, 1984; Lidderdale and St Pierre, 1990). To the authors' best knowledge, this is the only clinical case report with no recurrence was observed in a long-term follow up (Bauck and Hagan, 1984; Lidderdale and St Pierre, 1990; Johnson-Delaney, 1998; Capello, 2011a). In both cases reported in literature, the diagnosis was achieved by radiography showing a radiolucent cystolith and animals were both intact males showing hematuria, dysuria and incontinence (Bauck and Hagan, 1984; Lidderdale and St Pierre, 1990). Only in one of the two cases described the nature of the urolith was determined showing: magnesium, calcium and phosphate (Bauck and Hagan, 1984).

Normal urinary pH of rodents is basic therefore, uroliths composed by calcium and phosphate would be expected (Wagner and Mohebbi, 2010). For this reason in one case reported, acidification of urine with ammonium chloride administration was used to dissolve uroliths but no positive results were observed (Bauck and Hagan, 1984).

Although it is not demonstrated in hamster, interactions among dietary calcium, magnesium and phosphorus seem to affect the incidence, severity and type of uroliths in rats (Chow et al., 1980).

The etiology of urolithiasis in Syrian hamsters is still unknown but dry food diet has been suggested as a possible predisposing factor (Capello, 2011b).

Palmitoylethanolamide is an endogenous fatty acid amide, exerting biological effects on chronic pain and inflammation, used to control hyper-reactivity of the urinary tract. Since its discovery, PEA has been considered to negatively modulate the inflammatory process. Its effects have been extensively investigated in vitro, in vivo, and in clinical studies. Notwithstanding some discrepancy, nowadays the efficacy of PEA in modulating mast cells, which may likely account for its anti-inflammatory, anti-angiogenic and analgesic properties, is well recognized (De Filippis et al., 2013). In fact, it has been demonstrated that PEA significantly attenuates the degree of renal dysfunction, injury, and inflammation caused by ischemia-reperfusion injury in mice, that lowers arterial blood pressure, and can protect against hypertensive renal injury by increasing

the antioxidant defense and anti-inflammatory response (Di Paola et al., 2012). It also has been shown that PEA can modulate the renin-angiotensin system in rats (Mattace Raso et al., 2013). Glucosamine is an amino sugar and a prominent precursor in the synthesis of glycosylated proteins and lipids that plays an important role in the protection of the urothelium. Its efficacy in the treatment of feline idiopathic cystitis has been demonstrated (Farquhar-Smith and Rice, 2001; Panchaphanpong et al., 2011). Furthermore, it has been shown to attenuate referred hyperalgesia in a dose-dependent fashion (Farquhar-Smith and Rice, 2001). The importance of glucosamine in this specific case is also supported by its presence in a specific nutritional support made for urinary tract health of hamsters (Natural Science Urinary Support Oxbow®). Unfortunately, the aforementioned product was not available on the Italian market when the reported clinical case was presented. The dose suggested by the manufacturer for one hamster is around 5 mg of glucosamine per day. The same dose of glucosamine was administered to the subject of this case report. Hesperidin is a flavanone glycoside found in citrus fruits that has chemopreventive effects. It effectively inhibits chemical carcinogenesis of the bladder in mice, and it has been suggested that such inhibition might be partly related to suppression of cell proliferation (Yang et al., 1997).

Although this is the report of a single clinical case, this outcome differs from the results reported in the available literature. Considering the positive outcome, and the beneficial properties of dietary supplementation with palmitoylethanolamide, glucosamine and hesperidin, the authors encourage the use of these nutritional elements in Syrian hamsters to reduce recurrence after surgical treatment of urolithiasis.

References

Bauck, L.A. and Hagan, R.J. 1984. Cystotomy for treatment of urolithiasis in a hamster. J. Am. Vet. Med. Assoc. 184, 99-100.

Capello, V. 2011a. Common Surgical Procedures in Pet Rodents. J. Exotic Pet Med. 20, 294-307.

Capello, V. 2011b. Pet hamster medicine and surgery, part III: infectious, parasitic and metabolic diseases. Exotic DVM 3, 27-32.

Chow, F.H., Taton, G.F., Boulay, J.P., Lewis, L.D., Remmenga, E.E. and Hamar, D.W. 1980. Effect of dietary calcium, magnesium, and phosphorus on phosphate urolithiasis in rats. Invest. Urol. 17: 273-276.

De Filippis, D., Negro. L., Vaia, M., Cinelli, M.P. and Iuvone, T. 2013. New insights in mast cell modulation by palmitoylethanolamide. CNS Neurol. Disord. Drug Targets 12, 78-83.

Di Paola, R., Impellizzeri, D., Mondello, P., Velardi, E., Aloisi, C., Cappellani, A., Esposito, E. and

Cuzzocrea, S. 2012. Palmitoylethanolamide reduces early renal dysfunction and injury caused by experimental ischemia and reperfusion in mice. Shock, 38, 356-366.

Farquhar-Smith, P.W. and Rice, A.S.C. 2001. Administration of endocannabinoids prevents a referred hyperalgesia associated with inflammation of the urinary bladder. Anesthesiology 94, 507-513.

Johnson-Delaney, C.J. 1998. Disease of the Urinary System of Commonly Kept Rodents: Diagnosis and Treatment. Seminars Avian Exotic Pet Med. 7, 81-88.

Lidderdale, J.A. and St Pierre, S.J. 1990. Cystotomy for treatment of urolithiasis in a hamster. Vet. Rec. 127, 364.

Mattace Raso, G., Simeoli, R., Russo, R., Santoro, A., Pirozzi, C., d'Emmanuele di Villa Bianca, R., Mitidieri, E., Paciello, O., Pagano, T.B.,

Orefice, N.S., Meli, R. and Calignano, A. 2013. N-Palmitoylethanolamide protects the kidney from hypertensive injury in spontaneously hypertensive rats via inhibition of oxidative stress. Pharmacol. Res. 76, 67-76.

Panchaphanpong, J., Asawakarn, T. and Pusoonthornthum, R. 2011. Effects of oral administration of N-acetyl-D-glucosamine on plasma and urine concentrations of glycosaminoglycans in cats with idiopathic cystitis. Am. J. Vet. Res. 72, 843-850.

Yang, M., Tanaka, T., Hirose, Y., Deguchi, T., Mori, H. and Kawada, Y. 1997. Chemopreventive effects of diosmin and hesperidin on N-butyl-N-(4-hydroxybutyl) nitrosamine-induced urinary-bladder carcinogenesis in male ICR mice. Int. J. Cancer 73, 719-724.

24

Comparison between fish and linseed oils administered orally for the treatment of experimentally induced keratoconjunctivitis sicca in rabbits

Danielle Alves Silva[1], Gisele Alborgetti Nai[2], Rogério Giuffrida[3], Rafael Cabral Barbero[3], Jacqueline Marcussi Pereira Kuhn[3], Andressa Caroline da Silva[3], Ricardo Henrique Zakir Pereira[3], Maria Fernanda Abbade[3], Luiz Felipe da Costa Zulim[4], Carolina Silva Guimarães Pereira[4] and Silvia Franco Andrade[5,*]

[1]*Animal Science Post Graduate Program, Oeste Paulista University (UNOESTE), Presidente Prudente, SP, Brazil*
[2]*Department of Anatomy Pathology, Faculty of Medicine (UNOESTE), Brazil*
[3]*Faculty of Veterinary Medicine (UNOESTE), Brazil*
[4]*Resident in Small Animal Medicine of the Veterinary Hospital (UNOESTE), Brazil*
[5]*Department of Small Animal Medicine of the Veterinary Hospital (UNOESTE), Brazil*

Abstract

The objective of this study was to compare the efficacy of two sources of omega 3 and 6, fish oil (FO) and linseed oil (LO), orally administered, alone or in combination, for treating experimentally induced keratoconjunctivitis sicca (KCS) in rabbits. Twenty-eight New Zealand rabbits were used in this study. Seven animals were allocated to the C group (negative control), and KCS was induced in 21 animals by topically applying 1% atropine sulfate drops for 7 days. Treatment with atropine was maintained throughout the study period (12 weeks). The rabbits were divided into 3 treatment groups containing 7 animals each: FO group, LO group and FLO group (FO and LO). The animals were evaluated using the Schirmer Tear Test I (STT I), Rose Bengal Test (RBT), fluorescein test (FT), tear film break-up time (TBUT), and conjunctival and histopathological analysis. There was a significant increase in STT I and TBUT values in treatment groups, but the increase occurred earlier in the FO group. The results of the RBT and FT were similar among treatment groups, except FT, in the FLO group, negative staining was only in 12 weeks. There was a significant decrease in the number of goblet cells in the FLO group compared with the other groups. The results demonstrated that orally administered of FO and LO improved the clinical signs of KCS. However, improvement occurred earlier in the FO group. Using oils in combination did not provide additional benefits. These results contribute to the future development of new oral formulations as adjuvant therapies for KCS.

Keywords: Fish oil, Keratoconjunctivitis sicca, Linseed oil, Omega 3 and 6, Oral.

Introduction

Keratoconjunctivitis sicca (KCS) is a chronic inflammatory disease that is common in dogs and humans and that result from a deficiency in the production of the aqueous portion of tear film (quantitative deficiency) and/or excessive tear evaporation (qualitative deficiency). It mainly affects the cornea and conjunctiva (Miller, 2008a,b; McGinnigle et al., 2012; Stevenson et al., 2012). In the literature, many therapies for KCS have been described, including tear substitutes, immunosuppressive drugs (e.g., cyclosporine, tacrolimus and pimecrolimus), steroidal and nonsteroidal anti-inflammatory drugs, and topical antibiotics to control secondary infections. Other drugs, such as essential fatty acids (EFAs), mucolytics and pilocarpine, are used as adjunctive therapies (Izci et al., 2002; Grahn and Storey, 2004; Berdoulay et al., 2005; Miller, 2008b; Ofri et al., 2009; McGinnigle et al., 2012; Stevenson et al., 2012). Studies in human medicine and veterinary medicine (Sullivan et al., 2002; Barabino et al., 2003; Rashid et al., 2008; Wojtowicz et al., 2011; Neves et al., 2013) have demonstrated that omega-3 (ω-3) and omega-6 (ω-6) can be used to control dry eye because of the derivation of anti-inflammatory agents from these EFAs. In human medicine, orally administered ω-3 and ω-6 has been shown to be an effective alternative treatment for patients with various forms of tear deficiency and those with Sjögren's syndrome (Sullivan et al., 2002; Rashid et al., 2008; Wojtowicz et al., 2011). The principal anti-inflammatory agents, prostaglandins (PGs), leukotrienes (LTs) and thromboxanes (TXs) of series 1, 3 and 5, are derived from the actions of the enzymes cyclooxygenase (COX) 1 and lipoxygenase (LOX) on EFAs (Barabino et al., 2003). ω-3 is derived from linolenic acid (ALA), eicosapentaenoic acid (EPA) and docosahexaenoic acid (DHA), and ω-6 is derived from linoleic acid (LA), γ-linolenic acid (GLA) and dihomo-γ-linolenic acid (DGLA) (Sullivan et al., 2002; Barabino et al., 2003; Neves et al., 2013). Although ω-3 and ω-6 are found in many foods, such as nuts, cold-water fish, soybean

*****Corresponding Author:** Silvia Franco Andrade. Small Animal Medicine Department of the Veterinary Hospital (UNOESTE), Rodovia Raposos Tavares, Km 572, CEP 19001-970, Presidente Prudente, SP, Brazil. E-mail: *silviafranco@unoeste.br*

seeds, canola oil, olive oil and linseed oil (LO), there are differences in the concentrations of these EFAs between natural sources (Sullivan *et al.*, 2002; Rashid *et al.*, 2008; Wojtowicz *et al.*, 2011). Fish oil (FO) is an important source of ω-3 that also contains essential elements, such as selenium, iodine, and vitamins A, B, D and E. This oil is obtained from cold-water fish, such as salmon, tuna and herring (Oehlenschläger, 2012). FO is classified as a functional food because it facilitates the prevention and treatment of cardiovascular and neurological diseases, general inflammation, asthma, arthritis, psoriasis, and various types of cancer (Kris-Etherton *et al.*, 2002; Harris, 2004; Mahaffey, 2004; Mozaffarian and Rimm, 2006; Jenkins and Josse, 2008; Rand and Asbell, 2011; Oehlenschläger, 2012). A study that tested the effects of a diet rich in ω-3 (obtained by consuming fish) demonstrated a protective effect against macular degeneration in humans (Chong *et al.*, 2008).

LO, which is obtained from the seeds of the *Linum usitatissimum* plant, is an important source of ω-3 and ω-6 and has an ω-3:ω-6 ratio of 3:1, which is considered ideal, because higher proportions of ω-6 can lead to the formation of pro-inflammatory mediators, such as those derived from arachidonic acid via the enzyme COX2 (PGE2, PGI2, and TXA2) and mediate pathogenic mechanisms, including the inflammatory response (Barabino *et al.*, 2003). LO exerts an immunomodulatory effect by inhibiting interleukin-1, which itself inhibits the production and release of tumor necrosis factor (TNF) by macrophages (Oomah, 2001; Roncone *et al.*, 2010). It also has an anti-inflammatory effect because it induces the formation of anti-inflammatory mediators that are derived from the EFAs ω-3 and ω-6 (Oomah, 2001; Covington, 2004; Roncone *et al.*, 2010). One principal difference between FO and LO is that LO requires ALA to be converted to EPA and DHA, whereas in FO, these essential EFAs are already pre-formed as a result of the ingestion of marine plants, which contain synthesized ω-3, by fish [15]. LO is a source of ω-6, from which DGLA, via COX1, produces PGE1 and TXA1 that are anti-inflammatory mediators (Jenkins and Josse, 2008; Rand and Asbell, 2011). Because FO and LO are sources of EFAs, but with differences in their composition and concentrations, and given that no previous studies have compared the efficacies of these compounds for treating KCS, the aim of this study was to compare the efficacy of orally administering each of these two major sources of ω-3 and ω-6 to treat experimentally induced KCS in rabbits.

Materials and Methods

This study was approved by the Ethics Committee on Animal Use (CEUA) of UNOESTE (Protocol No. 955) according to the rules of the Brazilian College of Animal Experimentation (COBEA) and the Federal Council of Veterinary Medicine of Brazil (CFMV) as well as the Association for Research in Vision and Ophthalmology (ARVO) – Statement for the Use of Animals in Ophthalmic and Vision Research. A total of 28 New Zealand adult female rabbits (*Oryctolagus cuniculus*) that were aged 18 to 22 months old and weighed between 3 and 4 kg were obtained from the Central Bioterium of the university. The animals were kept in individual cages, with food and water provided *ad libitum*. Only animals with normal eyes, as identified using ophthalmic exams (biomicroscopy slit-lamp examination, pupillary light reflex test, Schirmer Tear Test I (STT I), tear film break-up time (TBUT) test and fluorescein test (FT) were used in this study.

The KCS induction protocol was based on those described in previously published studies (Burgalassi *et al.*, 1999; El-Shazly *et al.*, 2008; Shafaa *et al.*, 2011). It involved applying one drop of 1% atropine (Atropina 1% colírio®, Legrand, São Paulo, Brazil) three times daily. Atropine is a muscarinic blocker, and because the lacrimal gland is innervated by facial nerve (cranial nerve VII) that has a general somatic efferent fibre within the ear canal, a general visceral efferent fibre acting under parasympathetic control to lacrimal glands (Sgrignoli *et al.*, 2013), topical atropine causes a decrease in tear production and consequent inflammation in a manner similar to that which occurs in KCS (Burgalassi *et al.*, 1999). Atropine was applied to both eyes until a diagnosis of KCS (STT I result ≤5 mm/min and/or TBUT ≤10 seconds) was achieved. This took an average of 7 days for all of the rabbits in the KCS induction groups. The protocol was maintained by applying atropine two times daily for 12 weeks.

A positive-control group without treatment was not included because of the regulations of the Committee for Experimentation and Use of Laboratory Animals (CEUA/Brazil) of COBEA and the ethical standards of CFMV/Brazil, which prohibits experiments that cause unnecessary suffering in experimental animals. Because the experiment only evaluated drugs that were administered orally, maintaining a positive-control group by applying atropine over 12 weeks without oral treatment would have caused unnecessary discomfort and pain as a result of the disease, the effects of which are well documented in the literature. In any case, time T1 was the time prior to treatment, and this time was used as the positive control.

Data were analyzed from both eyes of all 28 rabbits. Seven animals were allocated to the C group (control), in which KCS was not induced and 1 ml/day of NaCl 0.9% solution was orally administered as a placebo. KCS was induced in the remainder of the rabbits, which were then randomly divided into 3 treatment groups containing 7 animals each: an FO group (1 g/day of oral Omega 3 Dog®, Organnact, Paraná, Brazil), an LO group (1 g/day of oral DryLin®, Ophthalmos, São Paulo, Brazil), and an FLO group (FO and LO) (500 mg/day of oral Dog® Omega 3 + 500 mg/day of oral of DryLin®). The animals received their respective treatments for 12 weeks. The times at which the instillation of 1% atropine eye drops occurred were 6:00 AM, 2:00 PM and 10:00 PM, and the times at which the oral administration of oils (FO, LO or both oils) occurred was 8:00 AM. Ophthalmologic examinations were performed using a portable slit lamp (SL15, Kowa, Japan) to identify the presence or absence of conjunctivitis, ocular discharge and corneal opacity, with scores described in Table 1. Ocular examinations and tests were always conducted in the morning (10:00 AM) at the following time points: T0 (before the induction of KCS), T1 (1 week post-induction and prior to treatment), and T2, T4, T8 and T12 (1, 2, 4, 8 and 12 weeks post-induction, respectively, with treatment). One masked observer (SFA) evaluated the eye examinations and tests.

Table 1. Clinical scoring system.

Clinical sign	Score
Conjunctivitis	0 = None
	1 = Mild conjunctival hyperemia
	2 = Moderate to severe conjunctival hyperemia
	3 = Moderate to severe conjunctival hyperemia and chemosis
Ocular discharge	0 = None
	1 = Minor serous discharge
	2 = Moderate mucoid discharge
	3 = Marked mucopurulent discharge
Corneal opacity	0 = None
	1 = <25%
	2 = 25-50%
	3 = >50%

The STT I was performed without anesthetic eye drops and used to quantify tear production. Values of ≤5 mm/min were considered positive for KCS (Maggs, 2008). The TBUT test, which can be used to determine the stability of the tear film and to check for evaporative dry eye in patients who have a normal quantity of tears but unstable tear film, was also performed. This test can explain dry eye symptoms that result from an imbalance in the composition of tears that may be caused by tears evaporating too quickly or not adhering properly to the surface of the eye. The TBUT test was performed specifically to evaluate the quality of the tear film. Two consecutive TBUT evaluations were performed, and their results were averaged. One drop of 1% Fluorescein Eye Drops (Fluoresceína 1% colírio®, Allergan, São Paulo, Brazil) was placed into the lower conjunctival fornix. The eyelids were manually blinked one time, and the lids were then held

open. A slit lamp with a cobalt blue filter was used to determine the time required for the first dark spot, indicating the break-up of the tear film, to appear on the cornea. Values ≤10 seconds were considered diagnostic for KCS (Wei et al., 2013).

The FT, which reveals irregularities in the corneal epithelium, was performed by instillation of one drop of 1% Fluorescein Eye Drops (Fluoresceína 1% colírio®, Allergan, São Paulo, Brazil) into the lower conjunctival fornix. After the stain was distributed in the tear film, the cornea was evaluated in quadrants (superior temporal, inferior temporal, superior nasal and inferior nasal). The FT score ranged from 0-4 according to the quadrant, with 0 indicating no stain uptake in any quadrant and 4 indicating uptake in all 4 quadrants (Maggs, 2008). The Rose Bengal Test (RBT) was performed to stain tissue that was devoid of mucus. For these tests, Rosa Bengala 1% Eye Drops (Rosa Bengala®, Ophthalmos, São Paulo, Brazil) were applied prior to anesthetic eye drops. The RBT scores ranged from 0-3: (0) no staining, (1) only the conjunctiva was stained, (2) only the cornea was stained, and (3) both the conjunctiva and the cornea were stained (Maggs, 2008). Conjunctival and corneal cytology were assayed at T0, T1, T4, T8 and T12. After anesthetic eye drops were applied, slides were made from conjunctival cells (upper and lower) and the cornea that were harvested using a sterile swab that was moistened with saline solution. The slides were fixed in alcohol for 5 minutes and then stained using the periodic acid-Schiff (PAS) staining technique (Merck, USA) and hematoxylin (Dolles, São Paulo, Brazil). Hematoxylin-eosin (HE) staining was used to evaluate the morphology of the cytoplasm and the nucleus in the cells, and PAS staining was used to evaluate the presence of mucus in goblet cells. The following parameters were evaluated in the conjunctiva: the numbers of neutrophils, lymphocytes, metaplastic cells and anucleate squamous cells. The following parameters were evaluated in the cornea: the numbers of neutrophils, lymphocytes and anucleate squamous cells. Cell counts were determined in 10 fields (40x) that were approximately 1 mm^2 in each slide using an optical microscope (Eclipse E200®, Nikkon, Tokyo, Japan). One masked observer (GAN) evaluated the results of all cytological exams.

At the end of the experiment (T12), the rabbits were euthanized using 2.5% sodium thiopental (Abbott Laboratories, Chicago, IL, USA) in an intravenous dose of 200 mg/kg (Neves et al., 2013; Sgrignoli et al., 2013). After transpalpebral enucleation was performed, the eyeball was placed in a 10% formaldehyde solution (Chemical Kinetics, São Paulo, Brazil) for 24-48 hours. The eyeball was then stored in 70% alcohol and routinely processed and embedded in paraffin (Dynamic Analytical Reagents, São Paulo, Brazil). Each eyeball was cut in half across the sagittal plane for histological processing. Three (5 μm-thick) serial sections were obtained from the cornea and conjunctiva, and these were stained separately with HE (Dolles, São Paulo, Brazil), PAS (Merck, USA) and Masson trichrome (Merck, USA). The parameters that were evaluated in the conjunctiva included the numbers of polymorphonuclear neutrophils (PMNs), mononuclear neutrophils (MNs), and goblet cells; the presence of squamous metaplasia in the epithelium; edema; and vascular congestion (e.g., capillary dilation with an increase in the number of intravascular erythrocytes). In the cornea and the lacrimal gland, the presence of edema or vascular congestion and the numbers of PMNs and MNs were assessed. Cell counts were determined in 10 fields (40x) that were approximately 1 mm^2 on each slide using an optical microscope (Eclipse E200®, Nikkon, Tokyo, Japan). Goblet cell density (cells/mm^2) was determined in five high-power fields (40x) on each slide, with each field corresponding to an area of approximately 0.5 mm^2. One masked observer (GAN) evaluated the results of all histopathological exams. For the STT I and TBUT variables, the goblet cell density, and the numbers of PMNs and MNs, we used two-way analysis of variance (ANOVA) for paired samples with contrasts by Tukey's method. For the FT and RBT variables, we used the nonparametric Friedman test to compare moments and the Kruskal-Wallis test with contrasts by Dunn's method for comparisons of groups. A significance level of $P<0.05$ was adopted. The software used for statistical analysis was R version 3.2.2. (The R Foundation for Statistical Computing, 2015)

Results

The clinical signs that were observed are shown in Figure 1. Improvements in signs of conjunctival hyperemia, ocular discharge and corneal opacity were observed in the FO, LO and FLO groups from T1 to T12. Neither vascularization nor corneal pigmentation was observed in any group. There was a significant decrease ($P<0.05$) in STT I (Fig. 2A) and TBUT (Fig. 2B) values in the LO and FLO groups at T1, T2 and T4, but only at T1 and T2 in the FO group. The FT was negative at T0 in all groups, at T8 and T12 in the FO and LO groups, and at T12 in only the FLO group (Fig. 3A). At all other times, the FT was positive (Fig. 3A). All irregularities of the cornea that arose as a result of KCS were found to be superficial (Fig. 4A). The results of the RBT were similar among all treatment groups (Fig. 3B), and all groups were positively stained (Fig. 4B) in the RBT from T1 to T8 and negatively stained at T0 and T12 (Fig. 3B). We obtained and analyzed 28 cytological samples in each group for a total of 112 samples. In 100% of the samples, conjunctival and corneal cytology at T0 revealed that there were no anuclate squamous cells or squamous metaplasia in any group (C, FO, LO and FLO). An analysis of

conjunctival samples at T1 (Fig. 5A) revealed that 57% of the samples from the FLO group, 35.7% from the FO group and 42.8% from the LO group presented a moderate number of anuclate squamous cells, whereas at T4, 78.5%, 85.7% and 92.8% of the samples in the FO, LO and FLO groups, respectively, presented a moderate number. At T8 and T12, the samples from the FO, LO and FLO groups presented a small number of anuclate squamous cells. Based on the number of anuclate squamous cells that were observed using corneal cytology, the samples from the FO, LO and FLO groups presented a small number of such cells at all time periods. Squamous metaplasia (Fig. 5B) was observed at T1 in the FO, LO, and FLO group samples. In the FLO group, at T1, 7.1% of the samples exhibited anuclate squamous cells (Fig. 5C), but these were not observed in the other groups. In general, there was no mucus in the evaluated groups except in some animals like at T4 in a rabbit of FO group (Fig. 5D). We obtained and analyzed 28 histological samples of conjunctiva, 28 of cornea and 28 of lacrimal gland, in each group. Based on an analysis of the histopathology of the conjunctiva, goblet cell density (cells/mm^2) (Fig. 6A and 6B), was significantly lower ($P<0.05$) in the FLO group (5.4 ± 2.2; $P=0.0012$) than in the C (8.9 ± 1.8), FO (9.6 ± 2.1) and LO (10.8 ± 2.0) groups. A moderate amount of squamous metaplasia was observed in 50% (14 out of 28 samples) of the FLO samples, and vascular congestion was observed in 28.5% (8 out of 28 samples) of the FLO samples. Edema of the conjunctiva was mild in 21.4% (6 out of 28 samples) and 35.7% (10 out of 28 samples) of the FO and LO samples, respectively, and moderate in 50% (14 out of 28 samples) of the FLO group samples. Based on an analysis of the histopathology of the cornea (Fig. 6C), edema (Fig. 6D) and vascular congestion were mild in 7.1% (2 out of 28 samples), 14.2% (4 out of 28 samples) and 21.4% (6 out of 28 samples) of the FO, LO and FLO samples, respectively. Based on the histopathology of the lacrimal gland (Fig. 6E), the FO and LO samples displayed no changes, whereas in the FLO group, 35.7% (10 out of 28 samples) demonstrated vascular congestion, and 7.1% (2 out of 28 samples) exhibited inflammatory infiltrates (Fig. 6F). The neutrophils counts (cells/mm^2) in the conjunctiva, cornea and lacrimal gland were zero in all of the evaluated groups. The lymphocytes counts were zero in all analyzed structures in the C group, and in all of the treatment groups, the counts in the cornea were also virtually zero. The lymphocytes counts (cells/mm^2) in the lacrimal gland was significantly higher ($P<0.05$) in the FLO group (7.7 ± 2.2; $P=0.0032$) than in the FO (2.7 ± 1.0) and LO (2.9 ± 1.1) groups, and there was no significant difference ($P>0.05$) in the lymphocytes count in the conjunctiva between the FO (1.7 ± 0.8), LO (2.2 ± 1) and FLO (2.4 ± 1.0) treatment groups.

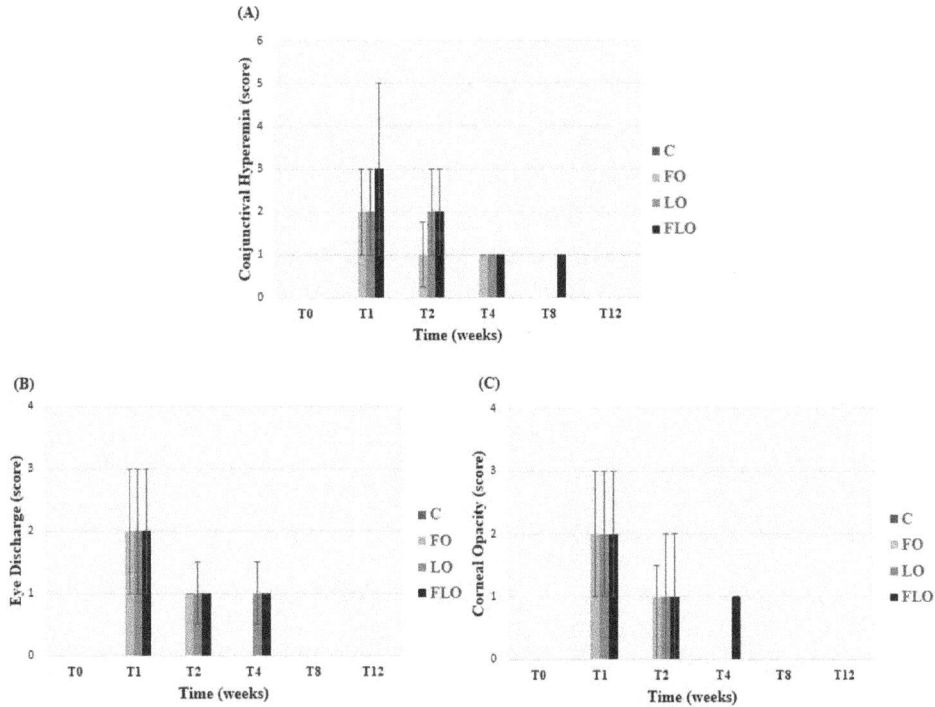

Fig. 1. Medians and interquartile deviations of observed clinical signs (Table 1). **(A)** Conjunctival hyperemia, **(B)** eye discharge and **(C)** corneal opacity in the eyes of rabbits with experimentally induced keratoconjunctivitis sicca (KCS) that were subjected to oral treatment with fish oil (FO), linseed oil (LO), or a combination of fish oil and linseed oil (FLO), and the control group (C).

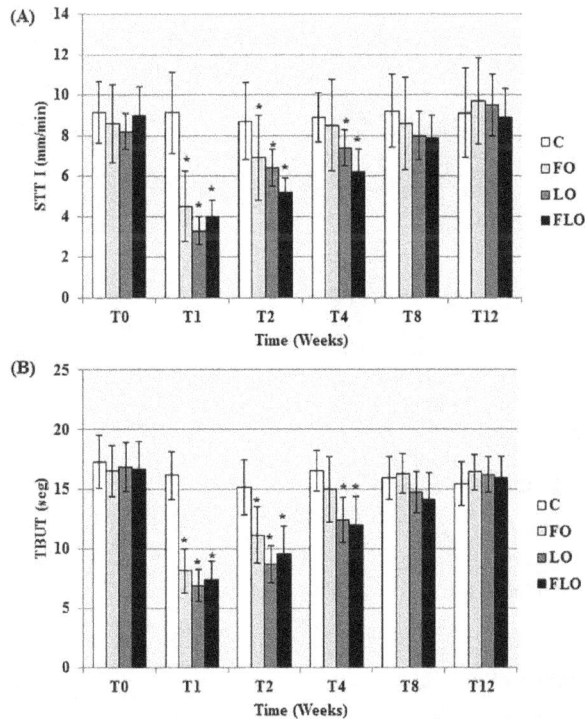

Fig. 2. Means and standard deviations of the values obtained from the **(A)** Schirmer Tear Test (STT I) [Values ≤ 5 mm/min (positive for KCS)] in mm/min and **(B)** the tear film break-up time (TBUT) test [TBUT ≤ 10 seconds (positive for KCS)] in seconds in rabbits with experimentally induced keratoconjunctivitis sicca (KCS) that were subjected to oral treatment with fish oil (FO), linseed oil (LO) or a combination of fish oil and linseed oil (FLO), and the control group (C). *: $P < 0.05$ (Tukey's test for comparisons with the control group at every time point).

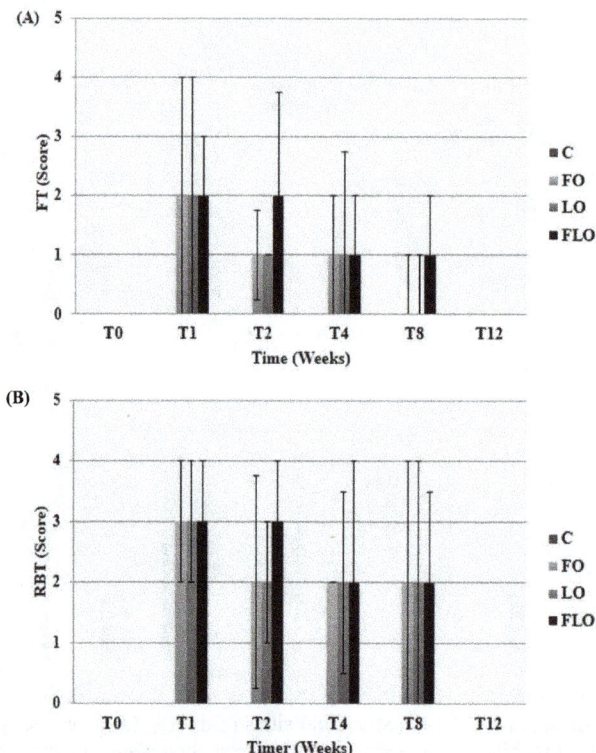

Fig. 3. Median and interquartile deviations of the values for the **(A)** fluorescein test (FT) [(0): without staining; (1): one stained quadrant; (2): two stained quadrants; (3): three stained quadrants; and (4): four stained quadrants] and **(B)** Rose Bengal Test (RBT) [(0): without staining; (1): only the conjunctiva was stained; (2): only the cornea was stained; and (3): both the conjunctiva and the cornea were stained] in rabbits with experimentally induced keratoconjunctivitis sicca (KCS) that were subjected to oral treatment with fish oil (FO), linseed oil (LO) or a combination of fish oil and linseed oil (FLO), and the control group (C).

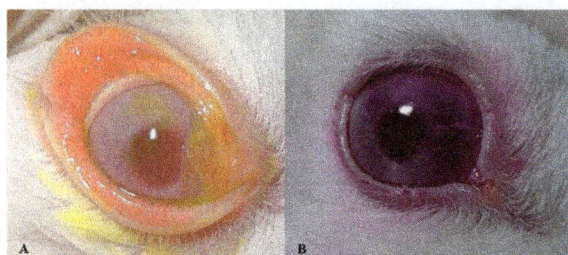

Fig. 4. (A) Right eye of rabbit No. 5 in the FLO group at T4 showing a conjunctival injection and a positive FT with superficial staining of the cornea. **(B)** Right eye of rabbit No. 2 in the LO group at T2 demonstrating a positive RBT result with staining in the superior quadrant of the cornea.

Discussion

In this study, orally administered FO and LO improved the clinical signs of experimentally induced KCS in rabbits, increased STT I and TBUT scores. This was possibly because these oils are rich in ω-3 and ω-6 fatty acids, which inhibit the formation of pro-inflammatory eicosanoids and increase the formation of anti-inflammatory mediators, primarily including EPA, DHA, PGE1 and TXA1 (Oomah, 2001; Covington, 2004).

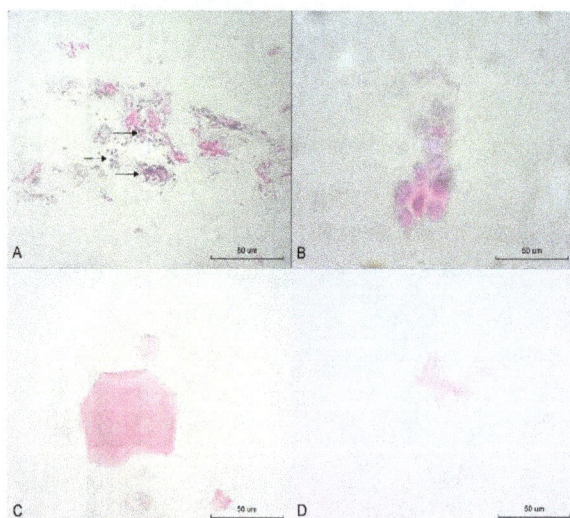

Fig. 5. Cytological smears: **(A)** T1 in the FLO group (OS): anucleate squamous cells and inflammatory cells in the conjunctiva (arrows) (hematoxylin-eosin (HE), 400x). **(B)** T1 in the FLO group (OS): metaplastic cells in the conjunctiva (HE, 400x). **(C)** T1 in the FLO group (OS): anucleate squamous cells of the cornea (HE, 400x). **(D)** T4 in the FO group (OD): neutral mucus (PAS-alcian blue, 400x).

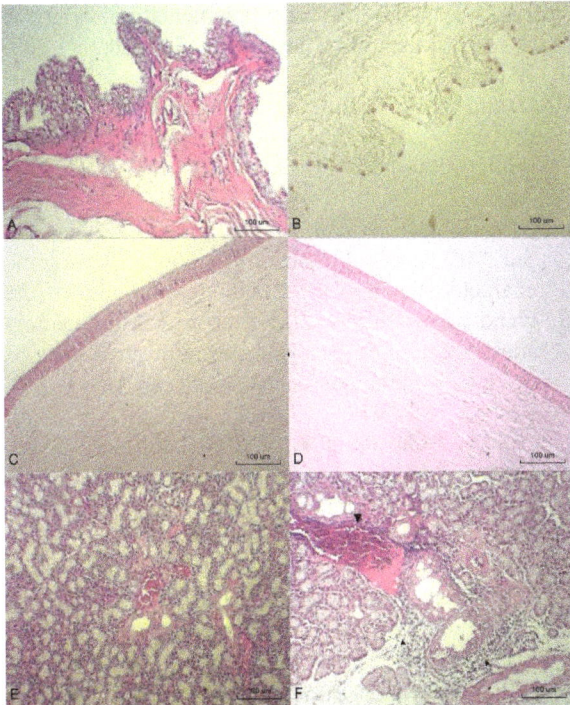

Fig. 6. Photomicrographs of the conjunctiva, cornea and lacrimal gland at T12. **(A)** LO group (OD): conjunctiva with large numbers of goblet cells (hematoxylin-eosin (HE), 100x). **(B)** LO group (OS): goblet cells (PAS-alcian blue, 100x). **(C)** LO group (OD): normal cornea (HE, 100x). **(D)** LO group (OD): cornea with edema (HE, 100x). **(E)** FO group (OD): normal lacrimal gland (HE, 100x). **(F)** FLO group (OS): lacrimal gland with inflammatory infiltration (arrows) and vascular congestion (arrowhead) (HE, 100x).

The consumption of LO and FO has also been demonstrated to control inflammation by decreasing the production of agents that promote inflammatory processes (e.g., cytokines, TNF and interleukin-1β) in studies involving healthy volunteers and patients with rheumatoid arthritis who were provided with dietary supplements containing these EFAs (James *et al.*, 2000).

A recent veterinary study concluded that LO, administered either orally or topically, was effective in treating induced KCS in rabbits (Neves *et al.*, 2013), although the experimental study used in this KCS induction protocol, topical atropine, was combined with third eyelid gland removal, which was different from our study, in which KCS was induced using topical atropine alone. However, these data (Neves *et al.*, 2013), show that even when a more aggressive induction protocol is used that results in the occurrence of severe ulcers, such as keratomalacia, which was not observed in our study, linseed oil was considered effective for treating KCS in rabbits.

Our study's result are also in agreement with the findings reported in a study that used a topical formulation containing ω-6 and ω-3 in mice that were

experimentally induced to develop KCS. In that study, the mice demonstrated improvement in the inflammatory symptoms associated with KCS (Rashid *et al.*, 2008). Another study by He and Bazan, also reported that the topical application of lipid derivatives containing ω-3, such as DHA, prevented complications related to KCS, such as erosion and corneal ulcers (He and Bazan, 2010).

In the present study, the FO group demonstrated earlier improvement in the analyzed parameters, possibly because this oil already contains EPA and DHA as a result of the ingestion by fish of marine plants that contain synthesized ω-3, whereas for LO, it is necessary to convert ALA to EPA and DHA (Jenkins and Josse, 2008). The human body can convert approximately 5% to 10% of ALA to EPA, but less than 2% to 5% of ALA it is converted to DHA (Burdge, 2006; Rand and Asbell, 2011). In rabbits, dogs and cats, the conversion of ALA to EPA and DHA is also limited (Bauer, 2008; Ander *et al.*, 2010).

In the present study, the combined oil treatment (the FLO group) did not result in additional benefits, demonstrating that this combination does not maximize the effects of these oils. Additionally, in this group, the number of goblet cells was lower. Because these cells are responsible for producing mucin in pre-tear film, which aids ocular lubrication, a reduction in the number of these cells could lead to deficient corneal lubrication (Davidson and Kuonen, 2004). In the cytological evaluation, the FLO group presented a higher incidence of inflammation and a higher number of keratinized corneal epithelial cells than were observed in the other groups at all time points. These data indicate that the cells produced more keratin to protect themselves from destruction. In the histopathological evaluation, edema and congestion were higher in the conjunctiva in the FLO group, possibly as a result of an inflammatory process (Kunert *et al.*, 2002; Davidson and Kuonen, 2004; Robbins *et al.*, 2015).

The combination therapy (the FLO group) was not as effective as either FO or LO alone, and a possible explanation for this result is that excess ω-3 and ω-6 results in an improper ratio of these two EFAs. This hypothesis was also suggested by Neves *et al.* (2013) that showed that LO, whether administered orally or topically, was effective in treating experimentally induced KCS in rabbits, while a combination of oral and topical LO did not result in additional benefits beyond those that were obtained from delivering LO via a single route.

We conclude that orally administered FO and LO effectively improved clinical signs of KCS in rabbits, possibly because these oils are rich in ω-3 and ω-6, which are both considered to be natural anti-inflammatory agents. FO induced these benefits earlier, possibly because it contains preformed EPA and DHA.

Combining the oils did not provide additional benefits. These results contribute to our ability to develop new oral formulations as an adjuvant therapy for KCS in the future.

Acknowledgments

We would like to thank the Post Graduate Program in Animal Science of UNOESTE, Laboratory Ophthalmos - SP and Laboratory Organnact – PR, for the donation of some of the materials necessary for the execution of the experiment.

Conflict of interest

The authors declare that they have no competing interests.

References

Ander, B.P., Edel, A.L., McCullough, R., Rodriguez-Leyva, D., Rampersad, P., Gilchrist, J.S.C., Lukas, A. and Pierce, G.N. 2010. Distribution of omega-3 fatty acids in tissues of rabbits fed a flaxseed-supplemented diet. Metabolism 59, 620-627.

Barabino, S., Rolando, M., Camicione, P., Ravera, G., Zanardi, S., Giuffrida, S. and Calabria, G. 2003. Systemic linoleic and g-linolenic acid therapy in dry eye syndrome with an inflammatory component. Cornea 22, 97-101.

Bauer, J.E. 2008. Essential fatty acid metabolism in dogs and cats. Rev. Bras. Zootecn. 37, 20-27.

Berdoulay, Y.A., English, R.V. and Naldelstein, B. 2005. Effect of topical 0.02% tacrolimus aqueous suspension on tear productin in dog with Keratoconjunctitis Sicca. Vet. Opthalmol. 8, 225-232.

Burdge, G.C. 2006. Metabolism of alpha-linoleic acid in humans. Prostag. Leukotr. Ess. 75, 161-168.

Burgalassi, S., Panichi, L., Chetoni, P., Saettone, M.F. and Boldrini, E. 1999. Development of a simple dry eye model in the albino rabbit and evaluation of some tear substitutes. Ophthalmic Res. 31, 229-235.

Chong, E.W., Kreis, A.J., Wong, T.Y., Simpson, J.A. and Guymer, R.H. 2008. Dietary-3 fatty acid and fish intake in the primary prevention of age related macular degeneration. A systematic review and meta-analysis. Arch. Ophthalmol. 126, 826-833.

Covington, M.B. 2004. Omega-3 fatty acids. Am. Fam. Physician. 70, 133-140.

Davidson, H.J. and Kuonen, V.J. 2004. The tear film and ocular mucin (Review). Vet. Ophthalmol. 7, 71-77.

El-Shazly, A.H., El-Gohrary, A.A., El-Shazly, L.H. and El-Hossary, G.G. 2008. Comparison between two cyclooxygenase inhibitors in an experimental dry eye model in albino rabbits. Acta. Pharm. 58, 163-173.

Grahn, B.H. and Storey, E.S. 2004. Lacrimomimetics and lacrimostimulants. Vet. Clin. North Am. Small Anim. Pract. 34, 739-753.

Harris, W.S. 2004. Fish oil supplementation: evidence for health benefits. Cleve. Clin. J. Med. 71, 208-221.

He, J. and Bazan, H.E.P. 2010. Omega-3 fatty acids in dry eye and corneal nerve regeneration after refractive surgery. Prostag. Leukotr. Ess. 82, 319-325.

Izci, C., Celik, I., Alkan, F., Ogurtan, Z., Ceylan, C., Sur, E. and Ozkan, Y. 2002. Histologic characteristics and local cellular immunity of the gland of the third eyelid after topical ophthalmic administration of 2% cyclosporine for treatment of dogs with keratoconjunctivitis sicca. Am. J. Vet. Res. 63, 688-694.

James, M.J., Gibson, R.A. and Cleland, L.G. 2000. Dietary polyunsaturated fatty acids and inflammatory mediator production. Am. J. Clin. Nutr. 71, 343-348.

Jenkins, D.J. and Josse, A.R. 2008. Fish oil and omega-3 fatty acids. Can. Med. Am. J. 178, 150.

Kris-Etherton, P.M., Harris, W.S. and Appel, L.J. 2002. Fish consumption, fish oil, omega-3 fatty acids, and cardiovascular disease. Circulation 106, 2747-2757.

Kunert, K.S., Tisdale, A.S. and Gipson, I.K. 2002. Goblet cell numbers and epithelial proliferation in the conjunctiva of patients with dry eye syndrome treated with cyclosporine. Arch. Ophthalmol. 120, 330-337.

Maggs, D.J. 2008. Basic diagnostic techiniques. In Slater's Fundamentas of Veterinary Ophthalmology, Eds., Maggs, D.J., Miller, P.E. and Ofri, R. Saunders Elsevier, St. Louis, pp: 81-106.

Mahaffey, K. 2004. Fish and shellfish as dietary sources of methylmercury and the omega-3 fatty acids, eicosahexaenoic acid and docosahexaenoic acid: risks and benefits. Environ. Res. 95, 414-428.

McGinnigle, S., Naroo, S.A. and Eperjesi, F. 2012. Evaluation of dry eye. Surv. Ophthalmol. 7, 293-316.

Miller, P.E. 2008a. Structure and function of the eye. In Slater's Fundamentas of Veterinary Ophthalmology, Eds., Maggs, D.J., Miller, P.E. and Ofri, R. Saunders Elsevier, St. Louis, pp: 1-19.

Miller, P.E. 2008b. Lacrimal system. In Slater's Fundamentas of Veterinary Ophthalmology, Eds., Maggs, D.J., Miller, P.E. and Ofri, R. Saunders Elsevier, St. Louis, pp: 157-174.

Mozaffarian, D. and Rimm, E.B. 2006. Fish intake, contaminants, and human health: evaluating the risks and the benefits. J. Am. Med. Assoc. 296, 1885-1899.

Neves, M.L., Yamasaki, L., Sanches, O.C., Amaral, M.S.P., Stevanin, H., Giuffrida, R., Candido, E.R., Goes, J.E., Zulim, L.F.C., Schweigert, A., Fukui, R.M., Meirelles, C.C, Sasaki, C.A. and Andrade, S.F. 2013. Use of linseed oil to treat experimentally induced keratoconjunctivitis sicca in rabbits. J. Ophthalmol. Inflamm. Infect. 3, 4.

Oehlenschläger, J. 2012. Seafood: nutritional benefits and risk aspects. Int. J. Vitam. Nutr. Res. 82, 168-176.

Ofri, R., Lambrou, G.N., Allgoewer, I., Graenitz, U., Pena, T.M., Spiess, B.M. and Latour, E. 2009. Clinical evaluation of pimecrolimus eye drops for treatment of canine keratoconjunctivitis sicca: a comparison with cyclosporine A. Vet. J. 179(1), 70-77.

Oomah, B.D. 2001. Flaxseed as functional source. J. Sci. Food Agric. 81, 889-894.

Rand, A.L. and Asbell, P.A. 2011. Current Opinion in Ophthalmology Nutritional Supplements for Dry Eye Syndrome. Curr. Opin. Ophthalmol. 22, 279-282.

Rashid, S., Jin, Y., Ecoiffer, T., Barabino, B., Schaumberg, D.A. and Dana, M.R. 2008. Topical omega-3 and omega-6 fatty acids for treatment of dry eye. Arch. Ophthalmol. 126, 210-225.

Robbins, S.L., Cotran, R.S. and Kumar, V. 2015. Robbins & Cotran: Pathologic Basis of Disease. Saunders Elsevier, St. Louis.

Roncone, M., Bartlett, H. and Eperjesi, F. 2010. Essential fatty acids for dry eye: A review. Cont. Lens Anterior Eye 33, 49-54.

Sgrignoli, M.R., Yamasaki, L., Sanches, O.C., Giuffrida, R., Ricci, C.L., Santos, G.C., Valle, H.F.D., Zulim, L.F.C., Silva, D.A., Basso, K.M., Silva, M.C.A. and Andrade, S.F. 2013. Comparison of topical 0.03% tacrolimus in almond and linseed oil to treat experimentally induced keratoconjunctivitis sicca in rabbits. Int. J. Ophthalmic. Pathol. 2, 3.

Shafaa, M.W., El Shazly, L.H., El Shazly, A.H., El Gohary, A.A. and El Hossary, G.G. 2011. Efficacy of topically applied liposome-bound tetracycline in the treatment of dry eye model. Vet. Opthalmol. 14, 18-25.

Stevenson, W., Chauhan, S.K. and Dana, R. 2012. Dry eye disease: an immune-mediated ocular surface disorder. Arch. Ophthalmol. 130, 90-100.

Sullivan, B.D., Cermak, J.M., Sullivan, R.M., Papas, A.S., Evans, J.E., Dana, M.R. and Sullivan, D.A. 2002. Correlation between nutrient intake and the polar lipid profiles of meibomian gland secretions in women with Sjogren's syndrome. Adv. Exp. Med. Biol. 506, 441-447.

Wei, X.E., Markoulli, M., Zhao, Z. and Willcox, M.D. 2013. Tear film break-up time in rabbits. Clin. Exp. Optom. 96, 70-75.

Wojtowicz, J.C., Butovich, I. and Uchiyama, E. 2011. Pilot, prospective, randomized, double-masked, placebo-controlled clinical trial of an omega-3 supplement for dry eye. Cornea 30, 308-314.

25

Ophthalmological abnormalities in wild European hedgehogs (*Erinaceus europaeus*): a survey of 300 animals

David Williams*, Nina Adeyeye and Erni Visser

Department of Veterinary Medicine, University of Cambridge, Madingley Road, Cambridge CB3 0ES, UK

Abstract

In this study we aimed to examine wild European hedgehogs (*Erinaceus europaeus)* in rescue centres and to determine ocular abnormalities in this animal population. Three hundred animals varying in age from 2 months to 5 years were examined, 147 being male and 153 female. All animals were evaluated with direct and indirect ophthalmoscopy and slit lamp biomicroscopy in animals where lesions were detected. Tonometry using the Tonovet rebound tonometer was undertaken in selected animals as was assessment of tear production using the Schirmer I tear test. Four animals were affected by orbital infection, 3 were anophthalmic, 2 unilaterally and one bilaterally, 3 by conjunctivitis, 3 by non-ulcerative keratitis and 4 by uveitis with corneal oedema. Fifty seven animals were affected by cataract, 54 with bilateral nuclear lens opacities. Twenty six of these animals were young animals considered too small to hibernate. This report documents the first prospective study of ocular disease in the European hedgehog. The predominant finding was bilateral nuclear cataract seen particularly in young poorly growing animals. Investigation into the potential causation of cataracts by poor nutrition or poor feeding ability by lens opacification requires further study.
Keywords: Cataract, Conservation, Eye abnormality, Hedgehog, Rehabilitation.

Introduction

The European hedgehog (*Erinaceus europaeus)* is a familiar creature among the rural hedgerows of Britain and, more recently, also in the urban environment. The species is postulated to have changed relatively little in the last 15 million years (Reiter and Gould, 1998) and thus the hedgehog visual system is considered relatively primitive. However, there is little reported data on the anatomy of physiology of the eye in this species (Dinopoulos *et al*., 1987).

The hedgehog is endemic in Europe (Morris, 1993; Amori *et al*., 2011) and has few natural predators, with the badger , fox and polecat among the few species with regular predatory success (Reeve, 1994). The increase in badger numbers in the UK over the past decades may be having an adverse effect on hedgehog numbers (Young, *et al*., 2006; Trewby *et al*., 2014) while changes in agricultural practice over the last half century with a decrease in pastureland and increase in pesticide use has influenced the invertebrate diet of the hedgehog with potential effects on hedgehog populations (Stoate *et al*., 2001).

Road traffic accidents are cited as the most common cause of death (Bunnell, 2001) with annual casualties are estimated between 100,000 to 1.3 million in the UK alone (Morris and Throughton, 1993). Together, these factors seem to be leading to an increase in injured and displaced hedgehogs that are subsequently rescued and rehabilitated. European hedgehogs, while not an endangered species under International Union for the Conservation of Nature (IUCN) criteria (Amori *et al*., 2011), are experiencing a significant reduction in population size and, given this, assessment of the health of wild and rescued hedgehogs is important. Prior to this study, there has been no information available relating to the prevalence of eye disease in wild hedgehogs. There are a small number of studies on animals in captivity mostly involving the African pygmy hedgehog, predominantly involving exophthalmos (Wheeler *et al*., 2001; Kuonen *et al*., 2002; Fukuzawa *et al*., 2004).

A recent study has documented Schirmer tear test and intraocular pressure measurements in the long-eared hedgehog (*Hemiechinus auritus*) (Ghaffari *et al*., 2012) a species found in Eastern Europe and Asia. None of the animals in that study had any ocular abnormalities and the small number of animals examined would have precluded assessment of prevalence of ocular disease in this population. The aim of the current study was to survey a sizeable number of 'rescued' wild European hedgehogs in the UK, to determine the prevalence of common ophthalmological diseases in this species and to investigate whether there may be a relationship between this and other factors such as weight, age or sex.

The hedgehog diet is primarily insectivorous, with 90% consisting of annelids (predominantly earthworms) and arthropods (mostly insects) and 6% accounted for by gastropods such as snails and slugs (Reeve, 1994). The fact that their favoured invertebrate prey is more

*Corresponding Author: David Williams. Department of Veterinary Medicine, University of Cambridge, Madingley Road, Cambridge CB3 0ES, UK. Email: *dlw33@cam.ac.uk*

abundant at night probably accounts for hedgehogs' crepuscular and nocturnal behaviour. Given this scotopic lifestyle, it has to be asked what relevance vision has to the species. The hedgehog retina, given the limited data available, appears predominantly rod rich, as one might expect, but 2% of photoreceptors in the nocturnal lesser hedgehog *Echinops telfairi* were middle to long-wave cones showing some degree of color vision (Peichl *et al.*, 2000).

Female hedgehogs produce one to two litters per year with an average of 4 hoglets per litter. These youngsters are independent by 8 weeks and must weigh a minimum of 450g by autumn as suggested by Robinson and Routh (1999) or 650g as suggested by Bunnell (2001) to survive the winter. Low weights are usually accompanied by large burdens of ectoparasites (fleas and ticks) (Thamm *et al.*, 2009) and endoparasites (most particularly lungworm) (Majeed *et al.*, 1989) which can fatally exacerbate any underlying problems. Most hedgehogs rescued are underweight, injured or found out during the day due to disease, dehydration or high parasite burden (Thamm *et al.*, 2009). The reasons for being found outside in the day vary between the age groups.

Young animals may have lost contact with their dam, juveniles may have been feeding insufficiently so are still foraging in an attempt to gain weight. Older animals and those of any age may have been unable to nest through systemic illness or injury and those that are blind may not be able distinguish day from night (Reeve, 1994).

It might thus be argued that the animals examined in this study do not constitute a normal wild population since they have been found during daylight hours. The high prevalence of lens opacities noted below may then represent a biased sample. Nevertheless it is hoped that this publication will be of interest both to veterinary ophthalmologists and those involved in wildlife conservation.

Materials and Methods

A total of 300 hedgehogs were examined from seven rescue centres ranging from large wildlife hospitals (St Tiggywinkles Wildlife Hospital, Aylesbury, Bucks UK and East Wynch Wildlife Hospital, Kings Lynn, UK) to five individuals caring for small groups of animals (<20) in their homes and gardens. Approximate age, gender and reason for rescue were ascertained. Age was estimated from information obtained from the rescue centre and from the appearance of the animal, following the criteria set out by Robinson and Routh (1999).

Each hedgehog underwent a non-dilated ophthalmological examination with direct and indirect ophthalmoscopy (Keeler Practitioner direct ophthalmoscope, Keeler Vantage All Pupil indirect ophthalmoscope, Keeler, Windsor UK) and slit lamp biomicroscopy (Kowa SL14 slit lamp, Nagoya, Aich,

Japan) where necessary. Photographic documentation was achieved with a Nikon Coolpix 4500 (Nikon, Tokyo, Japan) for adnexal lesions and a Genesis D fundus camera (Kowa, Nagoya, Aichi, Japan) Examination of retinal detail was thus somewhat compromised but in a darkened environment sufficient mydriasis occurred to allow evaluation of lens opacities although photography of lens lesions was somewhat difficult. The Schirmer tear test proved of little value due the relatively low fluid production of the eye compared to larger species but tonometry with the rebound tonometer (Tonovet, ICare, Helsinki) on calibration p was possible to provide a normal range of intraocular pressures in twenty normal eyes and values for animals with exophthalmos or uveitis. Anaesthesia, although reported as necessary in a previous study (Ghaffari *et al.*, 2012) was not required with careful gentle handling encouraging the animals to unroll onto a rough surface (Robinson and Routh, 1999). Globe size and pupil diameter was measured with a Vernier caliper. Ocular function was evaluated by assessing pupillary light reflexes and behavioural responses to objects in the accommodation in which animals were housed, although more precise assessment of vision was difficult.

Data was recorded using an Excel spreadsheet with differences in weight in animals with and without cataract compared using a Student's T test. Normality of globe and pupil size was determined using the Kolmogorov–Smirnov test.

Results

Three hundred animals were examined ranging in age from 2 months to 5 years with a median age of 12 months and a mean age of 12.6±9.2 months. One hundred and forty seven animals were male and 153 female. Intraocular pressure measurements on both eyes of 10 adult animals with unremarkable eyes gave a mean value of 12.6±1.8mmHg, this data being normally distributed. Schirmer I tear tests, undertaken in 20 animals with unremarkable eyes gave values of less than 1mm/min in normal eyes and thus were not considered particularly valuable.

Normal sighted animals often had eyes that appeared somewhat proptotic in the resting state (Fig. 1) but on handling all animals retracted their globes as they curled up. The globes, as measured with a Vernier calliper in 10 immature animals and 20 normal adult animals, had an average equator to equator diameter of 7.2±0.2 mm for the adult animals, this data being normally distributed with a range from 6.8 to 8.0mm, while smaller globes with a range from 5.5mm to 6.5mm were recorded in immature animals, these data not being normally distributed. The iris is brown with little variation between individuals with a pupil of maximum observed diameter in scotopic conditions of 3.0mm, again this measured in 20 normal adult animals.

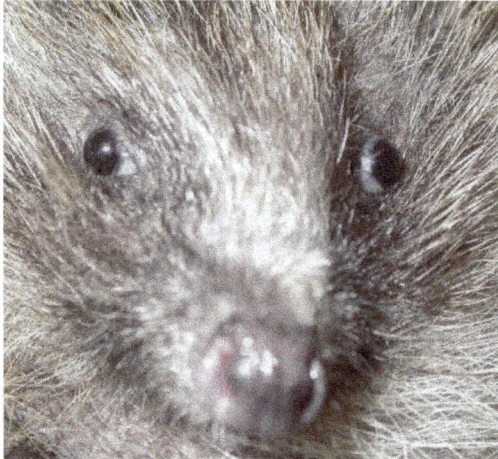

Fig. 1. The somewhat propototic eyes of a normal 2 year old male hedgehog.

Eighty seven hedgehogs (29%) had some degree of ocular abnormality. Three animals had orbital infection and abscessation (Fig. 2). In six no ocular structures visible in the orbit, two bilaterally, with inflammatory tissue filling the orbit (Fig. 3).

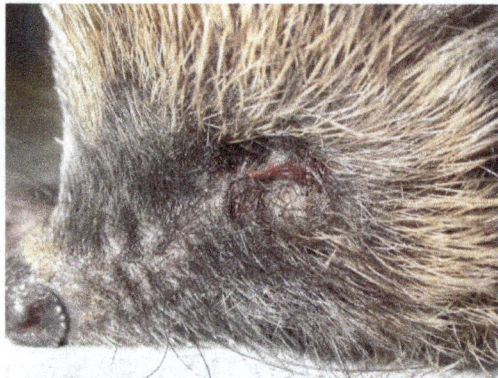

Fig. 2. Orbital infection and periorbital abscessation in a one year old male hedgehog.

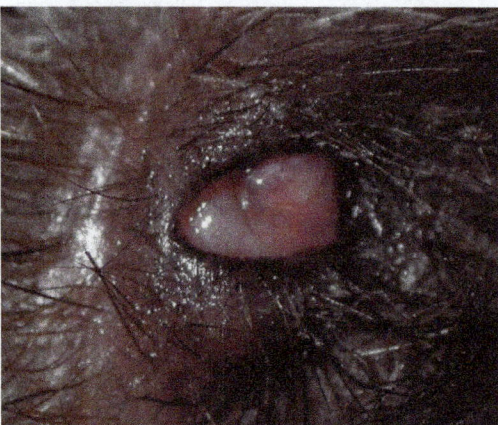

Fig. 3. A bilaterally anophthalmic hedgehog with inflammatory tissue filling the orbit.

Two of the three hedgehogs with orbital infection as defined by cytology and bacteriology (data not shown) and four animals with no ocular structures visible had previous histories of myiasis with eye loss after maggot infection, although none was affected with a viable infection at the time of examination.

Four animals exhibited blepharitis associated with periocular ringworm infection (Fig. 4), with *Trichopyton mentagrophytes* cultured on Sabaroud's dextrose agar after sampling with a standard bacteriology swab (English *et al.*, 1962).

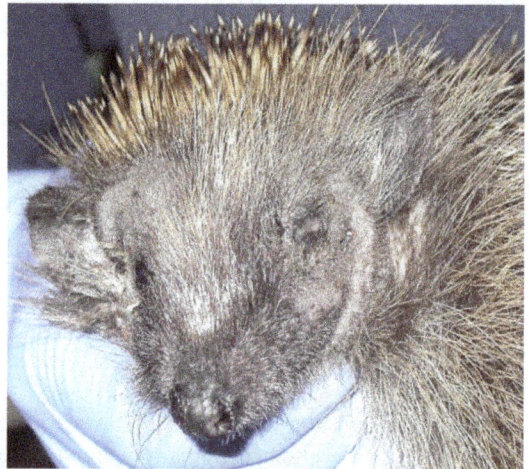

Fig. 4. Periorbital *Tricophyton* infection in an emaciated hedgehog.

Fourteen hedgehogs had ocular and adenexal injuries. Three animals had a non-ulcerative keratitis. These animals were affected with trichiasis but this finding was also evident in many animals with a normal ocular surface where normal periocular hair, with short and bristly spines impinged on the ocular surface (Fig. 5).

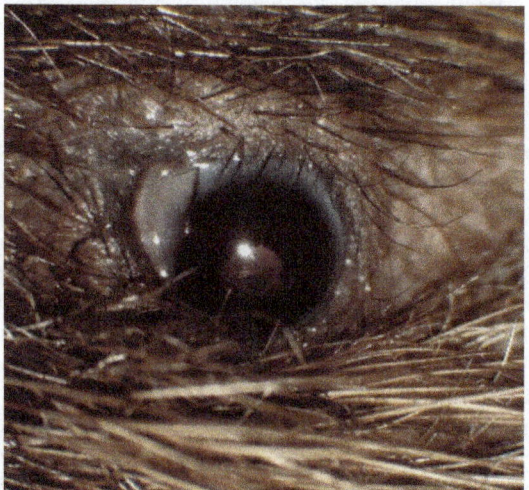

Fig. 5. A hedgehog with trichiasis, a common finding in otherwise normal eyes.

Many of these animals exhibited moderate to marked epiphora. Conjunctivitis with hyperaemia with or without a mucopurulent discharge was seen in six animals. Four hedgehogs had unilateral corneal oedema and central ulceration with presumed uveitis (Fig. 6). In these animals, although intraocular detail was difficult to observe, uveitis was presumed given that the eyes were hypotonous with a mean intraocular pressure 6.3±1.7mmHg compared with the intraocular pressures of 12.6±1.8mmHg in normal eyes as reported above.

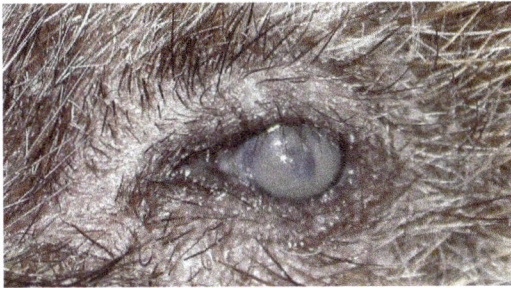

Fig. 6. Hedgehog with corneal oedema and presumed uveitis with a hypotonous globe.

The most common ocular condition was cataract with 57 animals (19%) exhibiting lens opacities, 54 of them bilateral and 51 nuclear (Fig. 7, Table 1).

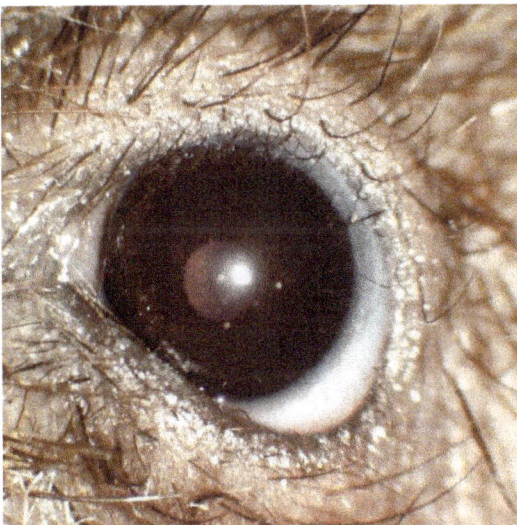

Fig. 7. Nuclear cataract in a 3 month old hedgehog.

There was no sex predeliction for presence of lens opacity with 20% of males and 17% of females affected. There was no significant difference in prevalence in animals of different ages (Fig. 8). The majority of animals examined (194 of 300) were under one year of age but the prevalence of cataract in this group was not higher than in older animals (64 estimated between 1 and 3 years and 42 hedgehogs estimated to be aged 3 years or older).

Table 1. Number of animals affected and overall prevalence of ocular conditions.

Condition	Number of animals affected (prevalence)
Orbital cellulitis/abscessation	4 (1.3%)
Anophthalmos	6 (2%)
Conjunctivitis	4 (1.3%)
Keratitis	3 (1%)
Uveitis	4 (1.3%)
Cataract	57 (19%)

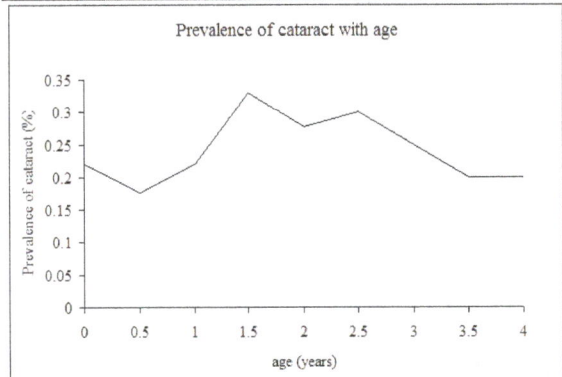

Fig. 8. Prevalence of cataract across age groups of hedgehogs in this study.

Considering all hedgehogs, there was no difference in weight of animals with and without lens opacity (mean weight of hedgehogs with cataract 596±271g, weight of hedgehogs without cataract 654±221g, not significant at p=0.11), while when evaluating only those under one year of age, the weight of hedgehogs with cataracts was substantially lower (384±275g) compared with those with clear lenses (510±258g) this difference significance at p=0.033. This is shown in the graph of weight at different ages (Fig. 9) where in juvenile hedgehogs the filled dots are at the lower end of the weight range while at later stages they are distributed more evenly across the weight range.

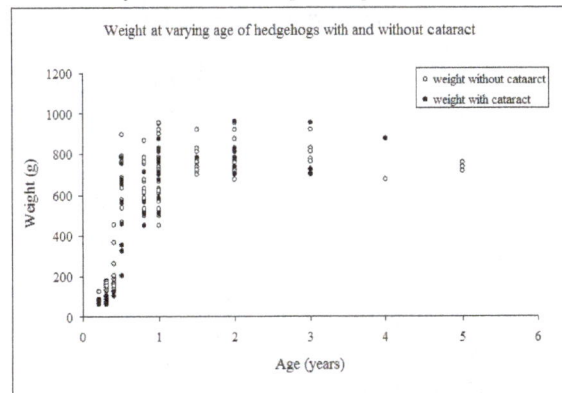

Fig. 9. Graphical representation of age and weight of hedgehogs with and without cataract.

Discussion

The detailed ocular anatomy of the European hedgehog has yet to be published but as a predominantly nocturnal mammal it is deemed to have a primitive optic system and no data on ophthalmic disease in the species has been available until now. However, the anatomically similar African pygmy hedgehog (*Atelerix albiventris*) is an increasingly popular pet, therefore published information relating to ocular procedures and disease is available (Fukuzawa, *et al.*, 2004; Johnson-Delaney, 2006). The European hedgehog *Erinaceus europaeus* belongs to a different genus *(Erinaceus)* from the African pigmy hedgehog which is from the genus *Atelerix* and although they are all from the same subfamily *Erinaceinae* they have quite different environmental requirements. Nevertheless we may be able to extrapolate somewhat from diseases of the African species to those of the European animals examined here.

The combination of wide palpebral fissure and shallow orbits occurring in both species predispose them to injury and proptosis (Wheeler *et al.*, 2001). Additionally, trauma from hedgehog spines, cages, tooth root infections, neoplasia and retrobulbar abscesses are considered contributory factors (Stocker, 1987). Captive obesity can lead to increases in the retrobulbar fat pad, further increasing the risk of proptosis (Stocker, personal communication, 2016), although this was not a problem in the wild animals examined here. In the European hedgehog, prolapse of the eyeball has been noted as a relatively common occurrence (Stocker, personal communication, 2016) and the prevalence of orbits devoid of ocular structures, presumably post-traumatic, in rescued wild hedgehogs here may give weight to concerns regarding the incidence of globe prolapse and subsequent injury. Infection and inflammation of the orbit and adnexa are also relatively commonly seen in the animals examined in this study together with ocular trauma. Injury to other parts of the animal was common in the rescued hedgehogs in the major rescue centres involved in this study with around 15% of the animals examined having some injury to the body (Stocker, personal communication, 2016). Causative factors in those animals included dog attacks, strimmer and lawnmower injuries and road traffic accidents. Many of the ocular conditions seen here, from adnexal defects through keratitis, corneal oedema and uveitis could quite conceivably have originated through trauma. Uveitis was associated with a lower intraocular pressure, although these findings must be interpreted with caution as the rebound tonometer has yet to be validated in this species.

The most striking finding seen in this study though, is one unlikely to have been caused by trauma. Finding nuclear cataracts in a sizeable minority (19%) of the animals examined was not at all expected. The prevalence of cataract did not vary with age, suggesting that these cataracts are congenital or early onset rather than age-related in which case the prevalence of cataract would have increased with age The apparent association with low weight and nuclear cataract could be explained either as a low weight juvenile developing nuclear cataract or as animals with early onset or congenital nuclear cataracts being unable to feed adequately. We consider this latter explanation to be unlikely, as these animals are nocturnal and probably need vision relatively little to search for their invertebrate prey. In addition the hedgehogs rescued which were completely blind were nevertheless in good or at least reasonable body condition suggesting that they were eating well before capture.

The association between poor nutrition and cataract development is acknowledged with regard to poor antioxidant status of the lens predisposing to cataractogenesis in humans and some laboratory rodent studies (Williams, 2006). But generally poor nutrition is correlated with pediatric cataract in several studies (Bamashmus and Al-Akily, 2010; Courtright *et al.*, 2011) often related to oxidative stress (Granot and Kohen, 2004). Other possibilities could involve specific nutritional deficiencies (Hall *et al.*, 1948; Tarwadi *et al.*, 2008), but in wild caught hedgehogs this is considered unlikely. Previous reports have noted cataracts in orphaned puppies fed on mild replacer (Martin and Chambreau, 1982), a factor which might have been significant in underweight juvenile hedgehogs in a rescue facility. Having said that there was no apparent correlation between cataract incidence and feeding of either goat's milk or Esbilac kitten mild replacer in the main rescue centre involved in this study, with all hoglets being fed one or other of these milk substitutes and only a proportion developing cataracts. We thus consider that a link between diet and these lens opacities is not likely, although clearly more work is needed in a prospective study to determine if this is indeed the case.

Other aetiological possibilities for such nuclear cataracts could be genetic with such lens opacities reported in the mouse (Arora *et al.*, 2008) the dog (Heinrich *et al.*, 2006) and the horse (Beech and Irby, 1985). While such a genetic trait is unlikely in a wild population, especially in animals seen in different areas of the country, an inherited agency cannot be ruled out. A final environmental factor which should be considered is ultraviolet light exposure. Animals brought in at a young age or born in captivity are more likely to experience higher levels of UV exposure than those in the wild. The rescue centres operate with artificial light and windows in most rooms which could be resulting in higher exposure to UV light on a daily basis. However UV bulbs or bright fluorescent lights were not used in the facilities where these animals were housed and thus this source of irradiation was not relevant in this study.

Each hedgehog is provided with a towel and nesting material, but despite this many sick hedgehogs may still experience higher exposure due to inability to roll up familiarisation with surroundings. As they become less timid they tend to spend more time waiting with their heads resting on the cage door, facing into the lighted rooms and giving significantly more illumination than they would be used to in the wild. Even so the level of UV-B illumination was very low in these facilities and the glass front of the cages filter out the vast majority of wavelengths which might be considered to cause lens opacification. In addition the cataracts which would be expected to result from excessive ultra-violet light exposure are not nuclear opacities, and so this agency is exceptionally unlikely to be central in their genesis. No mydriatics were used in this study due to unknown effects and safe dose rate in this small species where a single drop of parasympathomimetic absorbed across the conjunctiva into the small blood volume of the animal may have unforeseen effects. This might be considered a limitation of the study since it precluded evaluation of the peripheral lens and optimal fundoscopy, yet even so in a darkened room adequate ophthalmic examination was possible.

Intraocular pressure measurement was readily achieved using the Tonovet rebound tonometer designed initially for use in small eyes of laboratory rodents. The Schirmer tear test strip was, however, found to be too large for such a small globe with so limited a tear production. This limitation could have been overcome by use of the phenol red tear test strip as reported in other small mammals (Lange *et al.*, 2012; Rajaei *et al.*, 2013) but the test was not available to us at the time of this study and we look forward to evaluating it in due course. The major limitation in this study however in our opinion, is that the group of animals examined are in no way a representative sample of the wild population. The animals are likely to be a group biased towards those with disabling conditions both ocular and systemic, the very sort of features which render the hedgehogs liable to be 'rescued' and rehabilitated. Nevertheless given the gradually reducing number of hedgehogs in the British population, it is important to assess the population in rescue centres, to assess the prevalence of potentially debilitating ocular conditions in these animals. A key next step is examination of hedgehogs trapped in the wild to determine whether animals in the truly wild population have the same prevalence of ocular lesions, and particularly nuclear cataracts, than do the animals examined in this study.

Conflict of interest

The Authors declare that there is no conflict of interest.

References

Amori, G., Hutterer, R., Kryštufek, B., Yigit, N., Mitsain, G. and Muñoz, L.J.P. 2011. *Erinaceus europaeus*. In: IUCN 2011. IUCN Red List of Threatened Species. Version 2011.2. www.iucnredlist.org. Accessed on 28 April, 2016.

Arora, A., Minogue, P.J., Liu, X., Addison, P.K., Russel-Eggitt, I., Webster, A.R., Hunt, D.M., Ebihara, L., Beyer, E.C., Berthoud, V.M. and Moore, A.T. 2008. A novel connexin50 mutation associated with congenital nuclear pulverulent cataracts. J. Med. Genet. 45(3), 155-160.

Bamashmus, M.A. and Al-Akily, S.A. 2010. Profile of childhood blindness and low vision in Yemen: a hospital-based study. East Mediterr. Health J. 16(4), 425-428.

Beech, J. and Irby, N. 1985. Inherited nuclear cataracts in the Morgan horse. J. Hered. 76(5), 371-372

Bunnell, T. 2001. The incidence of disease and injury in displaced wild hedgehogs (*E. Eurpaeus*). Lutra 44, 3-14.

Courtright, P., Hutchinson, A.K. and Lewallen, S. 2011. Visual impairment in children in middle- and lower-income countries. Arch. Dis. Child. 96(12), 1129-1134.

Dinopoulos, A.N., Karamanlidis, H., Michaloudi, J., Antonopoulos, H. and Papadopoulos, G. 1987. Retinal projections in the hedgehog (*Erinaeeus europaeus*). An autoradiographic and horseradish peroxidase study. Anat. Embryol. 176, 65-70.

English, M.P., Evans, C.D., Hewitt, M. and Warin, R.P. 1962. Hedgehog ringworm. Brit. Med. J. 1, 149-151.

Fukuzawa, R., Fukuzawa, K., Abe, H., Nagai, T. and Kameyama, K. 2004. Acinic cell carcinoma in an African pygmy hedgehog (*Atelerix albiventris*). Vet. Clin. Pathol. 33(1), 39-42.

Ghaffari, M.S., Hajikhani, R., Sahebjam, F., Akbarein, H. and Golezardy, H. 2012. Intraocular pressure and Schirmer tear test results in clinically normal Long-Eared Hedgehogs (*Hemiechinus auritus*): reference values. Vet. Ophthalmol. 15(3), 206-209.

Granot, E. and Kohen, R. 2004. Oxidative stress in childhood--in health and disease states. Clin. Nutr. 23(1), 3-11.

Hall, W.K., Bowles, L.L., Sydenstricker, V.P. and Schmidt, H.L. 1948. Cataracts due to deficiencies of phenylalanine and of histidine in the rat. A comparison with other types of cataracts. J. Nutr. 36(2), 277-295.

Heinrich, C.L., Lakhani, K.H., Featherstone, H.J. and Barnett, K. 2006. Cataract in the UK Leonberger population. Vet. Ophthal. 9(5), 350-356.

Johnson-Delaney, C.A. 2006. Common procedures in hedgehogs, prairie dogs, exotic rodents, and companion marsupials. Vet. Clin. North Am. Exot. Anim. Pract. 9(2), 415-435.

Kuonen, V.J., Wilkie, D.A., Morreale, R.J., Oglesbee, B. and Barrett-Rephun, K. 2002. Unilateral exophthalmia in a European hedgehog (Erinaceus europaeus) caused by a lacrimal ductal carcinoma. Vet. Ophthal. 5(3), 161-165.

Lange, R.R., Lima, L. and Montiani-Ferreira, F. 2012. Measurement of tear production in black-tufted marmosets (Callithrix penicillata) using three different methods: modified Schirmer's I, phenol red thread and standardized endodontic absorbent paper points. Vet. Ophthalmol. 15(6), 376-382.

Majeed, S.K., Morris, P.A. and Cooper, J.E. 1989. Occurrence of the lungworms *Capillaria* and *Crenosoma* spp. in British hedgehogs (*Erinaceus europaeus*). J. Comp. Pathol. 100(1), 27-36.

Martin, C.L. and Chambreau, T. 1982. Cataract production in experimentally orphaned puppies fed a commercial replacement for bitch's milk. J. Am. Anim. Hosp. Assoc. 18, 115-122.

Morris, P. 1993. A Red Data Book for British Mammals. The Mammal Society, London.

Peichl, L., Künzle, H. and Vogel, P. 2000. Photoreceptor types and distributions in the retinae of insectivores. Vis. Neurosci. 17(6), 937-948.

Rajaei, S.M., Sadjadi, R., Sabzevari, A. and Ghaffari, M.S. 2013. Results of phenol red thread test in clinically normal Syrian hamsters (Mesocricetus auratus). Vet. Ophthalmol. 16(6), 436-439.

Reeve, N. 1994. Hedgehogs. Poyser Natural Histories. London, T&D Posyser.

Reiter, C. and Gould, G.C. 1998. Thirteen ways of looking at a hedgehog. Natural History (American Museum of Natural History, New York.

Robinson, I. and Routh, A. 1999. Veterinary care of the hedgehog. In Practice 21, 128-137.

Stoate, C., Boatman, N.D., Borralho, R.J., Carvalho, C.R., de Snoo, G.R. and Eden, P. 2001. Ecological impacts of arable intensification in Europe. J. Environ. Manage. 63(4), 337-365.

Stocker, L. 1987. The complete hedgehog. Chatto and Windlus, London.

Tarwadi, K.V., Chiplonkar, S.A. and Agte, V. 2008. Dietary and nutritional biomarkers of lens degeneration, oxidative stress and micronutrient inadequacies in Indian cataract patients. Clin. Nutr. 27(3), 464-472.

Thamm, S., Kalko, E.K. and Wells. K. 2009. Ectoparasite infestations of hedgehogs (*Erinaceus europaeus*) are associated with small-scale landscape structures in an urban-suburban environment. Ecohealth 6(3), 404-413

Trewby, I.D., Young, R., McDonald, R.A., Wilson, G.J., Davison, J., Walker, N., Robertson, A., Doncaster, C.P. and Delahay, R.J. 2014. Impacts of removing badgers on localised counts of hedgehogs. PLoS One. 9:e95477.

Wheeler, C.L., Grahn, B.H. and Pocknell, A.M. 2001. Unilateral proptosis and orbital cellulitis in eight African hedgehogs (*Atelerix albiventris*). J. Zoo Wildl. Med. 32(2), 236-241.

Williams, D.L. 2006. Oxidation, antioxidants and cataract formation: a literature review. Vet Ophthalmol. 9(5), 292-298.

Young, R.P., Davison, J., Trewby, I.D., Wilson, G.J., Delahay, R.J. and Doncaster, C.P. 2006. Abundance of hedgehogs (Erinaceus europaeus) in relation to the density and distribution of badgers (Meles meles). J. Zool. 2006;269(3), 349-356.

26

Environmentally toxicant exposures induced intragenerational transmission of liver abnormalities in mice

Mohamed A. Al-Griw[1], Soad A. Treesh[2], Rabia O. Alghazeer[3,*] and Sassia O. Regeai[1]

[1]*Developmental Biology Division, Zoology Department, Faculty of Science, University of Tripoli, Tripoli, Libya*
[2]*Department of Histology and Medical Genetics, Faculty of Medicine, University of Tripoli, Tripoli, Libya*
[3]*Chemistry Department, Faculty of Science, University of Tripoli, Tripoli, Libya*

Abstract

Environmental toxicants such as chemicals, heavy metals, and pesticides have been shown to promote transgenerational inheritance of abnormal phenotypes and/or diseases to multiple subsequent generations following parental and/ or ancestral exposures. This study was designed to examine the potential transgenerational action of the environmental toxicant trichloroethane (TCE) on transmission of liver abnormality, and to elucidate the molecular etiology of hepatocyte cell damage. A total of thirty two healthy immature female albino mice were randomly divided into three equal groups as follows: a sham group, which did not receive any treatment; a vehicle group, which received corn oil alone, and TCE treated group (3 weeks, 100 µg/kg i.p., every 4th day). The F0 and F1 generation control and TCE populations were sacrificed at the age of four months, and various abnormalities histpathologically investigated. Cell death and oxidative stress indices were also measured. The present study provides experimental evidence for the inheritance of environmentally induced liver abnormalities in mice. The results of this study show that exposure to the TCE promoted adult onset liver abnormalities in F0 female mice as well as unexposed F1 generation offspring. It is the first study to report a transgenerational liver abnormalities in the F1 generation mice through maternal line prior to gestation. This finding was based on careful evaluation of liver histopathological abnormalities, apoptosis of hepatocytes, and measurements of oxidative stress biomarkers (lipid peroxidation, protein carbonylation, and nitric oxide) in control and TCE populations. There was an increase in liver histopathological abnormalities, cell death, and oxidative lipid damage in F0 and F1 hepatic tissues of TCE treated group. In conclusion, this study showed that the biological and health impacts of environmental toxicant TCE do not end in maternal adults, but are passed on to offspring generations. Hence, linking observed liver abnormality in the offspring to environmental exposure of their parental line. This study also illustrated that oxidative stress and apoptosis appear to be a molecular component of the hepatocyte cell injury.

Keywords: Apoptosis, Hepatocyte cell injury, Oxidative stress, Parental transmission.

Introduction

In recent years, there is an increasing scientific evidence for the inheritance of environmentally induced abnormal phenotypes and/or diseases from parents to offspring (Skinner *et al.*, 2010). These abnormalities may not be only limited to first generation of descendents but to subsequent generations either exposed (multigenerational inheritance) or unexposed (transgenerational inheritance) (Skinner *et al.*, 2013; Nilsson and Skinner 2014, 2015).

Hence, the concept that today's environmental exposures can significantly affect later generations has been widely accepted under the term "epigenetic inheritance"; the transmission of phenotypic traits (e.g. molecular, cellular, organismal) that involve alterations in gene expression without changes in gene sequence (Nilsson and Skinner, 2014). Epigenetic inheritance has now been shown to be present in plants (Henderson and

Jacobsen, 2007), nematode worms (Greer *et al.*, 2011), flies (Ruden and Lu, 2008), rats (Manikkam *et al.*, 2012), mice (Guerrero-Bosagna *et al.*, 2012), and humans (Pembrey, 2010). Experimental studies in rodents indicate that exposure to environmental toxic substances during intrauterine life, postnatal life, early life, and/or germ cell exposures play a significant role in determining the mature phenotype and susceptibility to diseases in later life (Skinner *et al.*, 2010, 2013). Epigenetic abnormalities/diseases in humans have been documented for reproductive tract abnormalities, brain and behavior abnormalities, immune system abnormalities (Anway *et al.*, 2006a; Crews *et al.*, 2007) as well as kidney (Anway *et al.*, 2006b), ovarian, testis and prostate diseases (Salian *et al.*, 2009; Manikkam *et al.*, 2012; Nilsson *et al.*, 2012; Al-Griw *et al.*, 2015a). A number of environmental factors have been shown to induce transgenerational inheritance of adult onset disease and phenotypic variations (Skinner *et al.*,

*Corresponding Author: Rabia Alghazeer. Chemistry Department, Faculty of Sciences, University of Tripoli, P.O. Box: 13203, Tripoli, Libya. Email: Rabia_alghazeer@yahoo.com

2010). These include exposures to synthetic chemical agents (e.g. hydrocarbons, dioxin, trichloroethylene), pesticides (e.g. methoxychlor, permethrin, dichlorvos, vinclozolin), heavy metals (e.g. cadmium, mercury, arsenic, nickel), and plastics (e.g. bisphenol A, phthalates) (Aitken *et al*., 2004; Wong, 2010; Manikkam *et al.,* 2012; Easley *et al*., 2015).

These environmental exposures can act on both somatic and gamete (sperm or egg) genomes inducing specific altered epigenetic patterns such as DNA methylation, histone modification, and miRNA alterations (Hou *et al*., 2012; Guerrero-Bosagna and Skinner, 2012; Nilsson and Skinner, 2015); that can be transmitted to future generations in the absence of direct environmental exposure (Hou *et al.,* 2012; Skinner *et al*., 2013; Nilsson and Skinner, 2014). Therefore, the transmission of epigenetic variations rather than the direct induction of such variations is responsible for disease states through changes in gene expression and the establishment of heritable states of chromatin architecture (Kelly, 2014).

The transgenerational changes are specific and could be used as biomarkers of exposure and disease (Manikkam *et al.,* 2012; Skinner *et al*., 2013). The current study was designed to investigate the transgenerational actions of a specific environmental toxicant trichloroethane (TCE), an industrial solvent and a degreasing agent, to induce alteration in a somatic cell integrity that correlates to the induction of abnormality in the hepatic tissue.

Recently, it has been reported that TCE exposure environmentally (Al-Griw *et al*., 2015a, 2015c, 2016) or occupationally (Bruckner *et al*., 2001) on a daily basis is associated with increased risk of infertility, low fetal weight and early neonatal neurobehavioral abnormalities (Al-Griw *et al*., 2015b), as well as autoimmunity (Wang *et al*., 2013).

Epigenetic inheritance has been studied extensively in the germ line through *in utero* exposure (Skinner, 2007; Manikkam *et al.,* 2012; Skinner *et al*., 2013). Most studies expose the gestating female F0 generation mice to a toxicant at the time their embryo were undergoing sex determination, the F1 generation mice were exposed directly as a fetus. In addition, the germ cells present in the developing fetus were exposed directly. Furthermore, when F0 generation male is exposed to an environmental insult, his sperm is exposed directly. On the other hand, studies on the epigenetic changes in the somatic cells have been scarce. In addition, there are few studies (Skinner and Guerrero-Bosagna, 2009; Skinner *et al*., 2010) addressed the transgenerational aspects of the environmental toxicant exposures on the subsequent development of an adult somatic cells. Therefore, the purpose of this study was to investigate the ability of TCE to induce intragenerational inheritance of liver abnormalities in F1 generation mice

(offspring) through direct exposure of immature female F0 generation mice (dams); and to elucidate the molecular components of TCE-induced hepatocyte cell injury.

Materials and Methods
Animal Studies and Breeding

The protocol of the study was approved by Libyan National Committee for Biosafety and Bioethics on 2016. All efforts were made to fulfill the ethical experimentation standards such as minimizing the pain during animal handling and experiments as well as reducing the number of animals used. A total of twenty four animals used in this study were immature female Swiss albino mice (F0), 18 to 21 days old, weighing 12 to 15g. They were breed in the animal house of the Zoology Department (Faculty of Science, University of Tripoli, Tripoli, Libya), housed under standard conditions of light (12 hour cycle) and temperature (26 ± 2°C). The animals were fed with a standard mouse diet and *ad libitum* tap water for drinking.

Animals were divided into three groups of eight mice each. The mice were administered twice weekly for three weeks intraperitoneal (*i.p.*) injections of TCE (100 μg/kg body weight every [4]th day) or corn oil positive vehicle control, and the negative sham control did not receive any treatment. At ten weeks of age, treated F0 females were mated with fertility proofed control males. Mating was confirmed by the presence of vaginal plug, which was defined as gestation day-1 (GD-1). Once the vaginal plug was observed, F0 female mice were separated from males and individually caged. F0 pregnant dams were observed daily and total body weight (TBW) was measured daily to further confirm pregnancy. The dams were allowed to deliver naturally and the delivery day was designed as post-natal day 0 (PND-0).

After delivery, F1 litter weights, sex ratios, and percent of dead pups were recorded. Moreover, the size of each litter was standardized on PND-4 by eliminating extra pups through random selection within sex from litters with more than 10 pups to yield 10 pups, with five females and five males per litter. Control litters with 10 or fewer pups were not standardized. The treated female mice were designated as the F0 generation. The offspring of the F0 generation mice were the F1 generation. The control populations were larger than the TCE population due to the lower incidence of abnormality/disease in the control populations.

The increased number of control animals allowed for an increased ability to detect abnormality in the control populations that then allowed for more accurate statistical comparison of the control versus TCE populations. In consistence with our previous observations (Al-Griw *et al*., 2015c), we have found alterations in sex ratios, but not in litter size, in the F1 generations for the TCE, but not control animals.

Clinical Assessment

The clinical assessment included animal survival, TBW, weight gain/loss and locomotor activity. During the course of the exposure period, mice were observed twice daily for any abnormal clinical signs or behavior that may result from toxicity. Night deaths were recorded the next morning. Two independent observers confirmed the cause of death to exclude TCE-nonrelated mortality. A subset of F1 generation offspring of control and TCE populations was randomly selected to examine congenital malformations.

Tissue Harvest and Histopathology Processing

F0 and F1 generation mice (2 males and 2 females from each litter) were sacrificed at postnatal day 120 (four months) for tissue harvest. Body and organ (e.g. liver) weights were measured at dissection time. Livers were fixed in 10% formalin, and then processed for paraffin embedding by standard procedures for histopathology examination.

Six to eight micrometer tissue sections were made, stained and examined for histopathology. Portions of livers from control and TCE populations were stored at -20 °C for the measurment of oxidative stress biomarkers. Blood samples were also collected at the time of dissection, allowed to clot, centrifuged and serum samples stored for further analysis.

Histopathology

All histopathology was examined in randomly selected animals by three independent observers. H&E stain was used for general histopathological changes. For specific liver damage special stains: Mallory Trichrome (MTC) and Periodic Acid-Schiff stain (PAS) were used. Liver histopathology criteria included the presence of a vacuole, steatosis and inflammatory infiltrates and 'other' abnormalities including fibrotic and hepatocyte alterations (cell with vacuolated and pale-staining cytoplasm) as well as alterations in nuclear morphology.

A cut-off was established to declare a tissue 'diseased' based on the mean number of histopathological abnormalities plus two standard deviations from the mean of control tissues. This number was used to classify mice into those with and without liver abnormality in each population. A mouse tissue section was finally declared 'diseased' only when two of the three observers marked the same tissue section 'diseased'. The proportion of mice with obesity was obtained by counting those that had these conditions out of all the animals evaluated. The number of animals per litter (litter representation) mean ± SEM used for the control versus TCE population comparisons for each specific abnormality was found not to be statistically different ($P > 0.05$). Therefore, no litter representation differences or litter bias was detected for any of the specific abnormality assessed.

Scoring of Cell Death

To assess cell death, images of H&E-stained liver tissues were opened in ImageJ software (version 1.45) and a manual count was performed. Cell counts were expressed as a percentage of the number present for each treatment group and an overall percentage obtained by averaging the data for all cells within a treatment group. The hepatocellular apoptotic cells were then quantified. Hepatocytes undergoing apoptosis were identified by morphological criteria such as cell shrinkage, chromatin condensation and margination, and apoptotic bodies (Gujral et al., 2001). However, hepatocytes undergoing necrosis were determined using the criteria such as increased eosinophilia, cell swelling and lysis, loss of architecture, karyolysis, and karyorrhexis (Gujral et al., 2002). The percent of cell death was estimated by evaluating the number of microscopic fields with dead cells compared to the entire histologic section.

The scoring scale was set from 0 (worst) to 5 (best), with the following criteria: (0): no tissue damage; (1): mild; (2): mild to moderate; (3): moderate; (4): moderate to severe; and (5): severe. For each liver tissue, the eight scores were averaged, and this average was considered as a replicate.

Lipid Peroxidation Measurment

Lipid peroxidation levels in the livers from F0 and F1 generation control and TCE populations was determined spectrophotometrically as a concentration of final lipid peroxidation products, which in reaction with thiobarbituric acid (TBARS) form colour complex (thiobarbituric acid-reactive substances; TBARS). In brief, liver tissues were homogenized with a tissue homogenizer (IKA, RW 20.n, Germany) in ice-cold 10% (w/v) phosphate-buffered saline (PBS) solution. After centrifugation, a 500 µL aliquot of liver homogenate samples were added to 2 ml of TCA-TBA HCL reagent (thioarbituric acid 0.37%, 0.24 N HCL and 15% TCA) and then boiled at 100 °C for 15 min, and allowed to cool. After centrifugation (Sigma 2K15, Germany) at 3000 rpm for 10 min, the supernatant was removed and the absorbance was read at 532 nm. The calibration curve was obtained using different concentrations of 1, 1, 3, 3-tetramethoxypropane as standard to determine the concentration of TBA-MDA (malondialdehyde; MDA) adducts in the samples (Zhang et al., 2004).

Nitric Oxide Measurment

Nitric oxide in the livers from F1 generation control and TCE populations was determined as described previously (Xu et al., 2011) with some modification. The liver samples were homogenized in cold 0.9% saline. The homogenates were then centrifuged at 10,000 rpm for 5 min at 4 °C. 1 ml of the supernatant was mixed with an equal volume of Greiss reagent containing 1% sulphanilamide and 0.1%

naphthylethylenediamine in 5% phosphoric acid. The mixture was then allowed to stand at room temperature for 30 min. The absorbance of the mixture was measured against the corresponding blank solutions at 546 nm. Sodium nitrate solution was used to obtain a standard curve.

Isolation and Measurment of Total Protein

Livers from F0 and F1 generation control and TCE populations were homogenized in sodium phosphate buffer pH 7.4. The homogenate was then centrifuged at 6000 x g at 4 °C for 15 min, and the supernatants collected were used for protein assay (Goa, 1953; Bradford, 1976). Bovine serum albumin was used as a standard.

Protein Carbonyl Measurment

Carbonyl content in the in the livers from F1 generation control and TCE populations was quantitated by the protein carbonyl assay as previous described (Wang *et al.*, 2013).

Microscopy

The liver cytoarchitecture and cell death scoring were observed and imaged using a low-power objective under a light microscope (Leica, Germany).

Statistical analysis

Data are expressed as means ± SEM. A computerized Kolmogorov-Smirnov test was used to determine whether the data fitted a normal distribution. Statistical analysis was performed using one-way ANOVA followed by a post-hoc test for multiple comparisons within SPSS 20.0 for Windows. Two tailed Student's *t* test was used when only two independent groups were compared. *P*-values less than 0.05 were considered statistically significant.

Result

The present study provides experimental evidence for intragenerational transmission of liver abnormality. The results of this study show that exposure to the environmental toxicant TCE promoted adult onset liver abnormalities in F0 female mice as well as unexposed F1 generation offspring (Fig. 1). It is the first study to report a transgenerational liver abnormality in the F1 generation mice through maternal line prior to gestation. Transgenerational inheritance signifies that environmental toxic effects manifested in the exposed generation also appear in the unexposed future generation(s). This finding was based on careful evaluation of liver histopathological abnormalities, apoptosis of hepatocytes, and measurements of oxidative stress biomarkers (lipid peroxidation, nitric oxide and protein carbonylation) in control and TCE groups (as explained below). There was an increase in liver histopathological abnormalities, cell death, and oxidative lipid damage in F0 and F1 hepatic tissues. Therefore, these results indicate exposure of immature F0 female mice to TCE transgenerationally transmitted

liver histopathology to their F1 generation offspring implying transgenerational transmission.

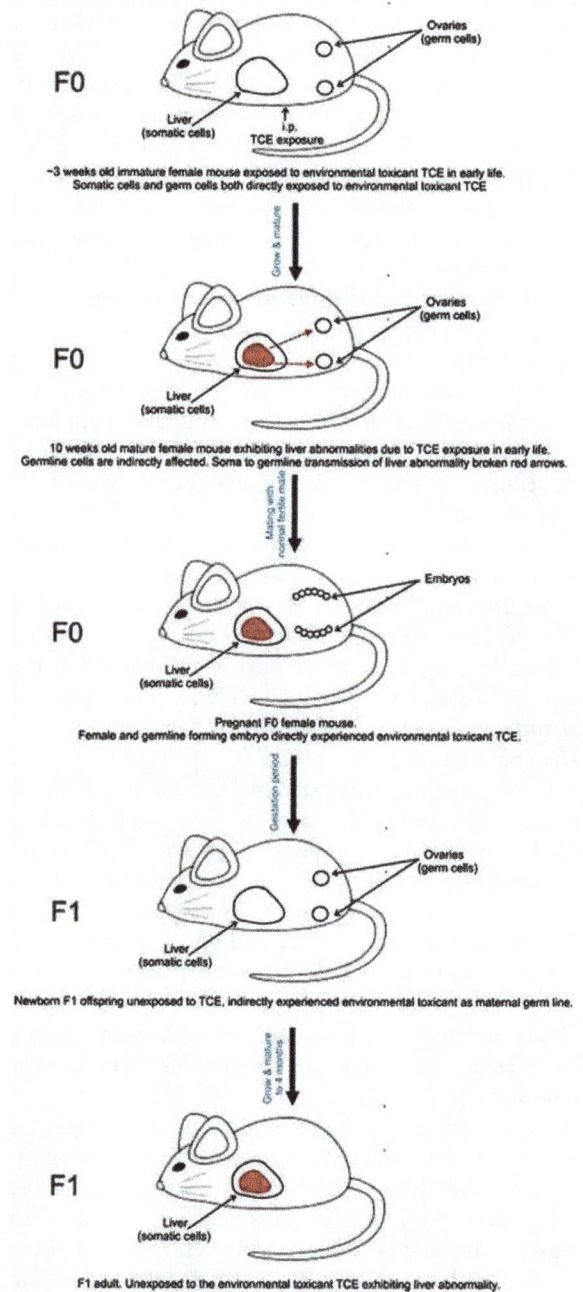

Fig. 1. Schematic early life exposures to the environmental toxicant TCE induce liver abnormality which leads to liver abnormality in later life. This is passed on to F1 generation indicating intragenerational inheritance of liver abnormalities and perhaps soma to germline transmission. In this study offspring (F1 generation) have never been exposed to environmental toxicant. F0 immature female somatic cells (e.g. ovaries) and germ cells (e.g. oocytes) were directly exposed to environmental toxicant in early life. TCE exposure caused epigenetic variations in the germline indirectly (red broken arrows) through its effect on somatic liver cells.

Liver Abnormality and Histopathology

Liver abnormalities were characterized by the presence of several histopathological lesions which included: disturbed parenchyma architecture of the hepatic lobules, infiltration of mononuclear cells (macrophages and lymphocytes) around central veins and in portal areas, some dilated congested blood vessels; severe cytoarchitectural distortions of the hepatocytes accompanied by steatosis and inflammatory infiltrates, and complete loss of nucleus (Fig. 2A) was found throughout hepatic tissue of TCE treated F0 and F1 mice. The incidence of liver abnormality in F0 and F1 of control and TCE l populations is presented in Figure 2B. There was a statistically significant increase in liver abnormality in TCE F0 generation compared to control F0 generation (Fig. 2B).

To further study the effect of TCE on liver histopathology, liver sections from F0 and F1 control and TCE groups were stained with two special stains Mallory's trichrome (MTC) and Periodic Acid-Schiff stain (PAS). The F0 and F1 control population showed normal liver architecture. Whereas the F1 generation mice of TCE populations showed destructed nuclei of hepatocytes, vacuolated cytoplasm; completely loss of the hepatocytes, mild pericellular fibrosis is present in lobule and periportal distribution and is associated with portal–portal linkage, massive accumulation of monocellular phagocytic cells around the blood vessels. There was also deposition of collagen fibers, the cytoplasmic vacuolation were still observed (Fig. 3).

In contrast to control populations, TCE F1 generation showed a remarkable reduction in the glycogen storage as well as carbohydrate content (Fig. 4).

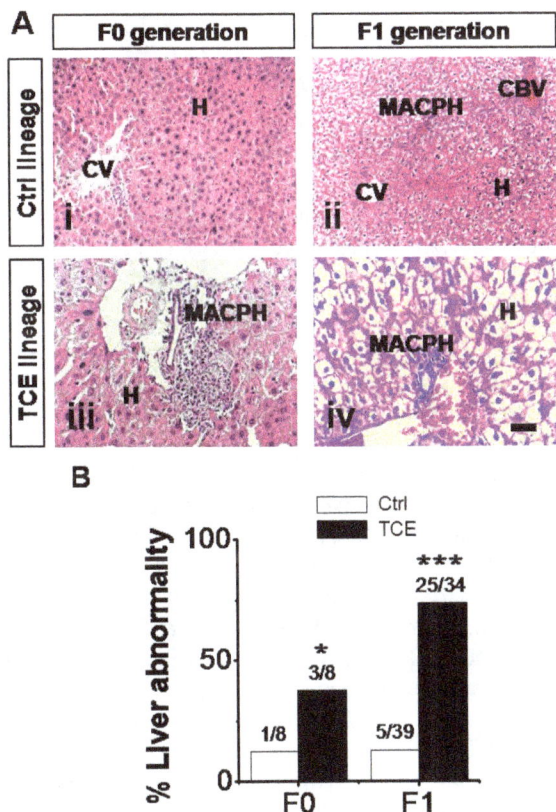

Fig. 2. Control (Ctrl) and TCE F0 and F1 generation adult-onset liver abnormality. (A) Micrographs H&E–stained sections show liver abnormality in F0 (panel iii) and F1 (panel iv) generation TCE animals compared to F0 (panel i) and (panel ii) Ctrl populations. Hepatocytes (H), central vein (CV), congested blood vessels (CBV), and macrophages (MACPH). Scale bar = 100 μm, 40X. (B) Percentages of mice with liver abnormality and number of diseased mice/total number of mice. Ctrl and TCE livers were examined with the mean ± SEM presented and asterisks (*) indicating a statistically significant difference ($P \leq 0.05$) vs. TCE-treated mice. Student's t-tests. *$P \leq 0.05$, ***$P \leq 0.001$.

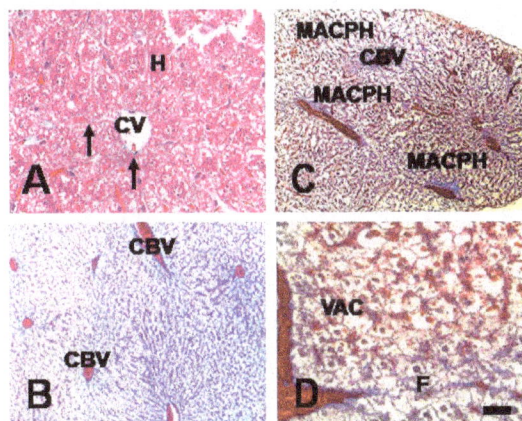

Fig. 3. Ctrl and TCE F1 generation adult-onset liver abnormality. Micrographs of MTC–stained liver sections show liver abnormality in F1 generation TCE populations (panel C and D) compared to that in F1 Ctrl population (panel A and B). Hepatocytes (H), central vein (CV), congested blood vessels (CBV), macrophages (MACPH), and vacuolated cytoplasm (VAC). Scale bar = 100 μm, 40X. To observe the location of hepatic glycogen granules and the glycogen density of hepatocytes, PAS stain was used.

Hepatocyte Nuclear Alterations

The percent of hepatocellular apoptosis was determined by strict morphological criteria. There was morphological evidence of apoptosis for individual hepatocyte cells in F0 and F1 generation of TCE population compared to control population. Nuclear morphological abnormality was characterized by prominent chromatin condensation, DNA fragmentation, and the formation of apoptotic bodies. This was accompanied by other degenerative changes (Fig. 5A), but no such changes were found in control populations. The quantitative analysis showed that the F0 and F1 generations of TCE populations had an increased percent of apoptotic hepatocyte cells compared to F0 and F1 generations control population (Fig. 5B).

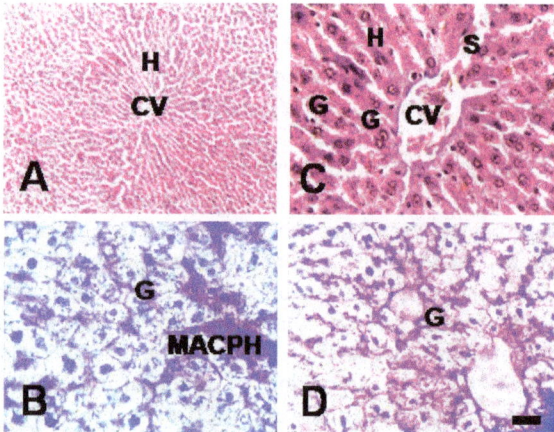

Fig. 4. Ctrl and TCE F1 generation adult-onset liver abnormality. Micrographs of PAS–stained sections show liver abnormality in F1 generation TCE populations (panel **C** and **D**) compared to Ctrl F1 generation (panel **A** and **B**). Hepatocytes (H), central vein (CV), congested blood vessels (CBV), macrophages (MACPH), glycogen (G), and vacuolated cytoplasm (VAC). Scale bar = 100 μm, 63X.

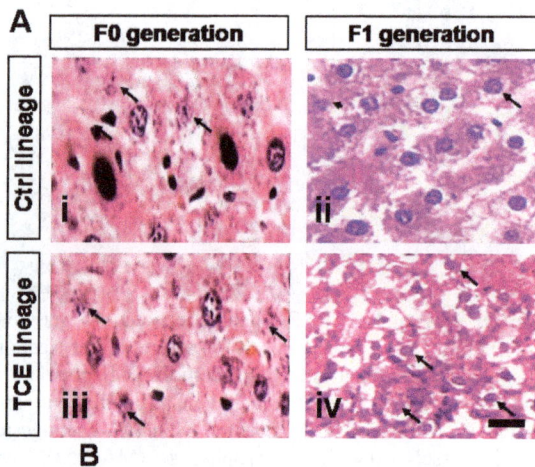

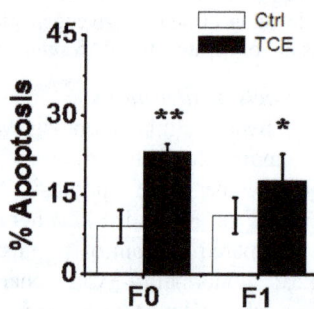

Fig. 5. Hepatocellular apoptosis in Ctrl and TCE F0 and F1 generation. (**A**) Micrographs H&E–stained sections show hepatocellular apoptosis in F0 (panel iii) and F1 (panel iv) generation TCE population compared to F0 (panel i) and (panel ii) Ctrl population. Scale bar = 100 μm, 63X. (**B**) Percentages of hepatocellular apoptosis. Ctrl and TCE livers were examined with the mean ± SEM presented and asterisks (*) indicating a statistically significant difference ($P \leq 0.05$) vs. TCE-treated mice. Student's t-tests. $*P \leq 0.05$, $**P \leq 0.01$.

Lipid Peroxidation in the Livers of the F0 and F1 Generations

Lipid peroxidation determination in hepatic tissues of control and TCE F0 and F1 generations was performed by the TBARS method. Levels of liver MDA formation in the four months old F0 and F1 generations of TCE population significantly increased compared to F0 and F1 generations of control, respectively, (Fig. 6), but no difference between sham and vehicle controls. Observations indicate that there were major F1 generation toxicological effects from the indirect TCE exposure.

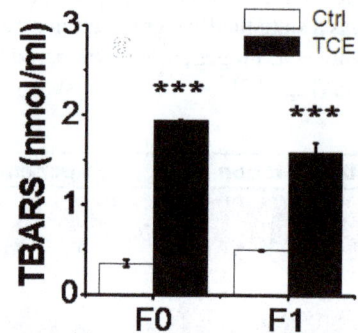

Fig. 6. Oxidative stress biomarker TBARS levels (nmol/ml) in Ctrl and TCE F0 and F1 generations. Ctrl and TCE liver TBARS levels were examined with the mean ± SEM presented and asterisks (*) indicating a statistically significant difference ($P \leq 0.05$) vs. TCE-treated mice. Student's t-tests. $***P \leq 0.001$.

Protein Carbonylation and Nitric Oxide in the Livers of the F1 Generation

Protein carbonyl content is not only a biomarker of oxidative stress, but also provides evidence of oxidative protein damage (Morgan et al., 2005). To evaluate the extent of protein oxidation in liver, protein carbonyls in this major organ, which is targets of TCE, was also analyzed. Our data showed that carbonyl protein content in the liver was significantly increased in TCE F1 generation compared to that in control F1 generation (Fig. 7A), suggesting increased protein oxidation (carbonylation) as a result of indirect exposure to TCE. Then we have assessed the status of inflammation in F1 generation livers by measuring nitric oxide levels in livers concerning markers of inflammation, levels of nitric oxide in livers were strongly increased in TCE F1 generation compared to that in control population F1 generation (Fig. 7B). These data correlated well with the increased oxidative lipid damage in F0 and F1 hepatic tissues. Observations indicate F0 generation parents exposed to TCE intragenerationally transmitted liver histopathology to their unexposed F1 generation descendants. Taken together, these observations indicate that maternal generation directly exposed to TCE transgenerationally transmitted liver abnormality to their unexposed F1 generation descendants.

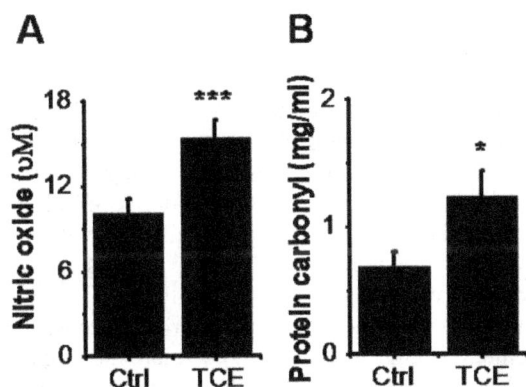

Fig. 7. Oxidative stress biomarkers in Ctrl and TCE F1 generations. (**A**) Nitric oxide (μM) in the livers of Ctrl and TCE F1 generations. (**B**) Protein carbonyl content (mg/ml) in the liver of Ctrl and TCE F1 generation. Liver oxidative stress biomarkers were examined in Ctrl and TCE groups with the mean $\pm$ SEM presented and asterisks (*) indicating a statistically significant difference ($P \leq 0.05$) vs. control. Student's t-tests. *$P \leq 0.05$, ***$P \leq 0.001$.

Discussion

The present study demonstrates that maternal exposure to the environmental toxicant TCE promoted the transmission of abnormal liver phenotypes between generations (intragenerational inheritance) based on nontoxic pharmacological dose 0.1% of the oral LD50 for TCE. This study provides evidence of the activation and/or inhibition of different proteins involved in oxidative stress and cell damage in an animal model of a chemically induced hepatotoxicity. Liver histology, biomarkers of oxidative stress and nuclear alterations related to molecular and cellular mechanisms of hepatocyte cell damage were measured in control and TCE F0 and F1 generations. Oxidative stress biomarker levels (e.g. lipid peroxidation, protein carbonyl, and nitric oxide), indicative of hepatic tissue damage and hepatocyte cell injury, as well as hepatocellular apoptosis were significantly increased in the TCE F0 and F1 generations compared to that in control, reaching values similar to those previously reported in other models of progressive cirrhosis induced in rat by repeated injections of diethyl nitrosamine (DEN) (Guiu et al., 2012).

Many studies reported that exposure to environmental insults may promote the transition of abnormal phenotypes between generations (Jones et al., 1996; Anway et al., 2005). The results of this study support our findings from previous studies in mice (Al-Griw et al., 2015b) by examining a variety of different abnormalities states in four-month-old male mice and characterizing the transgenerational changes in the F1 generation sperms (Al-Griw et al., 2015a). Early exposure to TCE reduces fertility and negatively affects pregnancy outcomes across multiple generations (Al-Griw et al., 2015c). Alterations in sperm quality and

testicular tissue architecture in the F1 generation offspring were observed after direct TCE exposure of the F0 generation parents. Other toxic effects of direct exposure to TCE included increase in relative liver weight and histopathological lesions (Xia and Yu, 1992; Al-Griw et al., 2016), weight loss (NTP, 2000; EPA, 2003), and kidney damage (NTP, 2000). Other studies showed evidence for the neurobehavioral and developmental teratogenicity of intermittent prenatal TCE exposure to high concentrations of TCE in rats (Jones et al., 1996; Coleman et al., 1999; Al-Griw et al., 2015b). Exposure of F0 generation gestating rats to environmental toxicant bisphenol-A (BPA) caused decreased fertility in F3 generation males (Salian et al., 2009). Vinclozolin exposure resulted in testis disease, prostate disease, kidney disease, immune system abnormalities, tumors, uterine hemorrhage during pregnancy and polycystic ovarian disease (Anway et al., 2005; Guerrero-Bosagna et al., 2012; Guerrero-Bosagna and Skinner, 2012; Nilsson et al., 2012); and alterations in the methylation patterns of imprinted genes in sperm of F3 generation male mice.

The transgenerational phenomena of toxic effects involve the transmission of abnormal phenotypes independently of direct exposure (Anway et al., 2006a,b). Two possible mechanisms induce abnormal phenotype through transgeneration of toxic effects, the first is alteration in genetic material structure such as DNA sequence change, the second one includes the changing in epigenetic information such as histone acetylation and methylation, or DNA methylation (Rakyan and Whitelaw, 2003; Skinner, 2007; Nadea, 2009). Animals studies show that parental exposure (F0 generation) to a variety of environmental factors can lead to observable effects (including both genetic and epigenetic) in the somatic cells of their offspring over several generations that are not attributable to the inheritance of a simple mutation through the parental germ line. Interestingly, we also demonstrate intragenerational inheritance of somatic (hepatocyte) effects induced by TCE in mice. This was accompanied by a significant decrease in the hepatocyte integrity. Perhaps, these findings indirectly support circumstantial evidence that hereditary information may transfer from soma to the germline. It has been reported that several environmental exposures can act on both somatic and germ cell genome replication and transcription, influencing the establishment and/or maintenance of specific epigenetic patterns (Guerrero-Bosagna and Skinner, 2012) that are transmitted to future generations in the absence of continued environmental exposures. The environmental exposures can cause heritable modifications (e.g. phenotypic variations) in the germline directly or indirectly through their primary effects on the soma (Jablonka, 2012; Sharma, 2013). Factors such as RNAs and hormones, including neurohormones and neuropeptides, have previously been considered to potentially mediate soma to germline communication in epigenetic inheritance (Jablonka, 2012). Cossetti *et al*. (2014) suggested that exosomes (extracellular vesicles) carrying various RNAs shed by somatic cells are carriers of flow of information from somatic cells to gametes (germ cells). It has been revealed that a flow of hereditary information can be transferred from the soma to the germline, escaping the principle of the Weismann barrier (Weismann, 1993) which postulates that somatically acquired genetic variations cannot be transferred to the germline (Cossetti *et al*., 2014). In consistent, we have demonstrated transgenerational inheritance of somatic effects induced by TCE in mice in the absence of continued TCE exposure. We have found that the vast majority of the livers in the F0 generation (parents) carried a hepatocyte (somatic) cell defect of increased apoptosis. This increased apoptosis persisted into the F1 generation (offspring), and in outcrossed offspring, exhibiting non-Mendelian genetic inheritance and affecting 90% of the mouse populations. Because the female F0-generation mice were directly exposed to the toxicant TCE before gestation, the F1-generation animals were not exposed directly. In addition, the germ cells present in the F0 generation were exposed directly to TCE. These exposed germ cells created the offspring (F1 generation). Therefore, the first generation without direct environmental exposure is the F1 generation, and this is the first generation said to exhibit transgenerational inheritance of disease susceptibility. Together, these findings suggest transgenerational inheritance of somatic effects.

In conclusion, environmental and/or occupational exposure to toxic substances (i.e. chemicals, pesticides, plastics, and heavy metals) continues to be a major worldwide public health concern. Many of these environmental toxicants are widely spread and difficult to degrade in the environment (Shi *et al*., 2008). It is estimated that approximately 24% of human diseases are caused by exposure to environmental toxicants (Hou *et al*., 2012); with the possibility of these diseases to be transmitted to future generations in the absence of direct exposure. In this study, we have shown that direct exposure of maternal generation to environmental toxicant TCE can promote inheritance of adult-onset liver abnormality. Associated with the occurrence of this transgenerational abnormality may be genetics/epigenetic alterations in mouse hepatocyte cell DNA. This transgenerational inheritance may be useful as early stage biomarkers of compound exposure and adult onset abnormality/disease. Although not designed for risk assessment, these findings have implications for the human populations that are exposed to a variety of toxicants. Especially to those who are experiencing

declines in fertility and increases in adult onset abnormality/disease, with a potential to transmit them to future offspring generations. The degree that environmentally induced transgenerational inheritance of phenotypic variations and/ or adult-onset disease is implicated in human disease etiology remains unknown. However, since the majority of chronic diseases have increased dramatically over the past decades, environmental exposures and transgenerational epigenetics will likely be a component of disease etiology to seriously consider in the future (Skinner *et al*., 2013). A more thorough and mechanistic understanding of the molecular etiology of disease, including the role of environmental epigenetics, is anticipated to provide insights into new diagnostics and therapeutics for specific diseases.

Conflict of interest
The authors declare that they have no competing interests.

Acknowledgements
This investigation was supported in part by the Division of Developmental Biology, Zoology Department, Faculty of Science, University of Tripoli, Tripoli, Libya.

References

Aitken, R.J., Koopman, P. and Lewis, S.E.M. 2004. Seeds of concern. Nature 432, 48-52.

Al-Griw, M.A., Al-Azreg, S.A., Bennour, E.M., El-Mahgiubi, S.A.M., Al-Attar, A.R., Salama, N.M. and Elnfati, A.S. 2015c. Fertility and Reproductive Outcome in Mice Following Trichloroethane (TCE) Exposure. Am. J. Life Sci. Res. 3, 293-303.

Al-Griw, M.A., Al-Ghazeer, R.O., Al-Azreg, S.A. and Bennour, E.M. 2016. Cellular and Molecular Etiology of Hepatocyte Injury in a Murine Model of Environmentally Induced Liver Abnormality. Open Vet. J. 6(3), 150-157.

Al-Griw, M.A., Maamar, M.S., Salama, N.M., Algadi, L.N., Elnfati, A.S. and Bennour, E.M. 2015b. Maternal Exposure of Mouse to Low-Dose of Trichloroethane is Associated with Increased Birth Weight and Early Neonatal Neurobehavioral abnormalities. Am. J. Biol. Life Sci. 3, 206-210.

Al-Griw, M.A., Salama, N.M., Treesh, S.A. and Elnfati, A.H. 2015a. Transgenerational Genetic Effect of Trichloroethane (TCE) on Phenotypic Variation of Acrosomal Proteolytic Enzyme and Male Infertility Risk. Int. J. Genet. Genomics 3(5), 43-49.

Anway, M.D., Cupp, A.S., Uzumcu, M. and Skinner, M.K. 2005. Epigenetic transgenerational actions of endocrine disruptors and male fertility. Sci. 308, 1466-1469.

Anway, M.D., Leathers, C. and Skinner, M.K. 2006a. Endocrine disruptor vinclozolin induced epigenetic transgenerational adult-onset disease. Endocrinology 147, 5515-5523.

Anway, M.D., Memon, M.A., Uzumcu, M. and Skinner, M.K. 2006b. Transgenerational effect of the endocrine disruptor vinclozolin on male spermatogenesis. J. Androl. 27, 868-879.

Bradford, M.M. 1976. A rapid and sensitive method for the quantification of microgram quantities of protein utilizing the principle of protein-dye binding. Anal. Biochem. 72, 248-254.

Bruckner, J.V., Kyle, G.M., Luthra, R., Acosta, D., Mehta, S.M., Sethuraman, S. and Muralidhara, S. 2001. Acute, short-term, and subchronic oral toxicity of 1,1,1-trichloroethane in rats. Toxicol. Sci. 60, 363-372.

Coleman, C.N., Mason, T. and Hooker, E.P. 1999. Developmental effects of intermittent prenatal exposure to 1,1,1-trichloroethane in the rat. Neurotoxicol. Teratol. 21, 699-708.

Cossetti, C., Lugini, L., Astrologo, L., Saggio, I., Fais, S. and Spadafora, C. 2014. Soma-to-Germline Transmission of RNA in Mice Xenografted with Human Tumour Cells: Possible Transport by Exosomes. PLoS One. 9: e101629.

Crews, D., Gore, A.C., Hsu, T.S., Dangleben, N.L. and Spinetta, M. 2007. Transgenerational epigenetic imprints on mate preference. Proc. Natl. Acad. Sci. U. S. A. 104, 5942-5946.

Easley, I.V., Bradner, J.M., Mosera, A., Rickmana, C.A., McEachina, Z.T., Merritt, M.M., Hansenc, J.M. and Caudle, W.M. 2015. Assessing reproductive toxicity of two environmental toxicants with a novel in vitro human spermatogenic model. Stem Cell Res. 14, 347-355.

EPA, U. S. 2003. Interpretation of body weight data; Health Effects Division (HED) Guidance Document #G2003.01. Prepared by the HED Toxicology Science Advisory Council, Health Effects Division, Office of Pesticide Programs (OPP), July 1.

Goa, J. 1953. A Micro Biuret Method for Protein Determination Determination of Total Protein in Cerebrospinal Fluid. Scand. J. Clin. Lab. Invest. 5, 218-222.

Greer, E.L., Maures, T.J., Ucar, D., Hauswirth, A.G. and Mancini, E. 2011. Transgenerational epigenetic inheritance of longevity in Caenorhabditis elegans . Nature 479, 365-371.

Guerrero-Bosagna, C., Covert, T., Haque, M.M., Settles, M. and Nilsson, E.E. 2012. Epigenetic Transgenerational Inheritance of Vinclozolin Induced Mouse Adult Onset Disease and Associated Sperm Epigenome Biomarkers. Reprod. Toxicol. 34, 694-707.

Guerrero-Bosagna, C. and Skinner, M.K. 2012. Environmentally induced epigenetic transgenerational inheritance of phenotype and disease. Mol. Cell Endocrinol. 354, 3-8.

Guiu, B., Deschamps, F., Boulin, M., Boige, V., Malka, D., Ducreux, M., Hillon, P. and de Baère, T. 2012. Serum gamma-glutamyl-transferase indepen-dently predicts outcome after transarterial chemoembolization ofhepatocellular carcinoma: external validation. Cardiovasc. Intervent. Radiol. 35, 1102-1108.

Gujral, J.S., Bucci, T.J., Farhood, A. and Jaeschke, H. 2001. Mechanism of Cell Death During Warm Hepatic Ischemia-Reperfusion in Rats: Apoptosis or Necrosis? Histol. 33, 397-405.

Gujral, J.S., Knight, T.R., Farhood, A., Bajt, M.L. and Jaeschke, H. 2002. Mode of cell death after acetaminophen overdose in mice: apoptosis or oncotic necrosis? Toxicol. Sci. 67, 322-328.

Henderson, I.R. and Jacobsen, S.E. 2007. Epigenetic inheritance in plants. Nature 447, 418-424.

Hou, L., Zhang, X., Wang, D. and Baccarelli, A. 2012. Environmental chemical exposures and human epigenetics. Int. J. Epidemiol. 41, 79-105.

Jablonka, E. 2012. Epigenetic inheritance and plasticity: the responsive germline. Prog. Biophys. Mol. Biol. 111(2-3), 99-107.

Jones, H.E., Kunko, P.M. and Robinson, S.E. 1996. Developmental consequences of intermittent and continuous prenatal exposure to 1,1,1-trichloroethane in mice. Pharmacol. Biochem. Behavior 55, 635-646.

Kelly, W.G. 2014. Transgenerational epigenetics in the germline cycle of Caenorhabditis elegans. Epigenetics Chromatin 7, 1-17.

Manikkam, M., Guerrero-Bosagna, C., Tracey, R., Haque, M.M. and Skinner, M.K. 2012. Transgenerational actions of environmental compounds on reproductive disease and identification of epigenetic biomarkers of ancestral exposures. PLoS One. 7: e31901.

Morgan, P.E., Sturgess, A.D. and Davies, M.J. 2005. Increased levels of serum protein oxidation and correlation with disease activity in systemic lupus erythematosus. Arthritis Rheum. 52, 2069-2079.

Nadea, J.H. 2009. Transgenerational genetic effects on phenotypic variation and disease risk. Hum. Mol. Genet. 18, R202-R210.

Nilsson, E., Larsen, G., Manikkam, M., Guerrero-Bosagna, C. and Savenkova, M. 2012. Environmentally Induced Epigenetic Transgenerational Inheritance of Ovarian Disease. PLoS One. 7: e36129.

Nilsson, E.E. and Skinner, M.K. 2014. Definition of Epigenetic Transgenerational Inheritance and Biological Impacts. Transgenerational Epigenetics. Washington State University, Pullman, WA, USA, pp: 11-16.

Nilsson, E.E. and Skinner, M.K. 2015. Environmentally induced epigenetic transgenerational inheritance of disease susceptibility. Transl. Res. 165, 12-17.

NTP. 2000. NTP technical report on the toxicity studies of 1,1,1-trichloroethane (CAS no.71-55-6) administered in microcapsules in feed to F344/N rats and B6C3F1 mice. Public Health Service, U.S. Department of Health and Human Services; NTP Toxicity Report Series No. 41. National Institute of Environmental Health Sciences, Research Triangle Park, NC, and National Technical Information Service, Springfield, VA; PB2001-100, 476 online: http://ntp.niehs.nih.gov/ntp/htdocs/ST_rpts/tox041.pdf.

Pembrey, M.E. 2010. Male-line transgenerational responses in humans. Hum. Fertil. (Camb). 13, 268-271.

Rakyan, V. and Whitelaw, E. 2003. Transgenerational epigenetic inheritance. Curr. Biol. 13, R6.

Ruden, D.M. and Lu, X. 2008. Hsp90 affecting chromatin remodeling might explain transgenerational epigenetic inheritance in Drosophila. Curr. Genomics 9, 500-508.

Salian, S., Doshi, T. and Vanage, G. 2009. Impairment in protein expression profile of testicular steroid receptor coregulators in male rat offspring perinatally exposed to Bisphenol A. Life Sci. 85, 11-18.

Sharma, A. 2013. Transgenerational epigenetic inheritance: Focus on soma to germline information transfer. Prog. Biophys. Mol. Biol. 113, 439-446.

Shi, X., Zhou, S., Wang, Z., Zhou, Z. and Wang, Z. 2008. CYP1A1 and GSTM1 polymorphisms and lung cancer risk in Chinese populations: A meta-analysis. Lung Cancer 59, 155-163.

Skinner, M.K. 2007. Endocrine disruptors and epigenetic transgenerational disease etiology.
Pediatr. Res. 61, 48R-50R.

Skinner, M.K. and Guerrero-Bosagna, C. 2009. Environmental signals and transgenerational epigenetics. Epigonomics 1, 111-117.

Skinner, M.K., Manikkam, M. and Guerrero-Bosagna, C. 2010. Epigenetic transgenerational actions of environmental factors in disease etiology. Trends Endocrinol. Metab. 21, 214-222.

Skinner, M.K., Manikkam, M., Tracey, R., Guerrero-Bosagna, C., Haque, M. and Nilsson, E.E. 2013. Ancestral dichlorodiphenyltrichloroethane (DDT) exposure promotes epigenetic transgenerational inheritance of obesity. BMC Medicine 11, 1-16.

Wang, G., Wang, J., Ma, H., Ansari, G.A.S. and Khan, M.F. 2013. N-Acetylcysteine protects against trichloroethene-mediated autoimmunity by attenuating oxidative stress. Toxicol. Appl. Pharmacol. 273, 189-195.

Weismann, A. 1993. The germ-plasm: a theory of heredity. Charles Scribner's Sons; New York, USA: Electronic Scholarly Publishing.

Wong, E.W. 2010. Cell junctions in the testis as targets for toxicants. In: Richburg, JH.; Hoyer, P.,editors. Comprehesive toxicology. Academic Press, pp: 167-188.

Xia, L. and Yu, T. 1992. Study of the relationship between hepatotoxicity and free radical induced by 1,1,2-trichloroethane and 1,l,1-trichloroethane in rat. Biomed. Environ. Sci. 5, 303-313.

Xu, Y., Zhao, H., Zhang, M., Li, C.J., Lin, X.Z., Sheng, J. and Shi, W. 2011. Variations of antioxidant properties and NO scavenging abilities during fermentation of tea. Int. J. Mol. Sci. 12, 4574-4590.

Zhang, Y.T., Zheng, Q.S., Pan, J. and Zheng, R.L. 2004. Oxidative damage of biomolecules in mouse liver induced by morphine and protected by antioxidants. Basic Clin. Pharmacol. Toxicol. 95, 53-58.

27

Encephalomyocarditis virus in a captive Malayan tapir (*Tapirus indicus*)

Francis Vercammen[1,*], Leslie Bosseler[2], Marylène Tignon[3] and Ann Brigitte Cay[3]

[1]Centre for Research and Conservation, Royal Zoological Society of Antwerp, K. Astridplein 26, B-2018 Antwerp, Belgium
[2]Department of Pathology, Bacteriology and Avian Medicine, Faculty of Veterinary Medicine, University of Ghent, Salisburylaan 133, B-9820 Merelbeke, Belgium
[3]Department of Virology, Veterinary and Agrochemical Research Centre, Groeselenberg 99, B-1180 Brussels, Belgium

Abstract
A 5-month-old female captive Malayan tapir (*Tapirus indicus*) died suddenly without preceding symptoms. Gross necropsy revealed numerous white circular and linear foci in the myocard. Differential diagnosis all turned out negative, except for encephalomyocarditis virus. Histopathology revealed mineralisation of myocardial cells and interstitial infiltration of lymphocytes, plasma cells and less neutrophils. Encephalomyocarditis virus was detected by PCR. Although encephalomyocarditis virus occurs in many mammals, this is the first published description of this virus in a Malayan tapir.
Keywords: Encephalomyocarditis virus, Malayan tapir, Myocard, *Tapirus indicus*.

Introduction

The Malayan tapir (*Tapirus indicus*) is one of the four tapir species and is currently endangered with less than 2500 animals remaining in the wild and only 164 captive animals in 81 institutions worldwide (Traeholt et al., 2016; Zoological Information Management System). Its major threats are habitat loss (deforestation) and increased hunting (Traeholt et al., 2016).

There is no descriptive report on encephalomyocarditis virus (EMCV) in tapirs in the international literature, but the occurrence of this disease is mentioned in the Tapir (Tapiridae) Care Manual of the Association of Zoos and Aquariums (2013) and two cases were mentioned briefly by Janssen et al. (1996). Yet, several publications exist of EMCV in other mammal species in zoological collections (Wells et al., 1989; Reddacliff et al., 1997; Vogelnest et al., 2006; Canelli et al., 2010; Liu et al., 2013; Yeo et al., 2013).

The present report describes the gross necropsy, histopathology and ancillary laboratory examinations of a fatal EMCV infection in a young captive Malayan tapir. This case is the first published description of this disease in this animal species.

Case details

At the Antwerp Zoo (Royal Zoological Society of Antwerp), a young, female Malayan tapir, 5 months old, was found dead in its inside enclosure without preceding clinical abnormalities. Gross post-mortem examination revealed a normal body condition (body weight of 130 kg) and the following salient findings: white foam in nostrils; about 1 litre abdominal serohaemorrhagic fluid containing some fibrin clots; spumeous liquid in the trachea; congestion of the lungs; large pale liver areas with central degeneration; areas of mucosal congestion in the duodenum and jejunum with a greyish to chocolate brown liquid content, but without visible blood present; congestion of the mesenterial lymph nodes; soft kidney consistency with a pale cortex; and with the most important findings was the presence of multiple white circular and linear foci of up to 0.5 cm diameter in the myocard (Fig. 1).

A set of tissue samples (liver, lung, kidney, duodenum, jejunum, mesenterial lymph node and heart) were collected and fixed in 10% neutral buffered formalin, embedded in paraffin, sectioned at 4 μm, and stained with haematoxylin and eosin for histologic examination at the Veterinary Pathology Lab (Faculty of Veterinary Medicine, University of Ghent, Belgium).

Samples of the abnormal myocardial tissue were sent to the National Reference Lab (Veterinary and Agrochemical Research Centre, Brussels, Belgium) and to the Laboratory for Exotics (Faculty of Veterinary Medicine, University of Ghent, Belgium) for the detection of encephalomyocarditis virus and herpes virus by polymerase chain reaction (PCR). A large piece of the liver was sent to the Toxicology Lab (Faculty of Veterinary Medicine, University of Ghent, Belgium) for the detection and quantification of ionophores (maduromicin, narasin, lasalocid, monensin, salinomycin and semduramicin), vitamin E and selenium.

*Corresponding Author: Francis Vercammen. Centre for Research and Conservation, Royal Zoological Society of Antwerp, K. Astridplein 26, B-2018 Antwerp, Belgium. Email: francis.vercammen@kmda.org

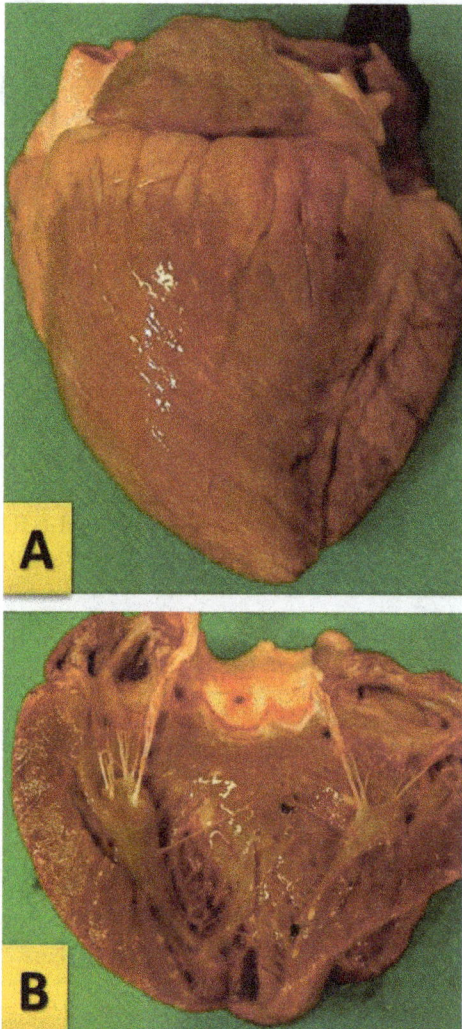

Fig. 1. Gross necropsy: Heart (A: External view; B: Internal view) of a Malayan tapir with encephalomyocarditis virus infection. Multiple circular to linear white foci (mineralisation) are present in the myocardium.

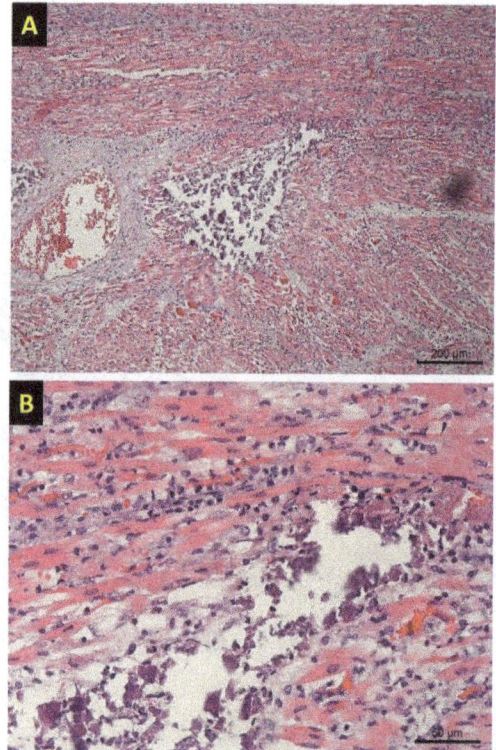

Fig. 2. Histopathology of the heart of a Malayan tapir with encephalomyocarditis virus infection. **(A):** Areas of basophilia (mineralisation) are surrounded by an intense interstitial inflammatory infiltrate. **(B):** Myocardial cells with a diffuse basophilic granulation (mineralisation), surrounded by interstitial infiltration of lymphocytes, plasma cells and a few neutrophils.

Histopathology of the lung showed diffuse mild to moderate congestion. The liver showed severe and diffuse congestion with centrolobular vacuolar degeneration. The duodenum showed severe congestion and a moderate infiltration of lymphocytes and plasma cells in its lamina propria. The lamina propria of the jejunum was mildly infiltrated with lymphocytes and plasma cells. Oedema was noticed in the mesenterial lymph nodes with the presence of blood in the subcapsular and medullary sinuses. The kidneys showed no histologic abnormalities. Multifocal large areas of myocardial cells with a diffuse basophilic granulation (mineralisation) were present. At the periphery of the mineralised areas, a few myocardial cells showed hypereosinophilia, loss of cross-striations and nuclear pyknosis (necrosis). Surrounding the mineralised areas was interstitial infiltration of lymphocytes, plasma cells and less neutrophils (Fig. 2).

The presence of encephalomyocarditis virus was confirmed by PCR amplification of 285 nucleotides located in the 3D polymerase-coding region with primers P1 and P2 (Koenen *et al.*, 1999). The sequence of the amplicon was compared with the reference strain VR-129 (AJ235699.1), the Belgian isolate BEL-279/95 (AJ235701.1), the typical Belgian porcine myocardial strain, and a Belgian field isolate circulating in the pig herds in the same period (data not published). The alignments were performed using the alignment tool Clustal O (Goujon *et al.*, 2010). The tapir isolate presented sequence identities of 86.4%, 97.4% and 100% with the VR-129, BEL-279/95 and the simultaneously circulating Belgian porcine isolate, respectively. Herpes virus was not be detected by PCR. Toxicological analysis of liver tissue was negative (< 2 µg/kg) for all examined ionophores and it contained 21.7% dry matter with 13.8 mg/kg vitamin E and 1.1 mg/kg selenium (all measurements in dry matter).

Tissue impression smears of heart, duodenum, mesenterial lymph node and liver were made for bacteriological examinations. Giemsa stain, Gram stain and Ziehl-Neelsen stain were all negative, except for the duodenum that contained a mixed flora. Cultivation on tryptone-soya-agar, blood agar and Sabouraud agar demonstrated *Escherichia coli* and *Enterococcus* sp. in the mesenterial lymph node, *E. coli* in the liver, a mixed flora with *Clostridium* sp. in the duodenum, but there was no growth of any bacteria in the heart. In addition, the cultivation of abdominal fluid did not yield any bacteria either.

Discussion

The observations in the myocardial macroscopy (white foci) and the histopathology (mineralisation) need some differential diagnosis especially for nutritional cardiomyopathy (vitamin E / selenium deficiency), ionophores intoxication and encephalomyocarditis virus.

Vitamin E / selenium deficiency is a well-known condition in domestic and zoo animals (Valentine *et al.*, 2002; Liesegang and Baumgartner, 2004; Katz *et al.*, 2009). Vitamin E and selenium values are unknown in normal tapir liver, but reference ranges for domestic horses are 10 – 40 µg/g and 0.7 – 2.0 µg/g dry weight, respectively (Yamini and Schillhorn van Veen, 1988; Finno *et al.*, 2006; Barigye *et al.*, 2007). A Brazilian tapir (*Tapirus terrestris*) with nutritional myopathy showing pale skeletal muscles and a pale myocard had a critically low hepatic vitamin E value of 1.3 µg/g and a normal selenium value of 1.20 µg/g dry weight (Yamini *et al.*, 1988). The authors considered the hepatic vitamin E value of 12.74 µg/g and the selenium value of 1.2 µg/g dry weight of a Quarter Horse with myocardial degeneration as suboptimal and normal, respectively (Barigye *et al.*, 2007). The tapir in the present case showed only the myocardial lesions while the skeletal muscles appeared normal with adequate hepatic dry weight values of 13.8 µg/g vitamin E and 1.1 µg/g selenium. Hence, vitamin E / selenium deficiency was excluded.

Since the toxicology lab did not find any of the ionophores that could be involved in Belgium (maduromicin, narasin, lasalocid, monensin, salinomycin, semduramicin) in the liver tissue, this possibility was also excluded.

Outbreaks of encephalomyocarditis virus are notorious for their suddenness and many cases occur as asymptomatic deaths both in zoo mammals and in young domestic pigs (Wells *et al.*, 1989; Reddacliff *et al.*, 1997; Gelmetti *et al.*, 2006; Vogelnest *et al.*, 2006; Canelli *et al.*, 2010; Yeo *et al.*, 2013). In our case, the Malayan tapir died suddenly without any predictive symptoms. The only reference in literature mentions one juvenile (1 - 4 years old) and one adult (4 - 20 years old), without specifying the tapir species, dying from EMCV during an observation period of 35 years (1960 - 1995) (Janssen *et al.*, 1996). In our case that aged 5 months, the animal was clearly much younger and more comparable to the young pigs that die due to EMCV in Belgium. Moreover, the viral sequences of our tapir

strain are identical to the porcine isolate, which was collected in the same period, and share a high (> 95%) identity with the typical Belgian porcine myocardial strain (Koenen *et al.*, 1999; Gelmetti *et al.*, 2006). Also the gross and histological lesions are comparable to the lesions described in young piglets with EMCV (Billinis *et al.*, 1999; Psychas *et al.*, 2001). Affected piglets typically show multiple circular or linear, white foci in the myocardium, excessive fluid in the pericardium, pleura and peritoneum, and pulmonary oedema. The tapir in this case showed similar myocardial lesions, peritoneal effusion, and pulmonary oedema and congestion.

Histologically, the cardiac lesions described in affected piglets consist of mainly mononuclear interstitial myocarditis, and multifocal zones of myocardial degeneration and necrosis with patchy mineralisation. The cardiac samples of the tapir in this case showed no massive myocardial degeneration and necrosis. Instead, the lesions consisted of large areas of mineralisation, minimal myocardial necrosis, and mononuclear interstitial myocarditis. However, since no other signs of hypercalcaemia were present in the tapir, the mineralisation is here interpreted to be of dystrophic nature. Why the mineralisation was so much more prominent in this case, compared to other EMCV cases, is not known.

Rodents, in particular rats and mice, are the natural hosts of encephalomyocarditis virus and excrete the virus in their faeces and urine (Quinn *et al.*, 2011). Therefore, a rigorous pest control programme is absolutely necessary and existing in our zoo. So far, the present case is still the only one that has been diagnosed in our zoo mammals, probably because of a thorough existing pest control. Whenever our zoo would experience a real epizootic, vaccination could be applied; yet, it remains unclear whether or not the vaccine will produce protective antibody titres in all the diverse zoo mammal species (Wells *et al.*, 1989; Vogelnest *et al.*, 2006).

Acknowledgements

The authors wish to thank the Flemish Government for structural support to the Centre for Research and Conservation.

Conflict of interests

The authors declare that there is no conflict of interest.

References

Association of Zoos and Aquariums Tapir Taxon Advisory Group (AZA Tapir TAG). 2013. Tapir (Tapiridae) Care Manual. Associations of Zoos and Aquariums, Silver Spring, Maryland, USA.

Barigye, R., Dyer, N.W. and Newel, T.K. 2007. Fatal Myocardial Degeneration in an Adult Quarter Horse with Vitamin E Deficiency. J. Equine Vet. Sci. 27, 405-408.

Billinis, C., Paschaleri-Papadopoulou, E., Anastasiadis, G., Psychas, V., Vlemmas, J., Leontides, S., Koumbati, M., Kyriakis, S.C. and Papadopoulos, O. 1999. A Comparative Study of the Pathogenic Properties and Transmissibility of a Greek and a Belgian Encephalomyocarditis Virus (EMVC) for Piglets. Vet. Microbiol. 70, 179-192.

Canelli, E., Luppi, A., Lavazza, A., Lelli, D., Sozzi, E., Moreno Martin, A.M., Gelmetti, D., Pascotto, E., Sandri, C., Magnone, W. and Cordioli, P. 2010. Encephalomyocarditis virus in an Italian zoo. Virol. J. 7, 64.

Finno, C.J., Valberg, S.J., Wünschmann, A. and Murphy, M.J. 2006. Seasonal pasture myopathy in horses in the midwestern United States: 14 cases (1998-2005). J. Am. Vet. Med. Assoc. 229, 1134-1141.

Gelmetti, D., Meroni, A., Brocchi, E., Koenen, F. and Cammarata, G. 2006. Pathogenesis of encephalomyocarditis experimental infection in young piglets: a potential animal model to study viral myocarditis. Vet. Res. 37, 15-23.

Goujon, M., McWilliam, H., Li, W., Valentin, F., Squizzato, S, Paern, J. and Lopez, R. 2010. A new bioinformatics analysis tools framework at EMBL-EBI. Nucleic Acids Res. 38, W695-699.

Janssen, D.L., Rideout, B.A. and Edwards, M.E. 1996. Medical management of captive tapirs (*Tapirus* spp.). Proc. Am. Assoc. Zoo Vet. 1-11.

Katz, L.M., O'Dwyer, S. and Pollock, P.J. 2009. Nutritional muscular dystrophy in a four-day-old Connemara foal. Irish Vet. J. 62, 119-124.

Koenen, F., Vanderhallen, H., Dickinson, N.D. and Knowles, N.J. 1999. Phylogenetic analysis of European encephalomyocarditis viruses: comparison of two genomic regions. Arch. Virol. 144, 893-903.

Liesegang, A. and Baumgartner, K. 2004. Liesegang L and Baumgartner K. 2004. Selenium and vitamin E deficiency in different species over a period of 8 years. European Association of Zoo- and Wildlife Veterinarians (EAZWV), 5th scientific meeting, Ebeltoft, Denmark.

Liu, H., Yan, Q. and He, H. 2013. Complete Nucleotide Sequence of Encephalomyocarditis Virus Isolated from South China Tigers in China. Genome Announc. 1, e00651-13.

Psychas, V., Papaioannou, N., Billinis, C., Paschaleri-Papadopoulou, E., Leontides, S., Papadopoulos, O., Tsangaris, T. and Vlemmas, J. 2001. Evaluation of Ultrastructural Changes Associated with Encephalomyocarditis Virus in the Myocardium of Experimentally Infected Piglets. Am. J. Vet. Res. 62, 1653-1657.

Quinn, P.J., Markey, B.K., Leonard, F.C., FitzPatrick, E.S., Fanning, S. and Hartigan, P.J. 2011. Veterinary Microbiology and Microbial Disease. Blackwell Publishing Ltd.

Reddacliff, L.A., Kirkland, P.D., Hartley, W.J. and Reece, R.L. 1997. Encephalomyocarditis virus infections in an Australian zoo. J. Zoo Wildl. Med. 28, 153-157.

Traeholt, C., Novarino, W., bin Saaban, S., Shwe, N.M., Lynam, A., Zainuddin, Z., Simpson, B. and bin Mohd, S. 2016. *Tapirus indicus*. The IUCN Red List of Threatened Species 2016: e.T21472A45173636. http://dx.doi.org/10.2305/IUCN.UK.2016-1.RLTS.T21472A45173636.en

Valentine, B.A., Hammock, P.D., Lemiski, D., Hughes, F.E., Gerstner, L. and Bird, K.E. 2002. Severe diaphragmatic necrosis in 4 horses with degenerative myopathy. Can. Vet. J. 43, 614-616.

Vogelnest, L., Hulst, F., Reiss, A. and Barnes, J. 2006. Efficacy of an inactivated vaccine in the prevention of encephalomyocarditis virus infection in chimpanzees (*Pan troglodytes*) and other species. Proc. Am. Assoc. Zoo Vet. 164-167.

Wells, S.K., Gutter, A.E., Soike, K.F. and Baskin, G.B. 1989. Encephalomyocarditis virus: epizootic in a zoological collection. J. Zoo Wildl. Med. 20, 291-296.

Yamini, B. and Schillhorn van Veen, T.W. 1988. Schistosomiasis and Nutritional Myopathy in a Brazilian Tapir (*Tapirus terrestris*). J. Wildl. Dis. 24, 703-707.

Yeo, D.S-Y., Lian, J.E., Fernandez, C.J., Lin, Y-N., Liaw, J.C-W., Soh, M-L., Lim, E. A-S., Chan, K-P., Ng, M-L., Tan, H-C., Oh, S., Ooi, E-E. and Tan, B-H. 2013. A highly divergent Encephalomyocarditis virus isolated from nonhuman primates in Singapore. Virol. J. 10, 248.

28

Effects of storage temperature on the quantity and integrity of genomic DNA extracted from mice tissues: A comparison of recovery methods

Huda H. Al-Griw[1,*], Zena A. Zraba[2], Salsabiel K. Al-Muntaser[2], Marwan M. Draid[3], Aisha M. Zaidi[4], Refaat M. Tabagh[2] and Mohamed A. Al-Griw[2]

[1]Department of Microbiology and Parasitology, Faculty of Veterinary Medicine, University of Tripoli, Tripoli, Libya
[2]Department of Forensic Biology, Faculty of Science, University of Tripoli. Tripoli, Libya
[3]Department of Pharmacology, Toxicology and Forensic Medicine, Faculty of Veterinary Medicine, University of Tripoli, Tripoli, Libya
[4]Department of Physiology, Biochemistry and Animal Nutrition, Faculty of Veterinary Medicine, University of Tripoli, Tripoli, Libya

Abstract
Efficient extraction of genomic DNA (gDNA) from biological materials found in harsh environments is the first step for successful forensic DNA profiling. This study aimed to evaluate two methods for DNA recovery from animal tissues (livers, muscles), focusing on the best storage temperature for DNA yield in term of quality, quantity, and integrity for use in several downstream molecular techniques. Six male Swiss albino mice were sacrificed, liver and muscle tissues (n=32) were then harvested and stored for one week in different temperatures, -20°C, 4°C, 25°C and 40°C. The conditioned animal tissues were used for DNA extraction by Chelex-100 method or NucleoSpin® Blood and Tissue kit. The extracted gDNA was visualized on 1.5% agarose gel electrophoresis to determine the quality of gDNA and analysed spectrophotometrically to determine the DNA concentration and the purity. Both methods, Chelex-100 and NucleoSpin® Blood and Tissue kit found to be appropriate for yielding high quantity of gDNA, with the Chelex®100 method yielding a greater quantity ($P < 0.045$) than the kit. At -20°C, 4°C, and 25°C temperatures, the concentration of DNA yield was numerically lower than at 40°C. The NucleoSpin® Blood and Tissue kit produced a higher ($P=0.031$) purity product than the Chelex-100 method, particularly for muscle tissues. The Chelex-100 method is cheap, fast, effective, and is a crucial tool for yielding DNA from animal tissues (livers, muscles) exposed to harsh environment with little limitations.
Keywords: DNA degradation, DNA extraction, DNA profiling, Purity, Temperature.

Introduction
In forensic science, purification of high quality and suitable quantity of DNA from challenged biological samples is a key tool for subsequent DNA profiling. Several organic and inorganic protocols are available for DNA extraction. They vary in their nucleic acids yield, processing time, and the ability of removing the Polymerase Chain Reaction inhibitors (PCR inhibitors) (Phillips et al., 2012). DNA can be successfully extracted from a wide range of biological samples, these include, blood residues, urine, semen, saliva, soft and hard tissues. These samples presented in several environmental conditions such as temperature, humidity changes, chemical, physical and microbial contamination, all of which require different extraction strategies to remove the inhibitors and ensure efficient DNA yields (Willard et al., 1998).
"Upon the death of an organism, internal nucleases contained within the cells cause autolysis, cellular organelles and nuclear DNA degradation over time"

(El-Harouny et al., 2008). Determining the quantity and quality of DNA may provide precise way to estimate the post mortem interval (Liu et al., 2001). Therefore, it is important to know which organ is most reliable for DNA extraction, and also to know the effect of post mortem interval on DNA degradation (El-Harouny et al., 2008).
Silica membranes and chelating resin are widely used for DNA extraction in forensic laboratory (Bogas et al., 2011). Silica membranes based technology provides reliable and reproducible DNA recovery. Its strategy follows four main steps: lysis of cellular membranes using a combination of enzymatic and mechanical approaches; selective binding of DNA on the designed silica membrane; washing away of contaminants and DNA elution (Phillips et al., 2012; Dhaliwal, 2013). Chelating resin such as Chelex®100 is simple and rapid DNA extraction method utilise inorganic solvent and do not require multiple tube transfer steps. It involves disruption of the cell membrane under boiling

*Corresponding Author: Dr. Huda H. Al-Griw. Department of Microbiology and Parasitology, Faculty of Veterinary Medicine, University of Tripoli, Libya. Email: h.Algriw@uot.edu.ly

temperature while preventing DNA degradation using chelex suspension. Chelex has been described as efficient method for removing of PCR inhibitors such as hem in porphyrin compounds from blood (Walsh *et al.*, 1991).

The aim of this work was to compare the efficiency of two extraction methods; Chelex-100 and NucleoSpin® Blood and Tissue kit for extraction of genomic DNA (gDNA) from mice tissue (liver and muscle) exposed to different temperature conditions, focusing on the best storage temperature for DNA yield in terms of quantity, purity, and integrity for forensic biology use.

Materials and Methods

Animals and tissue recovery

All experiments were performed in accordance with the regulation of the Animal Experimentation Committees of Faculty of Science, University of Tripoli (Tripoli, Libya). All efforts were made to fulfil the ethical experimentation standards such as minimizing the pain during animal handling and experiments as well as reducing the number of animals used. Six male Swiss albino mice, with an age range of four to five weeks and weight range of 11 g to 14 g, were used in this study. They were bred in the animal house of the Zoology Department, Faculty of Science, University of Tripoli, (Tripoli, Libya), and housed under natural conditions of light (12-hour cycle), temperature (24 ± 2°C) and 55 ± 5% relative humidity. During this period food and water were available *ad libitum*.

At the age of six weeks, mice were sacrificed by cervical dislocation and the intended tissue samples were removed (livers and muscles, n=32, 16 per each extraction method). The tissue samples were cut into small pieces (~ 1gm) and stored immediately in sterile Eppendorf tubes at -20°C (n=4), 4°C (n=4), 25°C (n=4) and 40°C (n=4) without using any preservative for one week.

gDNA extraction

Chelex-100 method

DNA was extracted using the Chelex-100 method as described previously. A homogenized tissue samples was added to 500 μL 5% Chelex-100 resin (Bio-Rad, US), with the subsequent addition of 10 μL proteinase K (QIAGEN, Venlo, Limburg, Netherlands) and 10μl of dithiothreitol (DTT; 1M). The mixture was vortexed, incubated at 56°C for 45 min, and boiled in a water bath for 8 min to inactivate proteinase K. After vigorous vortexing for 10 secs, the samples were centrifuged at 11,000 rpm for 5 min, and the supernatant was collected and stored in a new tube at -20°C until use.

NucleoSpin® Blood and Tissue kit

DNA was isolated from animal tissues (livers, muscles) using the NucleoSpin® Blood and Tissue kit (QIAGEN, Venlo, Limburg, Netherlands), according to manufacturer instructions, and the extracted gDNA were stored at -20°C until use.

Quantity and purity of gDNA

As described previously, the gDNA concentration and purity were assessed by optical density measurements using the NanoDrop™ 2000 Lite Spectrophotometer (Thermo Scientific, Wilmington. USA). For this purpose, DNA absorbance was measured at 260 nm to determine the quantity of DNA, and DNA purity was estimated by determining the A260/A280 ratio and comparing it to the reference value 1.8 (Desjardins and Conklin, 2010).

DNA visualization on agarose gel

The presence and quality/ integrity of gDNA extracted by the two methods were analysed on 1% agarose gel. Ten animal tissue DNA aliquots were stained with 1 μL RedGel fluorescence and subjected to electrophoresis on the agarose gel.

The gDNA was visualized under an UV transilluminator, and the image was digitalized. The degraded DNA of the samples was observed by the visibility of the bands compared against a known molecular weight marker.

Statistical analysis

The Statistical Package for the Social Sciences (IBM SPSS Statistics for Windows, Version 20.0. Armonk, NY: IBM Corp.) was used to perform the statistical analysis.

The gDNA quantity and purity values were statistically determined by one-way analysis of variance (ANOVA) test, and differences were compared with a two-way analysis of variance with post-hoc Tukey test. $P < 0.05$ was considered significant. The results are shown as means ± SD.

Results

Assessment of gDNA quality extracted from animal tissues

The spectrometric assay demonstrated that the quantity of DNA extracted from animal tissue samples was higher ($P < 0.05$) for the Chelex-100 method than for the NucleoSpin® Blood and Tissue kit, particularly for liver tissues.

Using Chelex-100 method, it was found that the quantities of the DNA extracted from liver samples stored at -20°C, 4°C, 25°C and 40°C were 1068.9±62.5, 507.8±118.51, 613.2±127.98 and 637.1±123.24, respectively. The greatest amount of DNA was obtained from tissue samples stored under -20°C ($P<0.05$).

However, there was no a significant difference between other conditions in terms of quantity of the gDNA extracted ($P > 0.05$) (Fig. 1). Furthermore, the results showed limited quantity of the DNA extracted from these samples using NucleoSpin® Blood and Tissue kit. It was found that the quantities of DNA extracted from liver tissues stored at -20°C, 4°C, 25°C and 40°C were 294.3±38.8, 18.05±4.31, 12.1±0.98 and 17.2±9.1, respectively (Fig. 1).

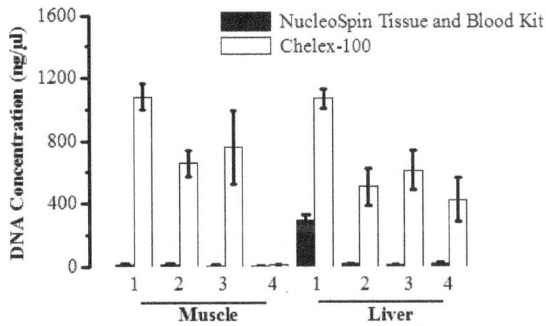

Fig. 1. Average concentration of DNA measured in ng/µl. DNA was extracted from animal tissues (muscles, livers) stored in different temperature conditions using NucleoSpin® Blood & Tissue kit (black bar) and Chelex-100 method (white bar). Data are expressed as mean ± S.D, $P < 0.05$ significant.

Similarly, to the results obtained by Chelex-100 method, the samples processed using NucleoSpin® Blood and Tissue kit immediately after one week storage at -20°C appear to have greatest amount of DNA (294.3 ± 38.8) although far less than result obtained by Chelex (1068.9 ± 62.5) (Fig. 1).

For muscle tissue samples, the total yields of extracted DNA using Chelex method for samples stored at -20°C, 4°C and 25°C was 1081.5±80.8, 659.6±82.7, and 759.1±236.3 respectively, that was comparable to the amount of DNA extracted from liver tissues using the same extraction technique.

However, the muscle samples stored under 40°C for a week gave low DNA copies (11.85±2.3) indicative degradation effect. All muscle tissue samples processed with NucleoSpin® Blood and Tissue kit recovered lower DNA concentration compared to Chelex-100 method (Fig. 1).

Assessment of gDNA purity extracted from animal tissues

The NucleoSpin® Blood and Tissue kit gave a higher ($P < 0.05$) DNA purity than did Chelex-100. Although there was a variation among the samples extracted, the kit yielded purities of nearly the reference value 1.8 (Desjardins and Conklin, 2010). The purity ratio (A260/A280) of DNA obtained by NucleoSpin® Blood and Tissue kit, particularly from liver samples, although it was not optimum, was higher than that extracted using Chelex-100 (0.9-1.9). DNA extracted from muscle tissues by Chelex-100 shown to have lower purity (0.7- 0.98) indicates contamination with protein (Fig. 2).

The integrity and quality of gDNA extracted by the two methods was also analysed on 1.5% agarose gel (Fig. 3). The quality of DNA observed by the visibility of the bands against a known molecular weight marker. Chelex produced DNA of minimum degradation from liver tissues stored at -20°C, 4°C, and 25°C as indicated by clear bands on the gel (Fig. 3).

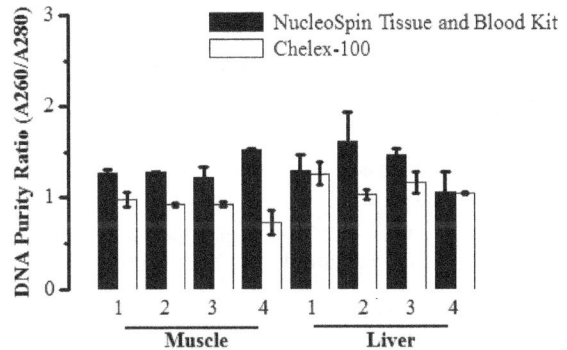

Fig. 2. Average purity of extracted gDNA. DNA was spectrophotometrically analysed to determine the purity (A260/A280) of extracted DNA from animal tissues (muscles, livers) stored in different temperature conditions using NucleoSpin® Blood & Tissue kit (black bar) and Chelex-100 method (white bar). Data are expressed as mean ± S.D, $P < 0.05$ significant.

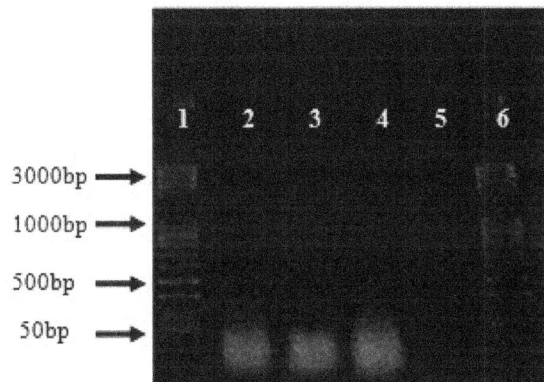

Fig. 3. Agarose gel electrophoresis results on 1% agarose gel with DNA extracted from four animal tissue samples (2-5) by using the Chelex-100 method. Lanes: 1 and 6 ladders; lanes 2-5 liver DNA samples stored in different temperatures, L4°C, L 25°C, L-20°C and L 40°C respectively.

However, Liver tissues kept under 40°C and all DNA samples extracted by Chelex from muscle tissues did not show bands on the gel indicates degradation of the DNA produced even though the quantity of DNA recovered were relatively high. The entire DNA samples extracted by the NucleoSpin® Blood and Tissue kit showed very shallow smearing, due to low copies of recovered DNA that could not have picked by the low-resolution camera used for documentation of the gel (data not shown).

Discussion

It has been well known that the best and efficient DNA extraction requires fresh tissue samples as a source material (Salman, 2000). Under some situations, particularly in case of criminal offences, fresh tissue cannot be obtained directly upon the crime occurrence. It is likely that the tissues in the field are present in several states of decomposition when exposed to different temperatures, humidity conditions, chemical, physical, and microbial contaminants (Willard *et al.*, 1998; Vass *et al.*, 2002).

This study was designed to keep the samples in different temperature settings, thus simulating different tissue states on the time of discovery at the crime scene. Such temperature settings (-20°C, 4°C, 25°C (room temperature), and 40°C) were maintained for one week, the amount of time assuming is adequate for transportation of the samples from the criminal scene into the forensic diagnostic laboratories where samples can then be store at -20°c for short-term manipulation or under -80°C for long-term storage.

Two protocols have been compared in this study for DNA extraction from the conditioned animal tissues in respect to the quantity, quality and time consumed for the extraction. The NucleoSpin® Blood and Tissue kit required less time (30 to 40min), compared to the Chelex protocol, which required 3.5 to 4 hrs, mostly for incubation time. However, the former protocol required multiple tubes transfer that made it laborious for manipulation of a large number of samples and subjecting to cross contamination and pipetting error.

Our preliminary results suggested that the amount of DNA extracted by Chelex from both muscle and liver tissues were far higher than the ones extracted by the NucleoSpin® Blood and Tissue kit for the same samples under the same conditions. However, the purity of the samples extracted by the later protocol was better than the ones extracted by Chelex.

Previously, it has been shown that typical DNA yield ranges from 1000–5000 ng·mg^{-1} in animal tissue (Pereira *et al.*, 2011). Our results showed that the quantity of DNA extracted from liver tissues that have been stored under 40°C using Chelex protocol was far higher (637.1 ± 123.24 ng/µl) comparing with the amount of DNA recovered from the muscle tissue stored under the same condition and extracted with the same technique (11.85±2.3 ng/µl). Such results could be explained by the ability of the liver to hold intact DNA longer than the muscle cells. In a comparative study by Ebuehi *et al.* (2015) for study of the effects of post mortem interval (PMI) on degradation of the DNA presented in the brain, liver, kidney, and heart tissues of male mice.

The results revealed that the degradation of gDNA was a time dependent process. While the brain showed slowest DNA, degradation compared to the other organs, the liver and brain tissues were similar rigidity when viewing the profile of random segments of gDNA on the agarose gel electrophoresis. Furthermore , the study suggested that at a later PMI, the brain, followed by the liver were preferred organs for forensic studies than the heart and kidney (Ebuehi *et al.*, 2015).

Our results agreed with Ebuehi and colleagues in term of quantity and the integrity of gDNA extracted from liver tissues which was prominent than the ones extracted from muscle tissues although we use muscle tissues rather than heart tissues, both which are multinucleated muscle tissues. Similarly, a study by Pooniya *et al.* (2014) suggested that muscle tissues were found to be the worst for gDNA extraction while the brain tissue preserved at -80°C and 4°C was the best among other soft tissue studied (Brain, Muscle, Kidney and heart) (Pooniya *et al.*, 2014).

One important reason regarding the needs for high purity of extracted gDNA is the suitability of the extract for long term banking for subsequence genotyping analysis, the time needed for collections and manipulation of all samples. It is well known that the Secondary compounds and heavy metals ions can result in gDNA damage (Psifidi *et al.*, 2015). The ability of Chelex to remove inhibitors remains controversial. Phillips *et al.* (2012) reported failure of the PCR to produce profile when Chelex was used for DNA extraction from blood samples suggesting that either the Chelex resin or haem were left within the samples, whereas a study by Walsh *et al.* (1991) suggested that gDNA extracted from bloodstain samples prepared by Chelex were less likely to have PCR inhibitors (Walsh *et al.*, 1991).

Our results showed that the gDNA recovered by Chelex was below the acceptable level of purity as indicated by the ratio of absorbance at 260nm and 280nm that should be ~ 1.8 (Desjardins and Conklin, 2010). These results suggested the presence of protein residue which can inhibit the subsequent PCR applications and hindered gDNA-banking, particularly for gDNA extracted from muscle tissue that have shown very low purity (0.7-0.98). DNA extracted by NucleoSpin® Blood and Tissue kit for all samples was far purer than the ones extracted by Chelex. However, the DNA concentration recovered by NucleoSpin® Blood and Tissue kit was very poor and below the adequate amount of DNA concentration required for genotyping studies (~ 50ng /µl) (Psifidi *et al.*, 2015). Furthermore, they were unable to produce visible bands on gel electrophoresis indicated the lower molecular weight of the yielded gDNA (Salman, 2000). The reason for poor quantity of gDNA produced from liver and muscle tissue when the NucleoSpin® Blood and Tissue kit was used for gDNA extraction could be explained by the fact that the technique failed to incorporate a vital step that takes into account the special feature of animal cells.

When using animal tissue, enzymatic lysis step or mechanical disruption of the tissue should be proceeding the separation of DNA from other cell components (Hofstetter *et al.*, 1997; Dhaliwal, 2013). However, we did not examine the performance of DNA extracts by the two methods for PCR applications to see whether a small amount of gDNA can be used for PCR profiling. Walsh *et al*. (1991) suggested, that native high molecular weight DNA is not required to amplify the target sequence and only the target sequences are required to be intact, thus partially degraded or denatured DNA could be successfully used for PCR applications (Walsh *et al*., 1991).

In conclusion, Chelex protocol appeared to be acceptable regarding the quantity of the DNA product whereas NucleoSpin® Blood and Tissue kit recovered purer gDNA. Furthermore, a lysis step should be incorporated before processing the tissue samples by NucleoSpin® Blood and Tissue kit to enhance the productivity of gDNA. Although the difference between the two extraction methods was clear, a small data set was used for this study. More samples are needed to be tested to make a solid conclusion.

Acknowledgments

Authors would like to thank the staff of the National Center of Disease Control Laboratory for their practical assistance. The authors also would like to thank Dr. Taher Shaibi, a staff member at the Faculty of Science, University of Tripoli, Tripoli-Libya, for his assistance.

Conflict of interest

The authors declare that there is no conflict of interests.

References

Bogas, V., Balsa, F., Carvalho, M., Anjos, M. J., Pinheiro, M. F. and Corte-Real, F. 2011. Comparison of four DNA extraction methods for forensic application. Forensic Science International: Genetics Supplement Series, 3(1), e194-e195.

Desjardins, P. and Conklin, D. 2010. NanoDrop microvolume quantitation of nucleic acids. J Vis Exp. (45), 2565. doi:10.3791/2565.

Dhaliwal, A. 2013. DNA Extraction and Purification. MATER METHODS [Online]. Available at: https://www.labome.com/method/DNA-Extraction-and-Purification.html

Ebuehi, O.A.T., Amode, M., Balogun, A. and Fowora, A. 2015. Postmortem Time Affects Brain, Liver, Kidney and Heart DNA in Male Rat. Am. J. Biochem. 5(1), 1-5.

El-Harouny, M., El-Dakroory, S., Attalla, S., Hasan, N. and Hassab El-Nabi, S.E. 2008. The relationship between postmortem interval and DNA degradation in different tissues of drowned rats. Mansoura J.

Forensic Med. Clin. Toxicol. 16(2), 45-61.

Hofstetter, J.R., Zhang, A., Mayeda, A.R., Guscar, T., Nurnberger, J.I.,Jr. and Lahiri, D.K. 1997. Genomic DNA from Mice: A Comparison of Recovery Methods and Tissue Sources. Biochem. Mol. Med. 62(2), 197-202.

Liu, L., Peng, D.B., Liu, Y., Deng, W.N., Liu, Y.L. and Li, J.J. 2001. A study on the relationship between postmortem interval and the changes of DNA content in the kidney cellule of rat. Fa. Yi. Xue. Za. Zhi. 17(2), 65-68.

Pereira, J.C., Chaves, R., Bastos, E., Leitão, A. and Guedes-Pinto, H. 2011. An Efficient Method for Genomic DNA Extraction from Different Molluscs Species. Int. J. Mol. Sci. 12, 8086-8095.

Phillips, K., McCallum, N. and Welch, L. 2012. A comparison of methods for forensic DNA extraction: Chelex-100(R) and the QIAGEN DNA Investigator Kit (manual and automated). Forensic Sci. Int. Genet. 6(2), 282-285.

Pooniya, S., Lalwani, S., Raina, A., Millo, T. and Dogra, T.D. 2014. Quality and quantity of extracted deoxyribonucleic Acid (DNA) from preserved soft tissues of putrefied unidentifiable human corpse. J. Lab. Physicians 6(1), 31-35.

Psifidi, A., Dovas, C.I., Bramis, G., Lazou, T., Russel, C.L., Arsenos, G. and Banos, G. 2015. Comparison of Eleven Methods for Genomic DNA Extraction Suitable for Large-Scale Whole-Genome Genotyping and Long-Term DNA Banking Using Blood Samples. PLoS One 10(1), e0115960.

Salman, A.H. 2000. Effect of Storage Temperature on the Quality and Quantity of DNA Extracted from Blood. Pakistan J. Biol. Sci. 3, 392-394.

Vass, A.A., Barshick, S.A., Sega, G., Caton, J., Skeen, J.T., Love, J.C. and Synstelien, J.A. 2002. Decomposition chemistry of human remains: a new methodology for determining the postmortem interval. J. Forensic Sci. 47, 542-553.

Walsh, P.S., Metzger, D.A. and Higuchi, R. 1991. Chelex 100 as a medium for simple extraction of DNA for PCR-based typing from forensic material. Biotechniques 10(4), 506-513.

Willard, J.M., Lee, D.A. and Holland, M.M. 1998. Recovery of DNA for PCR amplification from blood and forensic samples using a chelating resin. Methods Mol. Biol. 98, 9-18.

29

Tricuspid valve dysplasia: A retrospective study of clinical features and outcome in dogs in the UK

Xavier Navarro-Cubas[1,*], Valentina Palermo[2], Anne French[3], Sandra Sanchis-Mora[4] and Geoff Culshaw[5]

[1]*University of Liverpool, Small Animal Teaching Hospital, Leahurst Campus, Chester High Road, Neston, Wirral, CH64 7TE, UK*
[2]*Anderson and Moores Veterinary Specialists, The Granary, Bunstead Barns, Poles Lane, Hursley, Winchester, Hampshire, SO21 2LL, UK*
[3]*School of Veterinary Medicine, College of Medical, Veterinary and Life Sciences, University of Glasgow, Bearsden Road, Bearsden, Glasgow, G61 1QH, UK*
[4]*The Royal Veterinary College, Hawkshead Lane, North Mymms, Hatfield, Hertfordshire, AL9 7TA, UK*
[5]*R(D)SVS Hospital for Small Animals, The University of Edinburgh, Easter Bush Veterinary Centre, Roslin, Midlothian, EH25 9RG, UK*

Abstract

The objective of this study was to determine the demographic, clinical and survival characteristics and to identify risk factors for mortality due to tricuspid valve dysplasia in UK dogs. Records of client-owned dogs diagnosed with tricuspid valve dysplasia at a referral centre were retrospectively reviewed. Only dogs diagnosed with tricuspid valve dysplasia based on the presence of a right-sided heart murmur identified prior to one year of age, and confirmed with Doppler echocardiography, were included. Dogs with concomitant cardiac diseases, pulmonary hypertension and/or trivial tricuspid regurgitation were excluded. Analysed data included signalment, reason for presentation, clinical signs, electrocardiographic and echocardiographic features, survival status and cause of death. Survival times and risk factors for mortality were evaluated using Kaplan-Meier curves and Cox regression. Eighteen dogs met inclusion criteria. Border collies were over-represented (p= 0.014). Dogs were most frequently referred for investigation of heart murmur. The most common arrhythmia was atrial fibrillation (n=3). Median survival time from diagnosis of tricuspid valve dysplasia was 2775 days (range 1-3696 days; 95% CI 1542.41-4007.59) and from onset of right-sided congestive heart failure was 181 days (range 1-2130 days; 95% CI 0-455.59). Syncope was the sole risk factor for cardiac death. In this population of UK dogs, tricuspid valve dysplasia was uncommon but, when severe, frequently led to right-sided congestive heart failure. Prognosis was favourable for mild and moderate tricuspid dysplasia. Survival time was reduced with right-sided congestive heart failure but varied widely. Risk of cardiac death was significantly increased if syncope had occurred.

Keywords: Tricuspid valve dysplasia, Congestive heart failure, Atrial fibrillation, Survival time, Canine congenital heart disease.

Introduction

Tricuspid valve dysplasia (TVD) in dogs encompasses a spectrum of congenital malformations of the tricuspid valve (TV) apparatus including focal or diffuse thickening of the leaflets, underdevelopment or undifferentiated chordae tendineae (CT) and papillary muscles (PM), incomplete separation of valve components from the ventricular wall and focal agenesis of valvular tissue, resulting in valvular insufficiency or rarely stenosis (Famula *et al.*, 2002; Andelfinger *et al.*, 2003; MacDonald, 2006; Ohad *et al.*, 2013; Adin, 2014; Lake-Bakaar *et al.*, 2017) (Fig. 1).

In human cardiology, TVD is divided into two categories. "Ebstein's malformation (EM)" is characterised by the apical displacement of the basal attachment of the valvular leaflets (septal, mural or both), and atrialisation of the right ventricle (RV). Confirmation requires objective echocardiographic or post-mortem measurements of the valvular displacement indexed to body weight (Shiina *et al.*, 1984), cardiac catheterisation with an electrophysiology study (Choi *et al.*, 2009) or cardiac MRI (Said *et al.*, 2012). In "tricuspid valve dysplasia", the leaflets and tension apparatus are malformed but are not displaced (Becker *et al.*, 1971; Lang *et al.*, 1991). This terminology has been applied to veterinary cardiology (Eyster *et al.*, 1977; Cave, 2001; Andelfinger *et al.*, 2003; Takemura *et al.*, 2003; Sousa *et al.*, 2006; Choi *et al.*, 2009). In dogs, TVD is a rare congenital disease, affecting most commonly Labrador retriever (Wright *et al.*, 2001).

*Corresponding Author: Xavier Navarro-Cubas. University of Liverpool, Small Animal Teaching Hospital, Leahurst Campus, Chester High Road, Neston, Wirral, CH64 7TE, UK. Email: xncubas@gmail.com

Overall prevalence has been reported as between 2 and 7.4% in shelter and specialist referral populations (Tidholm, 1997; Oliveira *et al.*, 2011; Schrope, 2015). Heritability has been established in Labrador retrievers (Famula *et al.*, 2002) and Dogues de Bordeaux (Ohad *et al.*, 2013), and the disease has been mapped to chromosome 9 in Labrador retrievers (Andelfinger *et al.*, 2003).

EM in dogs is even more rarely reported, with only isolated case reports in the literature (Eyster *et al.*, 1977; Takemura *et al.*, 2003; Sousa *et al.*, 2006; Choi *et al.*, 2009). None of the published studies on canine TVD have included UK dogs.

Because TVD applies to a range of abnormalities and severities, valvular insufficiency is variable, although severe disease can lead to right-sided congestive heart failure (R-CHF) in both young and adult dogs (Adin, 2014).

Prognostication remains challenging, since, to the authors' knowledge, risk factors for disease progression and mortality have not been determined.

The aims of this study were to use retrospective data to describe demographic, clinical and survival characteristics and to identify risk factors for mortality due to TVD in UK dogs.

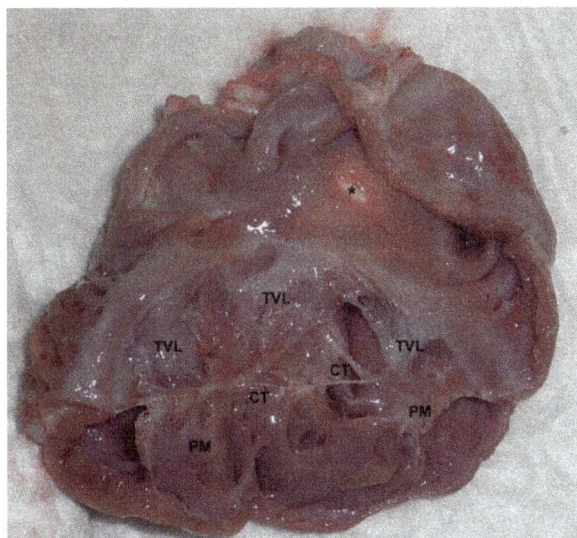

Fig. 1. Post-mortem image from a 3-month old Labrador retriever puppy diagnosed with TVD. There is diffuse marked thickening of the tricuspid leaflets (TVL), which exhibit irregular edges and are multifocally adhered to the endocardial surface. The chordae tendineae (CT) and papillary muscles (PM) are diffusely and severely shortened, fused and thickened. Marked right atrial enlargement is also observed. Please note the apparent defect (*) in the interatrial septum; this was an iatrogenic cut accidentally done during preparation of the specimen (Image courtesy of Prof. Joanna Dukes-McEwan and Dr Sonja Fonfara).

Materials and Methods

Medical records of client-owned dogs diagnosed with TVD between 1998-2011 were retrospectively reviewed. Data including signalment, clinical history, physical examination, electrocardiographic (ECG) and echocardiographic findings, diagnosis, survival status and date and cause of death were collected from all cases. Inclusion criteria were diagnosis of TVD based on presence of a right-sided systolic murmur that had been first identified prior to one year of age, and a comprehensive Doppler echocardiographic study. Exclusion criteria were incomplete case record and/or echocardiographic study, presence of trivial tricuspid regurgitation (TR) and/or pulmonary hypertension (TR vmax. >2.8 m/s) (Adams *et al.*, 2017). Dogs with concomitant cardiac diseases were included in order to identify conditions associated with TVD, and breed and sex predispositions, but, otherwise excluded from all other statistical analysis. Where collapse had been reported, and no non-cardiac cause had been identified on investigation, it was assumed to be cardiac syncope. Heart murmurs (HM) were categorised according to location and intensity (Grades I to VI). Standard six-lead electrocardiograms were reviewed.

Echocardiograms were performed on all dogs, without sedation, by an ECVIM-CA or RCVS-diplomate, or by a diplomate-supervised ECVIM-CA-enrolled resident. Measurements were made offline by the same echocardiographer. Echocardiographic findings consistent with a diagnosis of TVD, including valvular abnormalities, are listed in Table 1 (Boon, 2011a; Ohad *et al.*, 2013; Adin, 2014; Schrope, 2015; Bussadori and Pradelli, 2016) (Fig. 2). Tethering of the septal leaflet was only confirmed if the leaflet was attached to the septal wall by a short CT that was subjectively preventing its closure (Boon, 2011b) (Fig. 2).

Colour-flow Doppler was used to confirm TR, which was semi-quantitatively assessed by comparing jet area with right atrial size (Table 1). Trivial TR was not an inclusion criterion, as it is very common in healthy dogs (Boon, 2011c; Ohad *et al.*, 2013; Bussadori and Pradelli, 2016). Tricuspid stenosis was defined as the presence of diastolic doming or reduced diastolic excursion of the TV leaflets, reduced TV orifice diameter, increased diastolic pressure gradient between right atrium (RA) and RV (>3 mmHg), and/or presence of tricuspid inflow colour variance with Nyquist limit set at 0.7-1.0 m/s (Lake-Bakaar *et al.*, 2017).

Right-sided volume overload was subjectively assessed based on the right atrial and right ventricular size, viewed from the right parasternal long axis four chamber view, and by comparing chamber proportions with left atrial and left ventricular size (Lang *et al.*, 2006) as indicated in Table 1.

Table 1. Summary of the echocardiographic abnormalities associated with tricuspid valve dysplasia.

Tricuspid valve apparatus - morphological abnormalities	**Valve leaflets**	Dysplastic leaflets may be thickened, clubbed, shortened, elongated or fused.	
		Valvular leaflet elongation: more commonly observed in the parietal leaflet	
		Valvular tethering	Septal leaflet subjectively attached to the septal wall by short CT, preventing its normal closure.
			Can lead to non-coaptation of the valvular leaflets
		Tricuspid stenosis	Considered if presence of diastolic doming or reduced excursion of the TV leaflets, reduced TV orifice diameter, increased diastolic pressure gradient between RA and RV (>3 mmHg), and/or presence of tricuspid inflow colour variance with Nyquist limit set at 0.7-1.0 m/s
	Chordae tendineae	Dysplastic chordae include thickened, shortened or even absent chordae	
	Papillary muscles	Dysplastic papillary muscles include shortened, elongated, fused or with direct attachment to the valve leaflets	
Tricuspid regurgitation	Confirmed by Colour-flow and spectral Doppler echocardiography		
	Severity semi-quantitatively assessed by colour flow: TR jet size subjectively compared with right atrial size (left apical 4-chamber view optimised for RA & RV)	Mild	< quarter of the RA area
		Moderate	Quarter to half of the RA area
		Severe	Over half of the RA area
	Trivial TR: Small TR jet with narrow jet origin, extending only a short distance from the valve leaflets. Timing is brief, with TR early in systole.		
Right-sided volume overload (assessed from right parasternal long axis 4 chamber view, tipped to optimise RA & RV)	**RA enlargement**	Mild	RA subjectively remains smaller than LA
		Moderate	RA diameter subjectively is of similar size to the LA diameter
		Severe	RA subjectively has larger diameter than LA
	RV enlargement (normally RV > one third LV size)	Mild	RV subjectively remains smaller than LV
		Moderate	RV subjectively has similar size to the LV
		Severe	RV subjectively is larger than the LV

Severity of TVD was subjectively graded as mild, moderate or severe according to echocardiographic appearance of the TV apparatus, severity of right-sided volume overload and TR jet size (Zoghbi *et al.*, 2003). Cases compatible with EM were not categorised separately from the TVD population. This was because only subjective assessment of apical displacement of the valvular apparatus was available, and not objective assessment (indexing to body weight) (Kornreich and Moïse, 1997), cardiac catheterisation with an electrophysiology study (Choi *et al.*, 2009) or post-mortem confirmation (Kornreich and Moïse, 1997) were available.

Statistical analysis used SPSS Statistics (IBM 2013) and Microsoft Excel.

Demographic variables were explored and described using proportions for categorical data and median, range and 95% confidence interval (CI) for continuous data. For continuous data, normality of distribution was verified by Kolmogorov-Smirnov's test and visual assessment of Q-Q plots and histograms. Breed over-representation was calculated using Chi-square analysis, comparing the proportion of a breed between the TVD population and the entire hospital population. For this analysis, we included dogs with TVD and concomitant cardiac diseases.

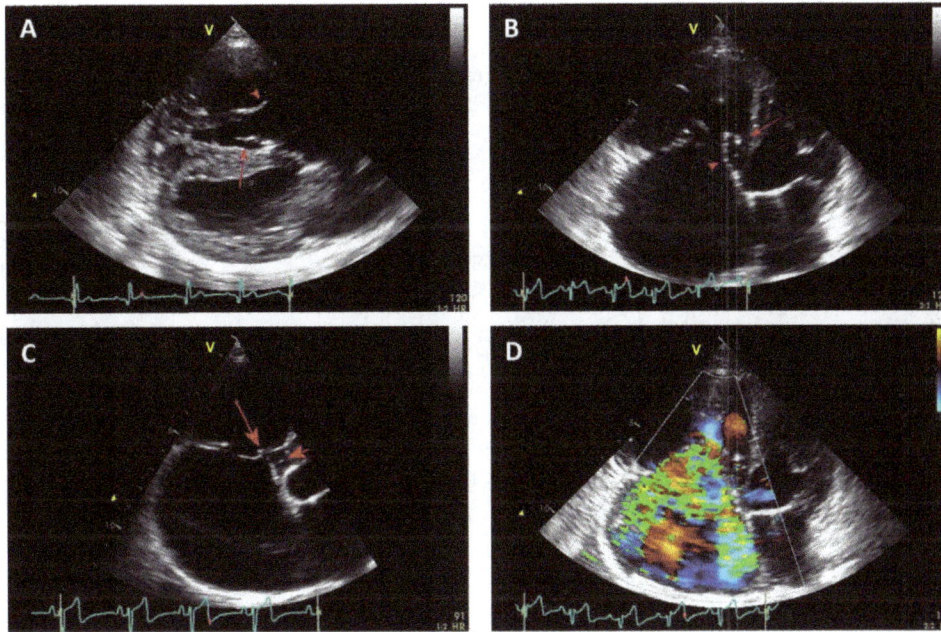

Fig. 2. (A): Right parasternal four-chamber long axis view showing right atrial and right ventricular dilation. The papillary muscle subjectively appears directly attached to the mural tricuspid valve leaflet (arrow head). The septal leaflet subjectively appears tethered to the septal wall (arrow) causing the incomplete occlusion of the tricuspid orifice in systole. **(B):** Left apical four-chamber view, optimised for the right atrium and right ventricle, showing severe right atrial and right ventricular dilation. The mural leaflet of the tricuspid valve subjectively appears markedly elongated. The septal leaflet appears tethered to the septal wall by short chordae tendineae (arrow), with the middle portion of the leaflet buckling away from the septum (arrow head). **(C):** Left apical four-chamber view, optimised for the right atrium and right ventricle, showing severe right atrial dilation. The mural leaflet of the tricuspid valve is markedly elongated, and is responsible for the occlusion of almost all the tricuspid valve orifice. The septal leaflet subjectively appears tethered to the septal wall by short chordae tendineae (arrow head), and the middle portion bows away from the interventricular septum. **(D):** Colour Doppler left apical four-chamber view, optimised for the right atrium and right ventricle, showing severe tricuspid regurgitation. Colour variance occupies the complete area of the right atrium.

The relationships between TVD severity, presence of an arrhythmia and heart murmur intensity were evaluated using a Fisher's exact test. The Kaplan-Meier method was used to estimate median survival times (MST) and plot time to event curves. The survival time (ST) study included two study periods: ST from diagnosis of TVD, and from diagnosis of R-CHF. The end-point for survival analysis was cardiac death, defined as euthanasia or natural death due to sudden death or worsening of R-CHF as a result of TVD. A questionnaire and telephone interview with referring veterinarians or the owners determined the status of each animal.

Dogs lost to follow-up (LTFU) were included in the survival analysis, left censored at the time of the last visit. Non-cardiac deaths and dogs still alive were also censored. Univariate analysis, using Cox regression, of the following risk factors was performed to determine whether there was any relationship with time to death from TVD diagnosis: age, sex, breed, TVD severity, HM intensity, R-CHF (at any point), syncope and arrhythmia. Multivariate analysis was not performed due to the low event rate. Significance of all tests was set at $p<0.05$.

Results

During the study period, a total of 29 dogs were identified with TVD, which was 1.1% of the population referred for cardiology evaluation. The two most common breeds with TVD were Labrador retrievers (n=7, 24%) and Border collies (n=5, 17%). Compared with the overall hospital population, only Border collies were over-represented (p=0.015) (Labradors p=0.219). Both sexes were diagnosed with the condition (female n=17, 59%; male n=12, 41%). TVD was the sole cardiac disease in 18 dogs (62% of all dogs with TVD, Table 2). In the remaining 11 dogs (38%), concomitant cardiac diseases were diagnosed including mitral valve dysplasia (n=4; 14%), pulmonic stenosis (n=3; 10%), atrial septal defect (n=2), and subaortic stenosis (n=1) and left-to-right patent ductus arteriosus (n=1) (Table 3). Dogs with isolated TVD were referred for investigation of a HM (n=14, 78%), syncope (n=3, 17%), presence of an arrhythmia (n=1), signs consistent with R-CHF (n=1), non-cardiac collapse (n=1) and vomiting (n=1) (Table 2). Age at diagnosis of TVD ranged between 50 days and 13 years (median=252.5 days). Twelve dogs (67%) were less than one-year-old at time of diagnosis (Table 2).

Table 2. Demographic information of dogs diagnosed with isolated TVD.

Dog	Breed	Reason for presentation	Heart murmur	Diagnosis	Age at TVD diagnosis (days)	RCHF	Age at RCHF diagnosis (days)	Signs of CHF	Status at the end of the study	Age at death (days)
Dog 1	Border collie	Heart murmur	IV/VI pansystolic right apical	Severe TVD	80	Yes	2713	Ascites	Euthanasia. Unresponsive RCHF	2855
Dog 2	Boxer	Non-Cardiac collapse	II/VI systolic right basilar	Moderate TVD	216	No		-	Euthanasia. Spleen rupture haemoabdomen.	3912
Dog 3	Doberman	Heart murmur	III/VI systolic right apical	Mild TVD	2535	No		-	Euthanasia. Lymphoma	4781
Dog 4	Border collie	Heart murmur, ascites, syncope, pleural effusion	V/VI pansystolic apical bilaterally	Severe TVD	318	Yes	322	Ascites, pleural effusion (mild), jugular distension/pulse	Euthanasia. Unresponsive RCHF	2297
Dog 5	Border collie	Heart murmur	V/VI pansystolic right apical	Severe TVD	2588	No		-	Natural death. Immune-mediated neutropenia.	5040
Dog 6	Pointer	Heart murmur	IV/VI systolic right basilar	Severe TVD	50	LTFU	LTFU	-	Lost to follow up	50
Dog 7	Labrador retriever	Heart murmur	IV/VI pansystolic right apical	Severe TVD	62	No		-	Alive	892
Dog 8	Golden retriever	Heart murmur	III/VI pansystolic right apical	Moderate TVD	1481	No		-	Euthanasia. Renal failure	2178
Dog 9	German shepherd	Heart murmur	V/VI pansystolic right apical	Severe TVD	199	Yes	2829	Ascites	Euthanasia. Unresponsive RCHF	3644
Dog 10	Golden retriever	Heart murmur	III/VI holosystolic right apical	Mild TVD	4745	No		-	Euthanasia. Hind limb weakness. Lumbosacral pain.	4988
Dog 11	Labrador retriever	Vomiting	II/VI holosystolic right apical	Mild TVD	858	No		-	Alive	2155
Dog 12	Golden retriever	Heart murmur	I/VI systolic right apical	Mild TVD	205	No		-	Alive	1393
Dog 13	Springer spaniel	Heart murmur	V/VI pansystolic right basilar	Severe TVD	109	Yes	749	Ascites	Euthanasia. Unresponsive RCHF	773
Dog 14	Border collie	Heart murmur, syncope	VI/VI pansystolic apical bilaterally	Severe TVD	60	Yes	61	Ascites	Euthanasia. Unresponsive RCHF	60
Dog 15	Bullmastiff	Arrhythmia	II/VI holosystolic right apical	Severe TVD	356	Yes	361	Ascites and pleural effusion	Natural death. Cardiorespiratory arrest	2486
Dog 16	Labrador retriever	Syncope	III/VI systolic right apical	Severe TVD	289	Yes	293	Ascites	Euthanasia. Unresponsive RCHF	363
Dog 17	Cross breed	Heart murmur	IV/VI pansystolic right basilar	Severe TVD	81	LTFU	LTFU		LTFU	841
Dog 18	Labrador retriever	Heart murmur	IV/VI systolic right apical	Mild TVD	2166	No			Alive	2761

Table 3. Demographic information of dogs diagnosed with TVD and other concomitant cardiac diseases*.

Dog	Breed	Reason for presentation	Heart murmur	Diagnosis	Status at the end of the study
Dog 19	Labrador retriever	Heart murmur	II/VI holosystolic left basilar	Mild TVD + mild SAS	Alive
Dog 20	Springer spaniel	Heart murmur	IV/VI systolic left apical	Mild TVD + Mild MVD	Lost to follow up
Dog 21	Labrador retriever	Ascites, pericardial effusion	III/VI holosystolic bilateral apical	Severe TVD + mild MVD	Euthanasia. Unresponsive CHF
Dog 22	Springer spaniel	Heart murmur, pulmonary oedema	III/VI pansystolic left apical	Severe TVD + Severe MVD	Euthanasia. Unresponsive CHF (left)
Dog 23	Bullmastiff	Arrhythmia, ascites, pulmonary oedema	III/VI systolic bilateral apical	Severe TVD + Severe MVD	Euthanasia. Unresponsive CHF (bilateral)
Dog 24	Rottweiler cross	Arrhythmia, firm head swelling	VI/VI continuous left basilar	Severe TVD + PDA (LtoR)	Euthanasia. Unresponsive seizures.
Dog 25	Labrador retriever	Heart murmur	III/VI pansystolic right apical	Mild TVD + small ASD	Euthanasia. Unresponsive seizures. Suspected meningioma
Dog 26	Border collie	Heart murmur	V/VI pansystolic right apical	Severe TVD + small ASD	Alive
Dog 27	German shepherd	Heart murmur	VI/VI pansystolic right apical	Severe TVD + severe PS	Euthanasia. Meningeal tumour.
Dog 28	Boxer	Ascites, arrhythmia	II/VI systolic right apical	Severe TVD + moderate PS	Natural. Cardiorespiratory arrest
Dog 29	English bulldog	Heart murmur, ascites, arrhythmia, pleural and pericardial effusion	III/VI holosystolic right apical	Severe TVD + severe PS	Natural. Cardiorespiratory arrest

(ASD): Atrial septal defect; (TVD): Tricuspid valve dysplasia; (SAS): Subaortic stenosis; (PS): Pulmonic stenosis; (MVD): Mitral valve dysplasia; (PDA): Patent ductus arteriosus; (LtoR): Left to right; (LTFU): Lost to follow up.
*Excluded from the descriptive and statistical analysis.

During initial clinical assessment, a systolic murmur was auscultated in all dogs, and ranged from grade I to VI out of VI (Table 2). In 16 dogs (89%) the murmur was louder over the right thorax, while in two dogs (11%), it had the same intensity bilaterally. The location of maximal intensity was right apical in 14 dogs (78%) and right basilar in four dogs (22%).

Standard electrocardiography was performed at least once in 14 dogs (78%). Configuration abnormalities were identified in nine dogs (50%) and consisted of a right axis shift (n=5, 28%), P *pulmonale* (n=4, 22%) and splintered QRS (n=3, 17%). Cardiac arrhythmias were reported at some point during the course of the disease in a total of four dogs (22%). Atrial fibrillation was recorded in three dogs (17%) and paroxysmal supraventricular tachycardia in 1/18 dogs (border collie).

Echocardiography identified thickened (n=16, 89%), shortened (n=4, 22%) and elongated (n=2, 11%) TV leaflets. The septal leaflet appeared tethered in five dogs (28%). Tricuspid stenosis was not observed in any dog. Other abnormalities of the TV apparatus included elongated PM (n=1) and shortened CT (n=1). TR was graded as severe in 11 dogs (61%), moderate in two dogs (11%) and mild in five dogs (28%). The RA was severely enlarged in 11 dogs (61%) and moderately enlarged in two dogs (11%). RV enlargement was severe in four dogs (22%), moderate in six dogs (33%) and mild in two dogs (11%). Chamber dimensions were within reference ranges in five dogs (28%). Overall, TVD was graded as mild (n=5, 28%), moderate (n=2, 11%) or severe (n=11, 61%). EM was suspected in four dogs (22%) based on the subjective apical displacement of the TV apparatus, but post-mortem diagnosis was not undertaken.

No association was observed between TVD severity and murmur intensity (p=0.198) or presence of an arrhythmia (p=0.371) (Fig. 3); all dogs with arrhythmias had severe TVD.

Age at diagnosis of R-CHF ranged from 61 days to 7.8 years (median=361 days). Three dogs (17%) were more than one year old. Seven dogs were diagnosed with R-CHF either on first presentation (n=4, 22%) or subsequently (n=3, 17%), and all of them were diagnosed initially with severe TVD (Table 2). When R-CHF occurred, ascites was always present, pleural effusion (modified transudate) occurred in two dogs (11%) and jugular distension/pulsation was reported in only one dog out of 18 (6%). Thoracocentesis was required in one dog with pleural effusion to alleviate severe dyspnoea (modified transudate).

At the time of analysis, 12 out of 18 dogs (67%) had died, four dogs were still alive (22%) and two dogs (11%) were LTFU.

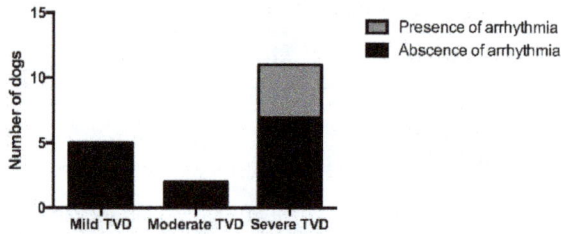

Fig. 3. Severity of TVD and presence of arrhythmias.

The seven dogs (39%) diagnosed with R-CHF suffered cardiac death: six of them were euthanased (Table 2) due to unresponsive R-CHF, and one dog, with severe pleural effusion, died suddenly during thoracocentesis. Age at death ranged between 50 days and 13.8 years (median=2237.5 days). The MST from diagnosis of TVD (censored dogs n=11, 61%) was 2775 days (range 1-3696 days; 95% CI 1542.41-4007.59). However, once R-CHF developed (censored dogs n=0), MST was 181 days (range 1-2130 days; 95% CI 0-455.59) (Fig. 4). None of the dogs without R-CHF suffered a cardiac-related death. Dogs that suffered syncope were more likely to have shorter survival times (Hazard ratio=21.814; 95% CI 2.213-215.008, p=0.008) (Fig. 4). The rest of the factors analysed, including age, sex, breed, TVD severity, HM intensity, R-CHF (at any point) and arrhythmia, were not significantly associated with survival time (p>0.05).

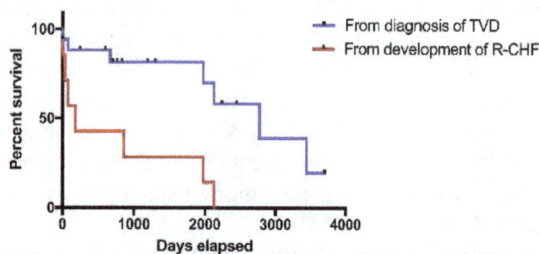

A

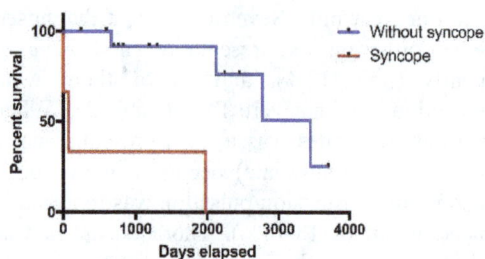

B

Fig. 4. Kaplan-Meier survival curves. **(A):** From diagnosis of TVD (n=7) and from diagnosis of R-CHF (n=7). **(B):** Dogs with (n=3) and without (n=4) syncope.

Discussion

This is the first study to document the demographic, clinical and survival characteristics of a UK population of dogs diagnosed with TVD. The prevalence was lower (1.1% of our cardiology cases) than the 2-7.4% of congenital heart disease reported previously in non-UK populations (Tidholm, 1997; Oliveira et al., 2011; Schrope, 2015), but our reference population included both congenital and acquired cardiac disease. In addition, the true prevalence in the general UK population of dogs may be lower, as we are reporting from a referral population. Previous studies have suggested that Labrador retrievers are over-represented (Wright et al., 2001). In contrast, in our study, Labradors were not over-represented compared with the hospital population, but Border collies were significantly over-represented.

To our knowledge, a predisposition to TVD in Border collies has not been previously reported. Additional studies attempting to identify a mode of inheritance and potential genetic locus are warranted. More than one third of cases in this study had concomitant congenital cardiac diseases. This is consistent with previous studies in non-UK dogs (Oliveira et al., 2011; Adin, 2014) and people (Formigari et al., 1993; Edwards, 1994; Webb et al., 2008; Luu et al., 2015). There was also broad agreement with the types of congenital diseases previously reported, suggesting that TV development may be adversely affected during embryonic development if loading conditions in the heart are abnormal (Formigari et al., 1993). Although dogs with additional cardiac abnormalities were excluded from statistical analysis to minimise confounding effects, this study still demonstrates the importance of performing a comprehensive echocardiographic study, when TVD is diagnosed, to ensure additional congenital cardiac disease is not missed. Unsurprisingly for a congenital disease, the majority of TVD-only dogs were less than one year of age at diagnosis. However, one third of the dogs were adults. Diagnosing TVD in adult dogs can be controversial, as differentiating it from acquired chronic valvular disease can be difficult. Furthermore, degenerative valvular changes can also be observed in young dogs (Michaëlson and Ho, 2000). It is not clear as to why TVD was not diagnosed in so many dogs until adulthood, although this has been previously reported (Kittleson, 1998). Since inclusion criteria included the detection of a heart murmur before 1 year of age, it is possible that these dogs were not referred until the appearance of clinical signs or until the heart murmur intensity had increased. Only including dogs with a detectable heart murmur before of one year of age, may have precluded the inclusion of dogs with TVD but very low or undetectable heart murmurs, which is recognised in TVD cases (Famula et al., 2002). These dogs could even have had severe TVD since our study failed to demonstrate a correlation between murmur intensity and severity of TVD, as reported by previous authors (Bonagura and Lehmkuhl, 1999). Non-arrhythmic electrocardiographic abnormalities were relatively common. Although *P mitrale* was not observed and splintering of the QRS complex was observed less frequently than in other studies (Kornreich and Moïse, 1997), *P pulmonale* and right axial shifts occurred at frequencies similar to those previously reported despite none of the dogs having precordial recordings (Kornreich and Moïse, 1997).

Cardiac arrhythmias were not frequently reported in our dogs. Neither ventricular pre-excitation nor the SVT typical of a macro re-entrant circuit was identified, despite an association between EM and Wolff-Parkinson-White syndrome in people (Misaki *et al.*, 1995), and the predisposition of Labradors to orthodromic atrioventricular reciprocating tachycardia (OAVRT) (Santilli *et al.*, 2007). The only case in this study with SVT was a border collie, a breed not considered to be of increased risk for OAVRT. However, features of OAVRT may be intermittent, and since no Holter monitoring or electrophysiological studies were performed, concurrent OAVRT could not be completely ruled out. The most common arrhythmia was atrial fibrillation which is unsurprising since right atrial enlargement is a feature of severe TVD. Indeed, all dogs with cardiac arrhythmias had severe TVD. Surprisingly, a relationship between TVD severity and presence of an arrhythmia could not be demonstrated although the low number of events may have underpowered this investigation. We conclude that while cardiac remodelling is important in arrhythmogenesis in TVD, other factors, as yet unidentified, may also contribute to the arrhythmia risk. Doppler echocardiography was used to confirm the diagnosis and severity of TVD. TVD constitutes a wide range of morphological abnormalities (Boon, 2011b; Adin, 2014; Bussadori and Pradelli, 2016). The accurate and objective echocardiographic examination of the TV apparatus is technically challenging, and is not always feasible (Boon, 2011a). For example, the relatively thick and nodular appearance of the septal leaflet of the TV, irrespective of age, can mimic degenerative valvular disease (Michaëlson and Ho, 2000). Echocardiography cine loops were carefully re-reviewed and diagnosis of congenital disease was subjectively achieved, based on typical morphological changes previously discussed (Table 1). Whether or not tethering of the septal tricuspid leaflet constitutes TVD is controversial. Although described in veterinary and human literature (Lang *et al.*, 1991; Said *et al.*, 2012) as resulting from an embryonic failure of programmed cell degeneration and inadequate undermining of the leaflet (Netter, 1981), other authors believe it to be a

normal feature in dogs (Michaëlson and Ho, 2000). When we observed tethering to be preventing septal leaflet closure and in some occasions buckling away of the middle portion of the leaflet from the septum, it was considered part of TVD. This occurred in one third of our cases, although was not confirmed post-mortem. Similarly, a lack of post-mortem and/or electrophysiological data to demonstrate atrialisation of the RV, meant that EM, an unusual form of TVD (Eyster *et al.*, 1977; Tilley and Liu, 1977; Cave, 2001; Takemura *et al.*, 2003; Sousa *et al.*, 2006; Choi *et al.*, 2009), could not be confirmed in the four cases in which it was suspected. In agreement with Michaëlson and Ho (2000), we believe that a clearer distinction between EM and isolated TVD is required, and so these dogs were included as TVD-only dogs in statistical analysis. Overall, TVD had a favourable prognosis, with a MST, from diagnosis of TVD, of over 7 years. None of the mild-to-moderate cases (approximately two thirds of cases) suffered cardiac death. Only those cases diagnosed with severe TVD developed R-CHF, in the form of ascites, jugular distension/pulsation or pleural effusion. R-CHF occurred over a wide age range, in senior adults as well as juveniles, demonstrating that, as in humans and non-UK dogs, severe TVD can be tolerated for many years (Arizmendi *et al.*, 2004; Webb *et al.*, 2008; Oyama *et al.*, 2010). Once R-CHF had developed, the MST was markedly reduced overall, although there was marked variation from a few days to over 5 years. Prolonged survival with TVD may reflect the capacity of the systemic venous vasculature to accommodate significant volume overload (MacDonald, 2006). Based on a small number of dogs reaching the end-point, syncope was the sole risk factor for reduced survival time. Syncope only occurred in young dogs with severe TVD and R-CHF but the mechanism could not be identified from the data available. The only arrhythmia recorded in the syncopal dogs was paroxysmal SVT which would not normally lead to loss of consciousness (Moïse, 1999). However, it is possible that profound weakness due to inadequate cardiac output with or without an arrhythmia may have been misinterpreted as syncope. There were limitations to this study, mainly due to its retrospective nature, which may have precluded homogeneity of the data, and its dependency on accuracy of record keeping. To minimise inclusion of dogs with acquired disease, diagnosis of TVD in adult dogs also required historical identification of a right-sided murmur at a young age. It is still possible that dogs with acquired TV degeneration were erroneously included. Furthermore, there may have been a selection bias against dogs with TVD in whom a low intensity murmur had not been noted before one year of age. Review of stored echocardiographic images was not performed in a blinded manner, which may have biased classification of severity of TVD. Tricuspid regurgitation severity was assessed by evaluation of the regurgitant jet size. Colour-flow Doppler mapping is a simple, highly sensitive, semi-quantitative method of assessment of TR severity, with good repeatability and reproducibility, used very commonly in both human and veterinary medicine (Jacob and Stewart, 2007; Lancellotti et al., 2010; Boon, 2011a; Badano et al., 2013). However, it can be significantly affected by technical (transducer frequency, gain, frame rate, depth and Nyquist settings) and loading conditions (Jacob and Stewart, 2007; Lancellotti et al., 2010; Badano et al., 2013). Although studies in people suggest an acceptable correlation with TR severity (Zoghbi et al., 2003; Badano et al., 2013), currently, vena contracta width (VC), PISA radius and effective regurgitant orifice area (EROA), early diastolic inflow wave velocity (Evel) and hepatic vein flow, are considered superior quantitative markers of TR severity in humans (Lancellotti et al., 2010; Badano et al., 2013), and avoidance of jet area as a marker of severity has been recommended (Lancellotti et al., 2010).

To the authors' knowledge, there are no published studies evaluating the accuracy of different echocardiographic methods to assess TR severity in dogs. Recently, Sargent et al. (2015) reported a poor correlation of mitral regurgitant jet area and mitral regurgitation severity, in dogs with myxomatous mitral valve disease (MMVD). The same study identified Evel and VC indexed to aortic diameter (VC:Ao) as having the tightest correlations with mitral regurgitant fraction determined by cardiac magnetic resonance imaging, but whether indices of MR in MMVD could be applied to canine TVD is not known. Unfortunately, because our retrospective study used cases dating as far back as 1998, the cine loops necessary to calculate Evel and VC:Ao were not always available. In our study, and in order to maintain continuity and permit comparison with published studies of canine TVD (Ohad et al., 2013), we opted to use a combination of methods of assessing TVD severity, including TV apparatus abnormalities, severity of the right heart volume overload and, lastly, severity of TR.

In conclusion, TVD in our UK population of dogs was associated with a prolonged MST, from diagnosis of the disease, of over 7 years. R-CHF occurred only when TVD was severe. Once R-CHF developed, MST decreased but syncope was the sole risk factor for cardiac death. Border collies were over-represented.

Acknowledgments

The author would like to show his gratitude to Prof. Joanna Dukes-McEwan BVMS (Hons) MVM PhD DVC DipECVIM-CA(Cardiology) MRCVS, for her assistance and constructive criticism of the manuscript.

Conflict of interest
The authors declare that there is no conflict of interest.

References

Adams, D.S., Marolf, A.J., Valdés-Martinez, A., Randall, E.K. and Bachand, A.M. 2017. Associations between thoracic radiographic changes and severity of pulmonary arterial hypertension diagnosed in 60 dogs via Doppler echocardiography: A retrospective study. Vet. Radiol. Ultrasound. 58, 454-462.

Adin, D. 2014. Tricuspid valve dysplasia. In Kirk's Current Veterinary Therapy, Eds., Bonagura, J.D. and Twedt, D.C. Saint Louis, MI: W.B. Saunders, pp: e332-e335.

Andelfinger, G., Wright, K.N., Lee, H.S., Siemens, L.M. and Benson, D.W. 2003. Canine tricuspid valve malformation, a model of human Ebstein anomaly, maps to dog chromosome 9. J. Med. Genet. 40, 320-324.

Arizmendi, A.F., Pineda, L.F., Jiménez, C.Q., Azcárate, M.J.M., Sarachaga, I.H., Urroz, E., de León, J.P., Moya, J.L. and Jiménez, M.Q. 2004. The clinical profile of Ebstein's malformation as seen from the fetus to the adult in 52 patients. Cardiol. Young. 14, 55-63.

Badano, L.P., Muraru, D. and Enriquez-Sarano, M. 2013. Assessment of functional tricuspid regurgitation. Eur. Heart J. 34, 1875-1884.

Becker, A.D., Becker, M.J. and Edwards, J.E. 1971. Pathologic spectrum of dysplasia of the tricuspid valve: features in common with Ebstein's malformation. Arch. Pathol. 91, 167-178.

Bonagura, J.D. and Lehmkuhl, L.B. 1999. Congenital heart disease. In Textbook of Canine and Feline Cardiology: Principles and Clinical Practice, Eds., Fox, P.R., Sisson, D. and Moïse, N.S. Philadelphia, PA: W.B. Saunders, pp: 471-535.

Boon, J.A. 2011a. Evaluation of size, function and haemodynamics. In Veterinary Echocardiography, Eds., Boon, J.A. Ames, IA: John Willey & Sons, pp: 153-266.

Boon, J.A. 2011b. Congenital shunts and AV dysplasia. In Veterinary Echocardiography, Eds., Boon, J.A. Ames, IA: John Willey & Sons, pp: 437-475.

Boon, J.A. 2011c. Acquired valvular disease. In Veterinary Echocardiography, Eds., Boon, J.A. Ames, IA: John Willey & Sons, pp: 267-333.

Bussadori, C. and Pradelli, D. 2016. Congenital cardiopathies. In Clinical Echocardiography of the Dog and Cat, Eds., Chetboul, V., Bussadori, C. and de Madron, E. St. Louis, MI: Elsevier, pp: 283-322.

Cave, T. 2001. What is your diagnosis? Congenital tricuspid dysplasia with concurrent Ebstein's anomaly. J. Small Anim. Pract. 42, 311-314.

Choi, R., Lee, S.K., Moon, H.S., Park, I.C. and Hyun, C. 2009. Ebstein's anomaly with an atrial septal defect in a jindo dog. Can. Vet. J. 50, 405-410.

Edwards, W.D. 1994. Embryology and pathologic features of Ebstein's anomaly. Progr. Pediatr. Cardiol. 2, 5-15.

Eyster, G.E., Anderson, L., Evans, A.T., Chaffee, A., Bender, G., Johnston, J., Muir, W. and Blanchard, G. 1977. Ebstein's anomaly: a report of 3 cases in the dog. J. Am. Vet. Med. Assoc. 170, 709-713.

Famula, T.R., Siemens, L.M., Davidson, A.P. and Packard, M. 2002. Evaluation of the genetic basis of tricuspid valve dysplasia in Labrador Retrievers. Am. J. Vet. Res. 63, 816-820.

Formigari, R., Francalanci, P., Gallo, P., D'Offizi, F., di Gioia, C., Hokayern, N.J., D'Alessandro, C. and Colloridi, V. 1993. Pathology of atrioventricular valve dysplasia. Cardiovasc. Pathol. 2, 137-144.

Jacob, R. and Stewart, W.J. 2007. A practical approach to the quantification of valvular regurgitation. Curr. Cardiol. Rep. 9, 105-111.

Kittleson, M.D. 1998. Congenital abnormalities of the atrioventricular valves. In Small Animal Cardiovascular Medicine, Eds., Kittleson M.D. and Kienle R.D. St. Louis, MI: Mosby, pp: 273-281.

Kornreich, B.G. and Moïse, N.S. 1997. Right atrioventricular valve malformation in dogs and cats: An electrocardiographic survey with emphasis on splintered QRS complexes. J. Vet. Intern. Med. 11, 226-230.

Lancellotti, P., Moura, L., Pierard, L.A., Agricola, E., Popescu, B.A., Tribouilloy, C., Hagendorff, A., Monin, J.L., Badano, L. and Zamorano, J.L. 2010. European Association of Echocardiography recommendations for the assessment of valvular regurgitation. Part 2: mitral and tricuspid regurgitation (native valve disease). Eur. J. Echocardiogr. 11, 307-332.

Lake-Bakaar, G.A., Griffiths, L.G. and Kittleson, M.D. 2017. Balloon Valvuloplasty of Tricuspid Stenosis: A Retrospective Study of 5 Labrador Retriever Dogs. J. Vet. Intern. Med. 31, 311-315.

Lang, D., Oberhoffer, R., Cook, A., Sharland, G., Allan, L., Fagg, N. and Anderson, R.H. 1991. Pathologic spectrum of malformations of the tricuspid valve in prenatal and neonatal life. J. Am. Coll. Cardiol. 17, 1161-1167.

Lang, R.M., Bierig, M., Devereux, R.B., Flachskampf, F.A., Foster, E., Pellikka, P.A., Picard, M.H., Roman, M.J., Seward, J., Shanewise, J., Solomon, S., Spencer, K.T., St John Sutton, M., Stewart, W.; American Society of Echocardiography's Nomenclature and Standards Committee; Task Force on Chamber Quantification; American College of Cardiology Echocardiography Committee; American Heart Association; European Association of Echocardiography, European Society of Cardiology. 2006. Recommendations for chamber quantification. Eur. J. Echocardiogr. 7(2), 79-108.

Luu, Q., Choudhary, P., Jackson, D., Canniffe, C., McGuire, M., Chard, R. and Celermajer, D.S. 2015. Ebstein's anomaly in those surviving to adult life – a single centre experience. Heart Lung Circ. 24, 996-1001.

MacDonald, K.A. 2006. Congenital heart diseases of puppies and kittens. Vet. Clin. North Am. Small Pract. 36, 503-531.

Michaëlson, M. and Ho, S.Y. 2000. Comparative aspects. In Congenital Heart Malformations in Mammals, Eds., Michaëlson, M. and Ho, S.Y. London: Imperial College Press, pp: 119-150.

Misaki, T., Watanabe, G., Iwa, T., Watanabe, Y., Mukai, K., Takahashi, M., Ohtake, H. and Yamamoto, K. 1995. Surgical treatment of patients with Wolff-Parkinson-White syndrome and associated Ebstein's anomaly. J. Thorac. Cardiovasc. Surg. 110, 1701-1707.

Moïse, N. S. 1999. Diagnosis and management of canine arrhythmias. In Textbook of Canine and Feline Cardiology: Principles and Clinical Practice, Eds., Fox, P.R., Sisson, D. and Moïse, N.S. Philadelphia, PA: W.B. Saunders, pp: 331-385.

Netter, F.H. 1981. The CIBA Collection of Medical Illustration. Vol 5: Heart. Ciba-Geigy Corporation.

Ohad, D.G., Avrahami, A., Waner, T. and David, L. 2013. The occurrence and suspected mode of inheritance of congenital subaortic stenosis and tricuspid valve dysplasia in Dogue de Bordeaux dogs. Vet. J. 197, 351-357.

Oyama, M.A., Sisson, D.D., Thomas, W.P. and Bonagura, J.D. 2010. Congenital heart disease. In Textbook of Veterinary Internal Medicine Vol. 2, Eds., Ettinger, S.J. and Feldman, E.C. St. Louis, MI: W.B. Saunders, pp: 1251-1298.

Oliveira, P., Domenech, O., Silva, J., Vannini, S., Bussadori, R. and Bussadori, C. 2011. Retrospective review of congenital heart disease in 976 dogs. J. Vet. Intern. Med. 25, 477-483.

Said, S.M., Burkhart, H.M. and Dearani, J.A. 2012. Surgical management of congenital (Non-Ebstein) tricuspid valve regurgitation. Semin. Thorac. Cardiovasc. Surg. Pediatr. Card. Surg. Annu. 15, 46-60.

Santilli, R.A., Spadacini, G., Moretti, P., Perego, M., Perini, A., Crosara, S. and Tarducci, A. 2007. Anatomic distribution and electrophysiologic properties of accessory pathways in dogs. J. Am. Vet. Med. Assoc. 231, 393-398.

Sargent, J., Connolly, D.J., Watts, V., Motsküla, P., Volk, H.A., Lamb, C.R. and Fuentes, V.L. 2015. Assessment of mitral regurgitation in dogs:

comparison of results of echocardiography with magnetic resonance imaging. J. Small Anim. Pract. 56, 641-650.

Schrope, D.P. 2015. Prevalence of congenital heart disease in 76,301 mixed-breed dogs and 57,025 mixed-breed cats. J. Vet. Cardiol. 17, 192-202.

Shiina, A., Seward, J.B. and Edwards, W.D. 1984. Two-dimensional echocardiographic spectrum of Ebstein's anomaly: detailed anatomic assessment. J. Am. Coll. Cardiol. 3, 356-357.

Sousa, M.G., Gerardi, D.G., Alves, R.O. and Camacho, A.A. 2006. Tricuspid valve dysplasia and Ebstein's anomaly in dogs: case report. Arq. Bras. Med. Vet. Zootec. 58, 762-767.

Takemura, N., Machida, N., Nakagawa, K., Amasaki, H., Washizu, M. and Hirose, H. 2003. Ebstein's anomaly in a beagle dog. J. Vet. Med. Sci. 65, 531-533.

Tidholm, A. 1997. Retrospective study of congenital heart defects in 151 dogs. J. Small Anim. Pract. 38, 94-98.

Tilley, L.P. and Liu, S.K. 1977. Ebstein's anomaly. J. Am. Med. Assoc. 171, 798-802.

Webb, G.D., Smallhorn, J.F., Therrien, J. and Redington, A.N. 2008. Disease of the heart, pericardium, and pulmonary vasculature bed. In Braunwald's Heart Disease: A Textbook of Cardiovascular Medicine, Eds., Libby, P., Bonow, R.O., Mann, D.L., Zipes, D.P., Braunwald, E. St. Louis, MI: W.B. Saunders, pp: 1561-1625.

Wright, K.N., Bleas, M.E. and Benson, D.W. 2001. Clinical spectrum of congenital tricuspid valve malformation in an extended family of Labrador retrievers. J. Vet. Intern. Med. 15, 280.

Zoghbi, W.A., Enriquez-Sarano, M., Foster, E., Grayburn, P.A., Kraft, C.D., Levine, R.A., Nihoyannopoulos, P., Otto, C.M., Quinones, M.A., Rakowski, H., Stewart, W.J., Waggoner, A., Weissman, N.J.; American Society of Echocardiography. 2003. Recommendations for evaluation of the severity of native valvular regurgitation with two-dimensional and Doppler echocardiography. J. Am. Soc. Echocardiogr. 16, 777-802.

Permissions

All chapters in this book were first published in OVJ, by Tripoli University; hereby published with permission under the Creative Commons Attribution License or equivalent. Every chapter published in this book has been scrutinized by our experts. Their significance has been extensively debated. The topics covered herein carry significant findings which will fuel the growth of the discipline. They may even be implemented as practical applications or may be referred to as a beginning point for another development.

The contributors of this book come from diverse backgrounds, making this book a truly international effort. This book will bring forth new frontiers with its revolutionizing research information and detailed analysis of the nascent developments around the world.

We would like to thank all the contributing authors for lending their expertise to make the book truly unique. They have played a crucial role in the development of this book. Without their invaluable contributions this book wouldn't have been possible. They have made vital efforts to compile up to date information on the varied aspects of this subject to make this book a valuable addition to the collection of many professionals and students.

This book was conceptualized with the vision of imparting up-to-date information and advanced data in this field. To ensure the same, a matchless editorial board was set up. Every individual on the board went through rigorous rounds of assessment to prove their worth. After which they invested a large part of their time researching and compiling the most relevant data for our readers.

The editorial board has been involved in producing this book since its inception. They have spent rigorous hours researching and exploring the diverse topics which have resulted in the successful publishing of this book. They have passed on their knowledge of decades through this book. To expedite this challenging task, the publisher supported the team at every step. A small team of assistant editors was also appointed to further simplify the editing procedure and attain best results for the readers.

Apart from the editorial board, the designing team has also invested a significant amount of their time in understanding the subject and creating the most relevant covers. They scrutinized every image to scout for the most suitable representation of the subject and create an appropriate cover for the book.

The publishing team has been an ardent support to the editorial, designing and production team. Their endless efforts to recruit the best for this project, has resulted in the accomplishment of this book. They are a veteran in the field of academics and their pool of knowledge is as vast as their experience in printing. Their expertise and guidance has proved useful at every step. Their uncompromising quality standards have made this book an exceptional effort. Their encouragement from time to time has been an inspiration for everyone.

The publisher and the editorial board hope that this book will prove to be a valuable piece of knowledge for researchers, students, practitioners and scholars across the globe.

List of Contributors

Y. Manat, E. Evtehova and S.Z. Eskendirova
Laboratory of Cell Biotechnology, National Centre for Biotechnology, Astana, 010000, Republic of Kazakhstan

A.V. Shustov
Laboratory of Genetic Engineering, National Centre for Biotechnology, Astana, 010000, Republic of Kazakhstan

M. David and R.M. Kartheek
Environmental and Molecular Toxicology Laboratory, Department of PG Studies and Research in Zoology, Karnatak University, Dharwad, Karnataka, India- 580003

A. Mariacher
Istituto Zooprofilattico Sperimentale delle Regioni Lazio e Toscana, Viale Europa 30, 58100 Grosseto, Italy
Dipartimento di Scienze Veterinarie, Viale delle Piagge 2, 56124 Pisa, Italy

F. Millanta, G. Guidi and S. Perrucci
Dipartimento di Scienze Veterinarie, Viale delle Piagge 2, 56124 Pisa, Italy

M.A. Al-Griw
Division of Developmental Biology, Zoology Department, Faculty of Science, University of Tripoli, Tripoli, Libya

R.O. Alghazeer
Chemistry Department, Faculty of Science, University of Tripoli, Tripoli, Libya

S.A. Al-Azreg
Department of Pathology and Clinical Pathology, Faculty of Veterinary Medicine, University of Tripoli, Tripoli, Libya

E.M. Bennour
Department of Internal Medicine, Faculty of Veterinary Medicine, University of Tripoli, Tripoli, Libya

N. Onkoba
College of Health Sciences, School of Nursing and Public Health, University of KwaZulu-Natal (UKZN), Howard Campus, Durban, South Africa
Tropical Infectious Diseases, Institute of Primate Research, Karen, Nairobi, Kenya

M.J. Chimbari
College of Health Sciences, School of Nursing and Public Health, University of KwaZulu-Natal (UKZN), Howard Campus, Durban, South Africa

J.M. Kamau
Tropical Infectious Diseases, Institute of Primate Research, Karen, Nairobi, Kenya
School of Medicine, Department of Biochemistry, University of Nairobi, Kenya
School of Life Sciences, University of KwaZulu-Natal, Westville Campus, Durban, South Africa

S. Mukaratirwa
School of Life Sciences, University of KwaZulu-Natal, Westville Campus, Durban, South Africa

L. Leigue
Department of Veterinary Medicine, Universidade Federal do Paraná; Curitiba, PR, Brazil
Department of Microbiology, Institute of Biomedical Sciences, Universidade de São Paulo; São Paulo, SP, Brazil

F. Montiani-Ferreira
Department of Veterinary Medicine, Universidade Federal do Paraná; Curitiba, PR, Brazil

B.A. Moore
Veterinary Specialty Hospital of San Diego, 10435 Sorrento Valley Road, San Diego, CA 92121, USA

A.D. Firdous, K. Massarat and M.A. Baba
Division of Veterinary Anatomy and Histology, FVSC & AH Shuhama Alusteng Jammu and Kashmir, India

S. Maya
Department of Veterinary Anatomy and Histology, CV & AS, Mannuthy, Kerala, India

F. Vercammen and J. Brandt
Centre for Research and Conservation, Royal Zoological Society of Antwerp, K. Astridplein 26, B-2018 Antwerp, Belgium

L. Van Brantegem, L. Bosseler and R. Ducatelle
Department of Pathology, Bacteriology and Avian Medicine, Faculty of Veterinary Medicine, University of Ghent, Salisburylaan 133, B-9820 Merelbeke, Belgium

M. Garvey
Department of Life Sciences, Institute of Technology Sligo, Sligo, Ireland

G. Coughlan
Department of Parasitology, National University of Ireland Maynooth, Maynooth, Ireland
Bioscience Research Institute, Athlone Institute of Technology, Athlone, Ireland

N. Murphy
Department of Parasitology, National University of Ireland Maynooth, Maynooth, Ireland

N. Rowan
Bioscience Research Institute, Athlone Institute of Technology, Athlone, Ireland

Mario Ricciardi
"Pingry" Veterinary Hospital, via Medaglie d'Oro 5, Bari, Italy

I.K. Wise
University of Cambridge, Department of Clinical Veterinary Medicine, Madingley Road, Cambridge, UK

S. Boveri
The University of Liverpool, School of Veterinary Science, Neston, UK

T. Rocha
Bacteriology Laboratory, National Reference Laboratory for CEM, Instituto Nacional de Investigação Agrária e Veterinária- INIAV (National Institute of Agrarian and Veterinary Research), Avenida da República, Quinta do Marquês, 2784-157 Oeiras, Portugal

A. Dellarupe, G. Moré and M. Rambeaud
Laboratorio de Inmunoparasitología, Facultad de Ciencias Veterinarias, Universidad Nacional de La Plata,60 y 118, 1900 La Plata, Argentina
Consejo Nacional de Investigaciones Científicas y Técnicas (CONICET), Buenos Aires, Argentina

J.M. Unzaga and M.C. Venturini
Laboratorio de Inmunoparasitología, Facultad de Ciencias Veterinarias, Universidad Nacional de La Plata, 60 y 118, 1900 La Plata, Argentina

M. Kienast
Instituto de Genética Veterinaria (IGEVET), CCT La Plata, CONICET, Facultad de Ciencias Veterinarias, Universidad Nacional de La Plata, La Plata, Argentina

A. Larsen
Cátedra de Inmunología Veterinaria, Facultad de Ciencias Veterinarias, Universidad Nacional de La Plata, La Plata, Argentina

C. Stiebel
Dpto. Zoonosis, Municipalidad Gral. San Martín, Prov. de Buenos Aires, Argentina

Ibrahim Eldaghayes, Abdunaser Dayhum and Abdulwahab Kammon
Faculty of Veterinary Medicine, University of Tripoli, Tripoli, Libya

Monier Sharif
Faculty of Veterinary Medicine, University of Omar Al-Mukhtar, Albeida, Libya

Giancarlo Ferrari
Food and Agriculture Organization of the United Nations (FAO), Rome, Italy

Christianus Bartels and Keith Sumption
European Commission for the Control of Foot-and-Mouth Disease (EuFMD), Food and Agriculture Organization of the United Nations (FAO), Rome, Italy

Donald P. King
The Pirbright Institute, Ash Road, Surrey, UK

Santina Grazioli and Emiliana Brocchi
Istituto Zooprofilattico Sperimentale della Lombardia e dell'Emilia Romagna (IZSLER), Brescia, Italy

Rogério Ribas Lange, Leandro Lima, Erika Frühvald and Fabiano Montiani-Ferreira
Universidade Federal do Paraná (UFPR), Departamento de Medicina Veterinária, Rua dos Funcionários, 1540, Bairro Juvevê, 80035-050, Curitiba – PR, Brazil

Vera Sônia Nunes da Silva and Aparecida Sônia de Souza
Universidade Estadual de Campina (UNICAMP), Centro de Ciência e Qualidade de Alimentos ITAL, Avenida Brasil, 2880, Campinas – SP, Brazil

Mario Ricciardi, Floriana Gernone and Pasquale Giannuzzi
"Pingry" Veterinary Hospital, via Medaglie d'Oro 5, 70126 Bari, Italy

Antonio De Simone
"Chisimaio" Veterinary Clinic, via Chisimaio 32, 00199 Roma, Italy

Alessandro Cirla
San Marco Veterinary Clinic, via Sorio 114/c – 35141 Padova, Italy
Department of Veterinary Science, University of Pisa, via Livornese Lato Monte – 56124 San Piero a Grado, Pisa, Italy

Marco Rondena
San Marco Veterinary Laboratory, via Sorio 114/c – 35141 Padova, Italy

Giovanna Bertolini
San Marco Veterinary Clinic, via Sorio 114/c – 35141 Padova, Italy

Giovanni Barsotti
Department of Veterinary Science, University of Pisa, via Livornese Lato Monte – 56124 San Piero a Grado, Pisa, Italy

F.B. Fulanetti, G.G.R. Camargo, M.C. Ferro and P. Randazzo-Moura
Pontifícia Universidade Católica de São Paulo. Rua Joubert Wey, 290 Sorocaba, SP. 18030-070, Brazil

Ana Paula Mestre
Laboratorio de Zoología Aplicada: Anexo Vertebrados, Facultad de Humanidades y Ciencias, Universidad Nacional del Litoral, (FHUC-UNL/MMA), Argentina
Consejo Nacional de Investigaciones Científicas y Técnicas (CONICET), Santa Fe, Argentina
Laboratorio de Genética, Departamento de Ciencias Naturales (FHUC-UNL), Santa Fe, Argentina

Patricia Susana Amavet
Consejo Nacional de Investigaciones Científicas y Técnicas (CONICET), Santa Fe, Argentina
Laboratorio de Genética, Departamento de Ciencias Naturales (FHUC-UNL), Santa Fe, Argentina

Pablo Ariel Siroski
Laboratorio de Zoología Aplicada: Anexo Vertebrados, Facultad de Humanidades y Ciencias, Universidad Nacional del Litoral, (FHUC-UNL/MMA), Argentina
Consejo Nacional de Investigaciones Científicas y Técnicas (CONICET), Santa Fe, Argentina
Laboratorio de Biología Celular y Molecular Aplicada, Instituto de Ciencias Veterinarias del Litoral (ICiVet-Litoral-UNL-CONICET), Esperanza, Santa Fe, Argentina

Wanderlei de Moraes
Universidade Federal do Paraná (UFPR), Departamento de Medicina Veterinária, Rua dos Funcionários, 1540, 80035-050, Curitiba - PR, Brazil
ITAIPU Binacional, Diretoria de Coordenação, Departamento de Áreas Protegidas, Refúgio Biológico Bela Vista, Rua Teresina, 62, Vila C,85870-280, Foz do Iguaçu - PR, Brazil

Thiago A.C. Ferreira, André T. Somma and Fabiano Montiani-Ferreira
Universidade Federal do Paraná (UFPR), Departamento de Medicina Veterinária, Rua dos Funcionários, 1540, 80035-050, Curitiba - PR, Brazil

Zalmir S. Cubas
ITAIPU Binacional, Diretoria de Coordenação, Departamento de Áreas Protegidas, Refúgio Biológico Bela Vista, Rua Teresina, 62, Vila C,85870-280, Foz do Iguaçu - PR, Brazil

Bret A. Moore
University of California-Davis, School of Veterinary Medicine, Ophthalmology, 1 Garrod Drive, Davis, CA, 95695, USA

Miguel Gallego
Centro Veterinario Madrid Exóticos, Madrid, Spain

Monier Sharif and Adel Mohamed
Department of Pathology and Anatomy, Faculty of Veterinary Medicine, University of Omar Al-Mukhtar, Al-Beida, Libya

Manfred Reinacher
Institute for Veterinary Pathology, Justus-Liebig-University, Frankfurter Str. 96, 35392 Giessen, Germany

D. Petrini
Freelance Veterinarian, Pisa, Italy

M. Di Giuseppe
Centro Veterinario per Animali Esotici, Viale Regione Siciliana Sud – Est 422-426, 90129 Palermo, Italy

G. Deli
Freelance Veterinarian, Roma, Italy

C. De Caro Carella
School of Veterinary Medicine, Louisiana State University, USA

Danielle Alves Silva
Animal Science Post Graduate Program, Oeste Paulista University (UNOESTE), Presidente Prudente, SP, Brazil

Gisele Alborgetti Nai
Department of Anatomy Pathology, Faculty of Medicine (UNOESTE), Brazil

Rogério Giuffrida, Rafael Cabral Barbero, Jacqueline Marcussi Pereira Kuhn, Andressa Caroline da Silva, Ricardo Henrique Zakir Pereira, and Maria Fernanda Abbade
Faculty of Veterinary Medicine (UNOESTE), Brazil

Luiz Felipe da Costa Zulim and Carolina Silva Guimarães Pereira
Resident in Small Animal Medicine of the Veterinary Hospital (UNOESTE), Brazil

Silvia Franco Andrade
Department of Small Animal Medicine of the Veterinary Hospital (UNOESTE), Brazil

David Williams, Nina Adeyeye and Erni Visser
Department of Veterinary Medicine, University of Cambridge, Madingley Road, Cambridge CB3 0ES, UK

Mohamed A. Al-Griw and Sassia O. Regeai
Developmental Biology Division, Zoology Department, Faculty of Science, University of Tripoli, Tripoli, Libya

Soad A. Treesh
Department of Histology and Medical Genetics, Faculty of Medicine, University of Tripoli, Tripoli, Libya

Rabia O. Alghazeer
Chemistry Department, Faculty of Science, University of Tripoli, Tripoli, Libya

Francis Vercammen
Centre for Research and Conservation, Royal Zoological Society of Antwerp, K. Astridplein 26, B-2018 Antwerp, Belgium

Leslie Bosseler
Department of Pathology, Bacteriology and Avian Medicine, Faculty of Veterinary Medicine, University of Ghent, Salisburylaan 133, B-9820 Merelbeke, Belgium

Marylène Tignon and Ann Brigitte Cay
Department of Virology, Veterinary and Agrochemical Research Centre, Groeselenberg 99, B-1180 Brussels, Belgium

Huda H. Al-Griw
Department of Microbiology and Parasitology, Faculty of Veterinary Medicine, University of Tripoli, Tripoli, Libya

Zena A. Zraba, Salsabiel K. Al-Muntaser, Refaat M. Tabagh and Mohamed A. Al-Griw
Department of Forensic Biology, Faculty of Science, University of Tripoli, Tripoli, Libya

Marwan M. Draid
Department of Pharmacology, Toxicology and Forensic Medicine, Faculty of Veterinary Medicine, University of Tripoli, Tripoli, Libya

Aisha M. Zaidi
Department of Physiology, Biochemistry and Animal Nutrition, Faculty of Veterinary Medicine, University of Tripoli, Tripoli, Libya

Xavier Navarro-Cubas
University of Liverpool, Small Animal Teaching Hospital, Leahurst Campus, Chester High Road, Neston, Wirral, CH64 7TE, UK

Valentina Palermo
Anderson and Moores Veterinary Specialists, The Granary, Bunstead Barns, Poles Lane, Hursley, Winchester, Hampshire, SO21 2LL, UK

Anne French
School of Veterinary Medicine, College of Medical, Veterinary and Life Sciences, University of Glasgow, Bearsden Road, Bearsden, Glasgow, G61 1QH, UK

Sandra Sanchis-Mora
The Royal Veterinary College, Hawkshead Lane, North Mymms, Hatfield, Hertfordshire, AL9 7TA, UK

Geoff Culshaw
R(D)SVS Hospital for Small Animals, The University of Edinburgh, Easter Bush Veterinary Centre, Roslin, Midlothian, EH25 9RG, UK

Index